# Practical Exam Preparation Guide of

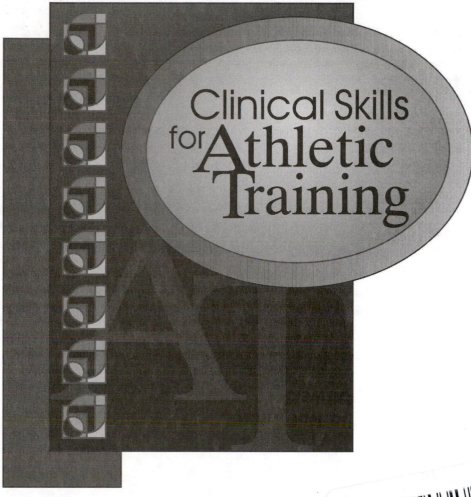

Clinical Skills for Athletic Training

HERB K. AMATO, DA, ATC
*James Madison University*
*Harrisonburg, Virginia*

CHRISTY VENABLE HAWKINS, MS, ATC
*Thomas Nelson Community College*
*Hampton, Virginia*

STEVEN L. COLE, MED, ATC, CSCS
*The College of William and Mary*
*Williamsburg, Virginia*

**SLACK**
INCORPORATED

*An innovative information, education, and management company*
6900 Grove Road • Thorofare, NJ 08086

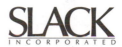

The procedures and practices described in this book should be implemented in a manner consistent with the professional standards set for the circumstances that apply in each specific situation. Every effort has been made to confirm the accuracy of the information presented and to correctly relate generally accepted practices. The author, editor, and publisher cannot accept responsibility for errors or exclusions or for the outcome of the application of the material presented herein. There is no expressed or implied warranty of this book or information imparted by it.

The work SLACK publishes is peer reviewed. Prior to publication, recognized leaders in the field, educators, and clinicians provide important feedback on the concepts and content that we publish. We welcome feedback on this work.

This book has been bound with a revolutionary adhesive process called lay flat binding. Using this binding results in a book with a free-floating cover and a flexible spine, allowing the book to open flat for greater ease of use.

Amato, Herb
  Practical exam preparation guide of clinical skills for athletic training / Herb Amato, Christy Venable Hawkins, Steven L. Cole.
    p. ; cm.
Includes bibliographical references.
  ISBN 1-55642-572-4 (pbk. : alk. paper)
  1. Physical education and training--Examinations, questions, etc. 2. Athletic trainers--Examinations, questions, etc. 3. Sports medicine--Examinations, questions, etc.
  [DNLM: 1. Physical Education and Training--Examination Questions. 2. Physical Education and Training--Outlines. 3. Sports--Examination Questions. 4. Sports--Outlines. QT 18.2 A488p 2002] I. Hawkins, Christy Venable, 1973- II. Cole, Steven L., 1954- III. Title.
  RC1210 .A435 2002
  613.7'076--dc21

                                                                                          2002006917


Printed in the United States of America

Published by:        SLACK Incorporated
                     6900 Grove Road
                     Thorofare, NJ 08086 USA
                     Telephone: 856-848-1000
                     Fax: 856-853-5991
                     www.slackbooks.com

Contact SLACK Incorporated for more information about other books in this field or about the availability of our books from distributors outside the United States.

For permission to reprint material in another publication, contact SLACK Incorporated. Authorization to photocopy items for internal, personal, or academic use is granted by SLACK Incorporated provided that the appropriate fee is paid directly to Copyright Clearance Center. Prior to photocopying items, please contact the Copyright Clearance Center at 222 Rosewood Drive, Danvers, MA 01923 USA; phone: 978-750-8400; website: www.copyright.com; email: info@copyright.com.

Last digit is print number: 10  9  8  7  6  5  4  3  2

# Contents

# Acknowledgments

Many thanks to our spouses, families, colleagues, students, and friends for their support in this endeavor. Special thanks to the NATABOC and all the athletic trainers who supervise athletic training students.

# About the Authors

Herb Amato, DA, ATC is the Athletic Training Program Director at James Madison University in Harrisonburg, Va. He has been involved in the education of athletic training students for 22 years at university and high school levels. He has an extensive public speaking and consulting background and has published several articles in the areas of athletic training education and clinical practice. Herb is also is active in service at community, university, and national levels.

An avid floor hockey player, Herb resides in Harrisonburg with his wife, Lori, and three daughters, Casey, Lyndy, and Jessy.

Christy Venable Hawkins, MS, ATC is the Program Manager for Workforce Training and Continuing Education at Thomas Nelson Community College in Hampton, Va. In this position, she develops and implements educational programs for the local workforce. For 6 years, Christy traveled to colleges and universities throughout the country as a workshop coordinator for Amato-Cole Educational Services (ACES Workshops). She has taught athletic training courses at the university level and coordinated leisure classes for both children and adults. Hawkins received a bachelor of science degree from James Madison University and a master of science degree from the University of South Carolina.

A newlywed, Christy resides in Newport News, Va with her husband, David, and a black lab, Jake.

Steven L. Cole, MEd, ATC, CSCS is the Director of Sports Medicine at the College of William and Mary, Williamsburg, Va. He oversees a staff of seven certified athletic trainers and coordinates a regional network of health care specialists to provide athletic health care for nearly 600 student-athletes annually. In addition to his local role with the college, he coordinates an on-site sports medicine program for Busch Entertainment Coporation in Williamsburg, aimed at educating entertainers in early recognition and self-management of common injuries. Steve is one of the co-founders of the ACES Preparatory Workshops for athletic training students who are eligible to sit for the National Athletic Trainers' Association Board of Certification exam.

Steve has served as a consultant to various athletic programs, medical practices, and industrial corporations. He is the sports medicine consultant to Tidewater Physical Therapy, Inc, a group of outpatient physical therapy clinics serving the Tidewater area of Virginia. He has extensive public speaking and consulting experience from local to international and has published several articles relevant to athletic health care and the administration of health care programs. Steve is a member of the Virginia High School League Sports Medicine Advisory Committee, the Legislative Committee for the Virginia Athletic Trainers' Association, and the Athletic Training Liaison to the Colonial Athletic Association.

A competitive triathlete, Steve resides in Williamsburg with his wife, Lana, and daughter, Sydney.

# Introduction

The purpose of this book is to provide the athletic training student and athletic training educator with a reference that focuses on clinical skills. This guidebook was written with both audiences in mind. The athletic training student working toward NATA Board of Certification (NATABOC) certification as an entry-level professional will find this book useful as both a learning tool and a study guide. As a learning tool, students may take notes on the individual skill sheets while listening to the instructor or reading from a reference text. As the student learns these practical skills in the classroom or clinical environment, this book can be used as a guide for practicing, with the final goal of mastery. As the student reviews skills acquired throughout his or her clinical experience in preparation for the NATABOC certification exam, he or she can also use this book as a study guide and evaluation tool. References and supplies needed are included on each skill sheet. These tips allow the student to focus on the task at hand, rather than wasting time figuring out what is needed or where to find additional information. Finally, the mock practical exam in the back of the book is a good resource to familiarize students with the length and weight of each task.

The athletic training educator or approved clinical instructor (ACI) in an athletic training program will also find this guide useful both in documenting student mastery of individual psychomotor skills and in helping students prepare for the certification exam. Since an ACI is a certified athletic trainer who is responsible for formal instruction and evaluation of clinical proficiencies, this book is designed to serve as a documentation instrument for learning over time. The building blocks of clinical proficiency are the individual skills. An example of a clinical proficiency may be the evaluation of an injured knee of a 17-year-old soccer player. There are many psychomotor skills needed in order to successfully evaluate that soccer player's knee.

In verifying student readiness to take the certification exam, the NATABOC no longer requires the logging of clinical hours. Instead, the NATABOC requires formal documentation of students' learning of specific clinical proficiencies over time. Thus, the ACI must document when a skill is taught, practiced, tested, and retested to verify student learning. The concept of learning over time views clinical proficiency as the "big picture"; however, each of the proficiencies has many subsets or psychomotor skills. This guidebook is designed with documentation requirements in mind. It provides a suitable format for recording individual skills to be used as part of a student portfolio to record a mastery of proficiencies.

Additionally, this book is formatted to record a student's progress in mastering psychomotor skills; therefore, it provides a history of that student's clinical strengths and weaknesses. The ACI can then review that history to prepare a study plan with the student. With the knowledge of the student's clinical strengths and weaknesses, the educator is better prepared to assist the student in exam preparation.

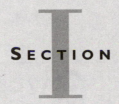

SECTION

I

INTRODUCTION

# OVERVIEW OF THE PRACTICAL EXAMINATION

In 1969, the National Athletic Trainers' Association (NATA) developed an examination to certify entry-level professionals. A function of any certification examination is to demonstrate to the public that an individual is qualified to perform specific duties without causing harm. The first certification exam included two sections: a written portion and an oral/practical portion. While the written portion of the exam strived to test the candidate's basic knowledge of athletic training domains, the oral/practical portion of the examination sought to test the clinical skills of the candidate. The candidate was asked to complete skills in four categories (taping/wrapping, evaluation, rehabilitation, and emergency management) within a given time frame. Examples included asking the candidate to explain and demonstrate his or her ability to tape an ankle, evaluate a shoulder, construct a rehabilitation program for an MCL sprain, or manage an athlete suspected of heat illness. While the intent of the oral/practical portion of the exam was to evaluate the clinical skills of a candidate, there was much concern over the discrepancy between what was "explained" and what was "demonstrated."

Every 5 years, a role delineation study is conducted as the initial step in updating each portion of the NATA Board of Certification (NATABOC) exam. The first step in this process is for the NATABOC to appoint a committee of subject matter experts. Through their work, performance domains for the practice of athletic training are defined. These performance domains are further broken down into tasks, knowledge areas, and skill abilities expected of a person working in the field of athletic training.

*The Role Delineation Study*, published in 1994, lead to changes in the design of the certification exam. The domain and task areas shifted from the previous study, which lead to a different configuration of the written exam. The oral/practical portion of the exam was eliminated, giving rise to the current "practical exam."

With the changes to the practical exam came an emphasis on the demonstration of *psychomotor skills*, rather than the explanation of the skill. Psychomotor skills are "physical activities associated with mental processes." In other words, candidates must apply their knowledge of athletic training skills by demonstrating those skills during the practical portion of the exam. The key term here is *demonstrate*. No longer are candidates asked to *explain* and demonstrate, and no longer are candidates' verbal explanations taken into account when scoring the practical exam. The current practical exam score is based solely on the skills demonstrated during the given response period.

The practical exam is worth a total of 50 points. Candidates are tested on 3 to 14 tasks; however, each task may be made up of a series of psychomotor skills. Candidates are given up to 4 minutes to demonstrate a response to each skill. The majority of the skills are given much less time. The total score received for the practical exam is based on the correct actions accumulated during the time allotted for all the skills combined.

A change in the scoring of the practical exam now includes disqualifiers for each skill. These disqualifiers are actions that are critical to the skill or may cause harm to the patient. Points accumulated for a specific skill will be eliminated if a disqualifier is left out or performed incorrectly.

## The Exam Room

The practical exam takes place in a room containing four people: a room captain, an examiner, a model, and a candidate. The primary role of the room captain is to oversee the tape recorder, read the instructions pertaining to the overall exam, and read each test question aloud to the candidate. The role of the examiner is to monitor the amount of time allocated for each response. Both the examiner and the room captain have the responsibility of recording skills demonstrated by the candidate during the practical exam. The model serves the role of an athlete and allows the candidate to demonstrate psychomotor skills.

The exam room is arranged to accommodate a treatment table, desks for both the examiner and the room captain, and a supply table. The treatment table can be used to perform skill demonstrations with the model as indicated. The supply table includes supplies for each skill the candidate is asked to perform. It may also contain additional materials *not* needed or used to complete the practical exam skills. The candidate cannot request additional or supplementary supplies. Thus, it is recommended that candidates take some time to review the supplies on the table upon entering the exam room.

A tape recorder is present on one of the desks in the exam room. The room captain tests the recorder and inserts a cassette tape to record the entire practical exam. While this feature of the test seems irrelevant since the exam has changed to demonstrating psychomotor skills, the tape recorder still serves the function of assuring that directions and responses are delivered to each candidate in a consistent and appropriate manner. The tape recorder runs from the time the door is opened until the model escorts the candidate out of the room.

## Exam Procedure

While the candidates are taking the written portion of the certification exam, they are summoned one at a time to the administrative area. At this time, the candidate is asked to turn in his or her written exam and proceed to the practical exam. This break serves as a transition from one test to the next and is an ideal time for the candidate to take a moment to get a drink or use the restroom. The model introduces him- or herself and accompanies the candidate to the practical exam room, where introductions to the examiner and room captain occur. Once introductions are complete, the practical examination officially begins.

The candidate is presented with a *candidate guidebook*. This allows the candidate to read along with the room captain as each question is read aloud. At the end of the question, a time limit is given for each response. The time starts immediately after the room captain has completed reading the question for the first time. The candidate may delay the starting of the clock by asking for the question to be reread. However, the *NATABOC Examiner Training Program Home Study Workbook* states that the examiner may start the clock when the candidate begins to respond to the question either by indicating directions to the model, touching supplies, or starting to demonstrate the skill. It is important to clarify upon arrival into the examination room *when* the examiner intends to start the clock. The candidate may use the entire allotment of time to demonstrate the skill, after which the examiner indicates that time is up. Any responses that occur after time runs out are not counted towards the candidate's score.

During each skill demonstration, candidates should have three expectations of the model. First, the model is to be treated as if he or she were your athlete. With regard to language, directions should be given to the model in layman's terms (eg, lie on your stomach on the table) as opposed to using medical terminology (eg, lie prone on the table). The same disrobing requirements should be assumed for the model that would be required of an athlete. For example, if an athlete would be asked to remove his or her shirt prior to evaluating her shoulder, the same procedure should be followed with the model. If an athlete would be asked to remove his or her shoes and socks prior to performing palpation of the foot, again the same procedure should be followed.

Second, the model has been directed not to respond to questions. If the candidate is asked to perform an anterior drawer test on the knee and poses the questions, "Does this hurt?" "Have you injured this knee previously?" or "How did it happen?", the candidate should not wait for the model to respond. The candidate is being evaluated on the performance of the skill, not questions asked of the model. It is expected that the candidate continue to follow procedure for the evaluation of the skill, disregarding the lack of response.

Third, the model will follow a candidate's directions. However, as with an athlete, the model may be asked to do something that he or she does not understand or may have difficulty performing. For example, if the model is asked to relax, it might be difficult for him or her to meet this request without assistance from the candidate. In this case, the candidate should repeat the instructions and/or help the model relax by tapping gently on the body part or by asking the model to shut his or her eyes and lie back on the table. The model should not be noncompliant; however, clear instructions from the candidate may be required to obtain cooperation.

The scoring sheets list several required tasks for each skill, along with boxes marked "yes" and "no" for the examiner and room captain to document when tasks are observed. Point values for each task within the same scenario may vary. For example, when taping an ankle, the following task list may apply:

- Applies prewrap = 1.0 point
- Proper positioning of the foot/ankle = 2.0 points
- Two/three anchors applied below the belly of the gastrocnemius = 0.5 point
- Two/three stirrups applied medial to lateral over the malleoli = 1.5 points

The candidate should have two goals for the practical exam. First, the candidate should aim to accumulate as many points as possible, especially for those tasks that are weighed more heavily. Since time is of the essence, the candidate should be certain that the key components are completed. However, rushing to complete a skill is not advised, as it could result in losing points for careless errors. Second, the candidate must remember that in order for the task to be observed and recorded by the examiner, it must be *demonstrated*! It is not sufficient to state, "The ankle should be placed in 0 degrees of dorsiflexion." The candidate must actually place the foot in that position and maintain it throughout the taping scenario. The evaluators should be able to see the actions of the candidate at all times.

## What If I Do Not Know the Answer?

What should a candidate do if faced with a skill that he or she does not entirely know how to demonstrate? First, remember that this test is an *accumulation* of points. The main objective is to gain as many points as possible by demonstrating skills. It is important to take a moment to think about the question, instead of immediately passing. Earning few points by demonstrating some of the tasks comprising a skill is better than the guaranteed zero points from passing on a scenario. Content clues can be used to determine the body area in question. Medical terminology may give clues to determine whether the question is about muscle (*myo-*), sensation (*derma-*), or nerves (*neuro-*).

Are there *aspects* of the question that are understood? If so, that portion should be demonstrated to gain points for those tasks. If the scenario presents a taping skill with which the candidate is unfamiliar, at least the points for components of *all* taping applications can be accumulated: prepare the skin, apply prewrap, and apply anchors overlapping halfway and to the skin. If the scenario presents an orthopedic test with which the candidate is unfamiliar, he or she should place the athlete in the most likely position (eg, prone). If the scenario addresses a muscle test and the candidate is uncertain of the "optimal procedure"

for manual muscle testing, he or she should use resistive range of motion to test the actions of that muscle.

The candidate must pay special attention to the order and correctness of any given response. The response should be contemplated and mentally outlined prior to demonstrating each skill. The examiners are instructed to grade only the first response. Common errors are usually the result of lack of concentration, such as mixing up skills or performing a series of tests to get to the requested one. An example of mixing up skills may occur when the candidate is asked to perform the Thomas test to determine the amount of flexibility of the iliopsoas muscle. Without thinking, he or she begins to perform the Thompson test. An example of performing a series of tests may occur when the candidate is asked to demonstrate a sensory test in order to rule out damage to the nerve root L4. The correct response would be to apply varied pressure to the medial side of the foot. However, if the candidate begins by applying pressure on the lateral side of the foot, then moves to the top of the foot, and finally the medial side of the foot, he or she would not receive credit for the correct response because the *initial response* was not aimed at the medial side of the foot. Knowing this information, the candidate is strongly encouraged to take advantage of the allotted time, to think the skill out in its entirety, and then to perform it correctly and in the proper sequence the *first* time. Without doing so, the results may be costly.

When faced with a skill that is unfamiliar, the candidate should take time to think about the task at hand. Pausing to refocus attention may help a candidate to stay calm and avoid the understandable—but performance-interfering—panic that can set in when it is realized that the entire skill is unknown. Rereading the question and using content clues as a guide to conclude what is being asked may help, as will trying to determine and perform skills that are congruent with the information provided.

The candidate should indicate that he or she has completed a skill by stating to the examiner, "My response is complete." However, the candidate should remember that once he or she states that a response is complete, he or she is not permitted to add anything to that skill demonstration. Once a candidate has expressed that he or she has completed the response to a scenario, the room captain immediately reads the next skill. If a little time is needed to regain composure after attempting a skill, especially one that is unfamiliar, it is recommended that the candidate let time expire. The examiner will call "time" and then move on to the next skill.

The candidate should remain focused on the task at hand. A previous skill or earlier section of the exam, especially one that did not go well, should not be allowed to influence performance on the next skill. Remember, the goal is to accumulate enough points to pass the practical exam, not to make an "A." Any early mistakes should be put aside to concentrate on the successful completion of as many skills as possible within the practical exam.

## Helpful Hints for the Candidate

- Carefully examine the supply table.
- Upon entering the room, clarify when time begins and how to indicate that a response is complete.
- Read the questions by following along in the *candidate guidebook*.
- Ask for the question to be read aloud a second time, if needed.
- Take your time—plenty of time is allotted for each skill (do not rush).
- Think the skill out in its entirety before starting your response.
- Perform tasks in a logical order and in the proper sequence.
- Treat the model as you would an athlete.
- Treat the exam room as you would the athletic training room or clinical setting.
- Focus on accumulating points.
- Remember to *demonstrate*! (what you *say* is not graded)
- Do not let previous tasks influence future parts of the exam.
- Do not be distracted by the examiners marking on their score sheets (avoid looking toward the examiners).
- While reviewing for the practical option of the exam at home, practice and demonstrate on a partner.

## Practical Exam Task Areas

- Ambulation assists
- Ligamentous stress tests
- Manual muscle testing
- Reflex testing
- Sensory testing
- Special tests
- Taping/wrapping

- Vital signs
- Protective device construction
- Other (anatomical landmarks, etc)

These task areas are listed in the revised version of the second edition of *The Study Guide for NATA Board of Certification: Entry-Level Athletic Trainer Certification Examination*. As stated in the NATABOC study guide, these are examples of entry-level tasks and are in no way all-inclusive. This version of the study guide is outdated in many aspects. However, these task areas may serve as a helpful guide to organize study time and optimize mastery for the practical portion of the NATABOC exam.

Other psychomotor skill areas that should be considered when reviewing for the exam are included in the "skill" sections under each task of the *1999 NATABOC Role Delineation Study* and in the sections entitled "Athletic Training Clinical Proficiencies" under each content area of the *1999 NATA Athletic Training Educational Competencies*. Many of the clinical skills listed in these sources are included as "skill proficiency assessments" within this publication. However, the provided assessments in the guidebook are not all-inclusive and the candidate is urged to review additional sources in preparation for the exam.

All information included in this chapter comes from published NATABOC materials and is considered to be public domain. Since what is said and done in the exam room is confidential, only when the NATABOC publicly announces changes can new information be incorporated into teaching and study materials. It is important for exam candidates, classroom teachers, and clinical instructors to continually seek current guidelines on the format and requirements of the NATABOC certification exam. The best source for current information is found by accessing the NATABOC website. The following links are most helpful:

- http://www.natoboc.org/atc/links/faq/
- http://www.nataboc.org/atc/exam/onlineexam/wb-test-anshe.pdf
- http://www.nataboc.org/news/developmentprocedures.pdf

Knowledge of the current format prevents surprises during the exam and helps lower stress levels on what is already a very stressful day.

*Chapter*

# HOW TO USE THIS BOOK

## *Skill Proficiency Assessments*

Skill proficiency assessments comprise the bulk of this book. They are organized into the task areas discussed in Chapter 1. For the most part, skill proficiency assessments are specific outcomes or psychomotor skills listed under "Athletic Training Clinical Proficiencies" within the *NATA Athletic Educational Competencies* (1999). In other words, the majority of the individual psychomotor skills contained herein are deemed necessary for the performance of athletic training clinical proficiencies. Thus, a candidate is likely to see many of these skills on the practical portion of the certification exam. In addition, these skills are used in the day-to-day duties of athletic training students as they progress toward mastering clinical proficiencies.

To gain the most from this practical exam guide, athletic training students and the ACI should review the following instructions on how to use the skill proficiency assessments (Figure 2-1). Each skill proficiency assessment is divided into four sections:

1. Introduction of the specific psychomotor skill
2. Score sheet of the specific tasks that comprise the skill
3. Evaluation box
4. Scale of skill mastery

The individual components of each section will be further dissected and explained so that both athletic training students and the ACI can gain maximum benefits from this guide.

## INTRODUCTION OF A SPECIFIC PSYCHOMOTOR SKILL

The introduction of a specific psychomotor skill is the first part of each skill proficiency assessment. This section focuses on the athletic training student's initial exposure to the skill. It also provides spaces to record peer review of the skill and dates of practice opportunities prior to testing.

The upper left corner of Figure 2-1 identifies the skill proficiency assessment classification by the place and unit in the study guide. Thus, in Figure 2-1A the title of the unit and the number of the test within that unit are indicated. *Sensory Testing* is the title of the unit and *SST-L-Test 1* identifies this skill proficiency assessment as being the first test for the lower extremity.

The remaining components of Section II allow the student and ACI to record exposure to and practice sessions of the skill. The spaces marked *Peer Review* should be initialed and dated by a peer who observes the skill being performed. The number of peer reviews may be increased or decreased depending on the difficulty of the skill and the amount of practice the instructor requires prior to testing. It should also be made clear that peer reviews are not part of the formal documentation for learning over time. Peer reviews should serve only as a learning tool.

*Skill Acquisition* refers to the student's initial exposure to the skill. Thus, this space should be completed with the class number (eg, AT 206) and the date the skill was introduced. The space marked *Practice Opportunities* allows for documentation of the structured opportunities

## SENSORY TESTING
# (SST-L-Test 1)    (A)

Peer Review SLC 10-20-01  Peer Review HKA 10-22-01

Skill Acquisition: AT 206 (10-4-01)          Practice Opportunities: 10-19-01, 10-23-01

*This problem allows you the opportunity to demonstrate a sensory test in order to rule out damage to the nerve root **L4**. You have 2 minutes to perform this task.*

| Tester places athlete and limb in appropriate position  (B) | YES | NO |
|---|---|---|
| Prone or seated | ●○○ | ○○○ |
| Shoes and socks off | ●○○ | ○○○ |

| Tester performs test according to accepted guidelines | YES | NO |
|---|---|---|
| Appropriate directions are given | ●○○ | ○○○ |
| Differences between varied pressure are explained | ●○○ | ○○○ |
| Directions/explanation given away from the injured area | ○○○ | ●○○ |
| Athlete is instructed to close eyes | ○○○ | ●○○ |
| Varied pressure used | ●○○ | ○○○ |
|   Sharp | ●○○ | ○○○ |
|   Dull | ●○○ | ○○○ |
|   No touch | ●○○ | ○○○ |
| Appropriate pressure is applied to the medial side of the lower leg | ○○○ | ●○○ |
| Tests bilaterally | ●○○ | ○○○ |

The psychomotor skill was performed completely and in the appropriate order    0 1 2 ③ 4 5

The tester had control of the subject and the situation (showed confidence)    0 1 2 3 ④ 5

Method of performing the skill allowed the tester the ability to determine:  (C)
severity, proper progression, and the *fit* in the overall picture (Oral)    0 1 2 3 ④ 5

In order for a grade of *minimum standard* to be given, the total must be ≥11    **TOTAL =**

(D)

                          10-24-01      2-22-02     3-21-03

|_____| L     A     P |

**Not Acceptable**      **Meets Minimum Standards**      **Exceeds Minimum Standards**

**L:** Laboratory/Classroom Testing
**C:** Clinical/Field Testing
**P:** Practicum Testing          (E)
**A:** Assessment/Mock Exam Testing
**S:** Self-Reporting

**Positive Finding:** No feeling, difficulty in distinguishing varied pressure
**Involved Structure:** Nerve root coming off L4
**Special Considerations:** N/A
**Reference(s):** Hoppenfeld
**Supplies Needed:** Table/chair, sharp/dull objects

**Figure 2-1.** Completed skill proficiency assessment.

by the student to practice the skill under the supervision of an instructor.

## THE SCORE SHEET FOR THE SPECIFIC TASKS THAT COMPRISE THE SKILL

The score sheet for the specific tasks that comprise the skill (Figure 2-1B) opens with the statement of the skill the student is being asked to perform. Following the initial statement of the skill, each individual task that contributes to that skill is listed. Blank circles, indicating *yes* or *no*, are provided next to each component of the skill. A response of *yes* indicates that component of the skill was performed correctly. A response of *no* indicates that component of the skill was either performed incorrectly or not at all. Note that the skill proficiency assessments in this section of the text are not weighted, but those assessments in Section III are weighted similarly to those on the certification exam.

The correct responses for each yes or no section are objective. The tester may want to use different colored markers and/or use the appropriate letters of the method for testing (L, C, P, A, or S), in order to document which circle was checked at a specific interval. The observed responses should be the same whether they were checked by a peer or by a clinical instructor. However, the level set for mastery is subjective and should be determined by the athletic trainer who is responsible for verifying (on the NATABOC application) that mastery has occurred. As a student preparing for entry into the athletic training profession, the goal for mastery should be 100%. As mentioned in Chapter 1, the student should strive to have as many *yes* boxes checked as possible because each point is important in tabulating the final score on the NATABOC exam.

This section may be used during the instruction, practice, or testing of a skill. During instruction, the student may use this score sheet, along with note taking from class and review of other recommended references, to learn the skill. Each score sheet was developed with the use of one or more appropriate references. However, total agreement between references does not occur in all cases, and, for the purposes of this book, when disagreements occurred between the references, a decision was made based on the knowledge of the authors. Very few score sheets have 100% agreement by multiple sources. It is important to understand that all references do not say the same thing. This fact may be frustrating to a young professional. However, when disagreements between references occur, discussion of these differences can enhance the learning experience between students and clinical instructors.

## EVALUATION BOX

The evaluation box (Figure 2-1C) begins to incorporate the individual psychomotor skill into the larger picture of the clinical proficiency. This section of the skill proficiency assessment is not part of the evaluation process for the NATABOC exam. It is strictly for student feedback. The higher the subjective score given, the greater the understanding of the overall skill. The first line of the evaluation box is directly related to the number of yes and no checks on the score sheet. The second line indicates the tester's confidence level in performing the skill. The third line is determined by verbal communication between the evaluator and the athletic training student. This communication is in a series of questions to determine whether the student understands the purpose of the skill being tested and where it fits into a clinical proficiency. The minimum standard score of 11 or higher is arbitrary; however, it does represent 73% of the total possible points. This section documents the essential concept of "learning over time," which is not assessed on the NATABOC exam.

## SCALE OF SKILL MASTERY

This section is designed to monitor the dates and methods used by the ACI when evaluation occurs. Figure 2-1D indicates that a student was tested three times over a 17-month period. In this example, the first testing situation was in a laboratory environment on 10-24-01. The placement of the *L* indicates that the score from the evaluation box meets minimum standards and was administrated in a laboratory or classroom environment. The second test of the same skill did not occur until the following semester during program assessment. The placement of the *A* has moved closer to exceeding minimum standards. The final test date (3-21-03) indicates that the student was tested a year later in a practicum class and scored very well, based on the placement of the *P*.

The letters *L*, *C*, *P*, *A*, and *S* are used to indicate the environment in which the skill proficiency assessment took place. While the following information indicates the authors' definitions for using these environmental indicators, these indicators may be adjusted to fit the testing methods used in individual athletic training programs.

### L: Laboratory or Classroom Testing

The letter *L* indicates that skill proficiency assessment took place during structured laboratory or classroom settings. These testing sessions may include formal lab tests, breakout sessions where testing occurs, or written exams that include practical testing.

### C: Clinical/Field Testing

The letter *C* indicates that skill proficiency assessment took place in the athletic training room, clinical setting, or on the athletic field and was performed by an ACI. This method of testing is based around the *teachable moment*. Practice occurs during down-time in the clinical setting or during the observation of a skill when the student is actually performing it.

### P: Practicum Testing

The letter P indicates that skill proficiency assessment took place during a scheduled testing at least one semester after the skill had been learned. This testing is included in practicum courses and the clinical packet associated with a practicum course.

### A: Assessment/Mock Exam Testing

The letter A indicates that skill proficiency assessment took place during assessment testing. This type of testing evaluates the same skill sets year after year. Program assessment gives students a baseline of strengths and weaknesses relative to their own performance in the previous year, their peers in the same class, and to previous student athletic trainers in the same program.

### S: Self-Reporting

The letter S indicates that skill proficiency assessment took place when the student evaluated him- or herself.

For example, if a student is asked whether he or she is confident in performing a specific skill and the answer is *no*, additional practice time is allotted to that student. This means of testing is not used as a replacement for formal testing or for documenting learning over time but is helpful in finding weaknesses in the curriculum and the individual student.

## ADDITIONAL INFORMATION

Finally, valuable information (Figure 2-1E) to assist the student in finding additional reading material on the skill proficiency assessment can be found on the bottom right corner of the page. This area includes the following information: positive finding of the skill, the structures being assessed, special considerations unique to the skill proficiency assessment, the primary reference book(s) used in developing the score sheet, and any supplies needed for the student to perform the skill.

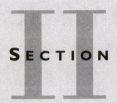

SECTION

II

PRACTICAL EXAM QUESTIONS BY TASK AREAS

# AMBULATION ASSISTS

# AMBULATION ASSISTS
## (AA-Test 1)

Peer Review _____    Peer Review _____

Skill Acquisition: _____     Practice Opportunities: _____

*This problem allows you the opportunity to demonstrate* **crutch fitting** *for an athlete. You have 4 minutes to complete this task.*

| Tester places athlete and limb in appropriate position | YES | NO |
|---|---|---|
| Standing with good posture | ○○○ | ○○○ |
| Feet shoulder width apart | ○○○ | ○○○ |
| Wearing low-heeled/flat shoes | ○○○ | ○○○ |
| **Tester measures athlete for ambulation device** | **YES** | **NO** |
| Places crutch slightly in front of the involved limb (2 to 4 inches) | ○○○ | ○○○ |
| Places crutch slightly to the side of the involved limb (4 to 6 inches) | ○○○ | ○○○ |
| Places axillary pad approximately 1 to 1.5 inches below axilla | ○○○ | ○○○ |
| Places elbow in approximately 30 degrees flexion | ○○○ | ○○○ |
| **Tester checks ambulatory device for safety** | **YES** | **NO** |
| Tightens all fasteners | ○○○ | ○○○ |
| Verifies axilla and hand grips are well-padded | ○○○ | ○○○ |
| Verifies that rubberized tips are not damaged | ○○○ | ○○○ |
| Instructs athlete to bear weight on hands, not axilla | ○○○ | ○○○ |

| | |
|---|---|
| The psychomotor skill was performed completely and in the appropriate order | **0  1  2  3  4  5** |
| The tester had control of the subject and the situation (showed confidence) | **0  1  2  3  4  5** |
| Method of performing the skill allowed the tester the ability to determine: severity, proper progression, and the *fit* in the overall picture (Oral) | **0  1  2  3  4  5** |

In order for a grade of *minimum standard* to be given, the total must be ≥11          **TOTAL =**

I_____I_____I

**Not Acceptable**          **Meets Minimum Standards**          **Exceeds Minimum Standards**

**Positive Finding:** N/A
**Involved Structure:** N/A
**Special Considerations:** Hand grips should be at the level of the greater trochanter
**Reference(s):** Arnheim et al; Anderson et al; Houglum
**Supplies Needed:** Crutches of various sizes

**L:** Laboratory/Classroom Testing
**C:** Clinical/Field Testing
**P:** Practicum Testing
**A:** Assessment/Mock Exam Testing
**S:** Self-Reporting

## AMBULATION ASSISTS
# (AA-Test 2)

Peer Review _____  Peer Review _____

Skill Acquisition: _____    Practice Opportunities: _____

*This problem allows you the opportunity to instruct an athlete in the nonweightbearing—tripod method of crutch walking. You have 4 minutes to complete this task.*

| Tester places athlete and limb in appropriate position | YES | NO |
|---|---|---|
| Standing with good posture | ○○○ | ○○○ |
| Feet shoulder width apart | ○○○ | ○○○ |
| Wearing low-heeled/flat shoes | ○○○ | ○○○ |
| **Tester verifies correct fit of ambulation device** | **YES** | **NO** |
| Places crutch slightly in front of the involved limb (2 to 4 inches) | ○○○ | ○○○ |
| Places crutch slightly to the side of the involved limb (4 to 6 inches) | ○○○ | ○○○ |
| Places axillary pad approximately 1 to 1.5 inches below axilla | ○○○ | ○○○ |
| Places elbow in approximately 30 degrees flexion | ○○○ | ○○○ |
| **Tester instructs athlete in walking with ambulatory device** | **YES** | **NO** |
| Weight evenly distributed on crutches | ○○○ | ○○○ |
| Instructs athlete not put weight on axilla | ○○○ | ○○○ |
| Involved limb is off the floor (flexed position) | ○○○ | ○○○ |
| Athlete moves both crutches forward (6 to 8 inches) | ○○○ | ○○○ |
| Athlete swings the noninjured limb forward (swing-to) or (swing-through) | ○○○ | ○○○ |
| Repeat the above two steps | ○○○ | ○○○ |

The psychomotor skill was performed completely and in the appropriate order    **0  1  2  3  4  5**

The tester had control of the subject and the situation (showed confidence)    **0  1  2  3  4  5**

Method of performing the skill allowed the tester the ability to determine:
severity, proper progression, and the *fit* in the overall picture (Oral)    **0  1  2  3  4  5**

In order for a grade of *minimum standard* to be given, the total must be ≥11    **TOTAL =**

I_____I_____I
**Not Acceptable**          **Meets Minimum Standards**          **Exceeds Minimum Standards**

**Positive Finding:** N/A
**Involved Structure:** N/A
**Special Considerations:**

**L:** Laboratory/Classroom Testing
**C:** Clinical/Field Testing
**P:** Practicum Testing
**A:** Assessment/Mock Exam Testing
**S:** Self-Reporting

**Reference(s):** Anderson et al

**Supplies Needed:** Crutches of various sizes

# AMBULATION ASSISTS
# (AA-Test 3)

Peer Review _____ Peer Review _____

Skill Acquisition: _____        Practice Opportunities: _____

*This problem allows you the opportunity to instruct an athlete in the* **nonweightbearing—ascending and descending stairs (without a handrail)** *method of crutch walking. You have 4 minutes to complete this task.*

| Tester places athlete and limb in appropriate position | YES | NO |
|---|---|---|
| Standing with good posture | ○○○ | ○○○ |
| Feet shoulder width apart | ○○○ | ○○○ |
| Wearing low-heeled/flat shoes | ○○○ | ○○○ |
| **Tester verifies correct fit of ambulation device** | **YES** | **NO** |
| Places crutch slightly in front of the involved limb (2 to 4 inches) | ○○○ | ○○○ |
| Places crutch slightly to the side of the involved limb (4 to 6 inches) | ○○○ | ○○○ |
| Places axillary pad approximately 1 to 1.5 inches below axilla | ○○○ | ○○○ |
| Places elbow in approximately 30 degrees flexion | ○○○ | ○○○ |
| **Tester instructs athlete in ascending stairs** | **YES** | **NO** |
| Weight evenly distributed on crutches | ○○○ | ○○○ |
| Athlete steps up with uninjured leg | ○○○ | ○○○ |
| Athlete follows with injured leg and crutches | ○○○ | ○○○ |
| **Tester instructs athlete in descending stairs** | **YES** | **NO** |
| Weight evenly distributed on crutches | ○○○ | ○○○ |
| Athlete steps down with injured leg and crutches | ○○○ | ○○○ |
| Athlete follows with uninjured leg | ○○○ | ○○○ |

The psychomotor skill was performed completely and in the appropriate order    0  1  2  3  4  5

The tester had control of the subject and the situation (showed confidence)    0  1  2  3  4  5

Method of performing the skill allowed the tester the ability to determine:
severity, proper progression, and the *fit* in the overall picture (Oral)    0  1  2  3  4  5

In order for a grade of *minimum standard* to be given, the total must be ≥11        **TOTAL =**

I_____I_____I

**Not Acceptable**        **Meets Minimum Standards**        **Exceeds Minimum Standards**

**L:** Laboratory/Classroom Testing
**C:** Clinical/Field Testing
**P:** Practicum Testing
**A:** Assessment/Mock Exam Testing
**S:** Self-Reporting

**Positive Finding:** N/A
**Involved Structure:** N/A
**Special Considerations:** If available, may use handrail
(see references)
**Reference(s):** Arnheim et al; Anderson et al; Houglum
**Supplies Needed:** Crutches of various sizes

## AMBULATION ASSISTS
# (AA-Test 4)

Peer Review _____ Peer Review _____

Skill Acquisition: _____    Practice Opportunities: _____

*This problem allows you the opportunity to demonstrate* **cane fitting** *for an athlete. This should include instruction on walking with a cane. You have 2 minutes to complete this task.*

| Tester places athlete and limb in appropriate position | YES | NO |
|---|---|---|
| Standing with good posture | OOO | OOO |
| Feet shoulder width apart | OOO | OOO |
| Wearing low-heeled/flat shoes | OOO | OOO |
| **Tester measures athlete for ambulation device** | **YES** | **NO** |
| Measure from greater trochanter of femur to the floor | OOO | OOO |
| Adjust cane to the measured length | OOO | OOO |
| **Tester instructs athlete in walking with ambulatory device** | **YES** | **NO** |
| Cane is placed on uninjured side | OOO | OOO |
| Athlete steps forward with cane and injured leg | OOO | OOO |
| Athlete follows with uninjured leg | OOO | OOO |

The psychomotor skill was performed completely and in the appropriate order      **0  1  2  3  4  5**

The tester had control of the subject and the situation (showed confidence)      **0  1  2  3  4  5**

Method of performing the skill allowed the tester the ability to determine:
severity, proper progression, and the *fit* in the overall picture (Oral)      **0  1  2  3  4  5**

In order for a grade of *minimum standard* to be given, the total must be ≥11      **TOTAL =**

I_____I_____I
**Not Acceptable**      **Meets Minimum Standards**      **Exceeds Minimum Standards**

**L:** Laboratory/Classroom Testing
**C:** Clinical/Field Testing
**P:** Practicum Testing
**A:** Assessment/Mock Exam Testing
**S:** Self-Reporting

**Positive Finding:** N/A
**Involved Structure:** N/A
**Special Considerations:** Instruct not to lean heavily on the cane (same instructions for the use of one crutch)
**Reference(s):** Arnheim et al; Anderson et al; Houglum
**Supplies Needed:** Canes of various sizes, measuring device

# AMBULATION ASSISTS
## (AA-Test 5)

Peer Review _____ Peer Review _____

Skill Acquisition: _____  Practice Opportunities: _____

*This problem allows you the opportunity to instruct an athlete in the **four-point gait method** of crutch walking. You have 4 minutes to complete this task.*

| Tester places athlete and limb in appropriate position | YES | NO |
|---|---|---|
| Standing with good posture | ○○○ | ○○○ |
| Feet shoulder width apart | ○○○ | ○○○ |
| Wearing low-heeled/flat shoes | ○○○ | ○○○ |
| **Tester verifies correct fit of ambulation device** | **YES** | **NO** |
| Places crutch slightly in front of the involved limb (2 to 4 inches) | ○○○ | ○○○ |
| Places crutch slightly to the side of the involved limb (4 to 6 inches) | ○○○ | ○○○ |
| Places axillary pad approximately 1 to 1.5 inches below axilla | ○○○ | ○○○ |
| Places elbow in approximately 30 degrees flexion | ○○○ | ○○○ |
| **Tester instructs athlete in walking with ambulatory device** | **YES** | **NO** |
| Weight evenly distributed on crutches | ○○○ | ○○○ |
| Athlete places one crutch tip forward | ○○○ | ○○○ |
| Athlete steps forward with opposite foot | ○○○ | ○○○ |
| Athlete places other crutch tip forward | ○○○ | ○○○ |
| Athlete steps forward with other foot | ○○○ | ○○○ |

The psychomotor skill was performed completely and in the appropriate order    0 1 2 3 4 5

The tester had control of the subject and the situation (showed confidence)    0 1 2 3 4 5

Method of performing the skill allowed the tester the ability to determine: severity, proper progression, and the *fit* in the overall picture (Oral)    0 1 2 3 4 5

In order for a grade of *minimum standard* to be given, the total must be ≥11    **TOTAL =**

I_____I_____I

**Not Acceptable**    **Meets Minimum Standards**    **Exceeds Minimum Standards**

**L:** Laboratory/Classroom Testing
**C:** Clinical/Field Testing
**P:** Practicum Testing
**A:** Assessment/Mock Exam Testing
**S:** Self-Reporting

**Positive Finding:** N/A
**Involved Structure:** N/A
**Special Considerations:** N/A
**Reference(s):** Arnheim et al; Houglum
**Supplies Needed:** Crutches of various sizes

# 4

# LIGAMENTOUS STRESS TESTS

# LIGAMENTOUS STRESS TESTS
## (LST-U-Test 1)

Peer Review _____ Peer Review _____

Skill Acquisition: _____    Practice Opportunities: _____

*Please demonstrate how you would perform the orthopedic test known as the* **Acromioclavicular Joint Distraction Test** *for the shoulder. You have 2 minutes to complete this task.*

| Tester places athlete and limb in appropriate position | YES | NO |
|---|---|---|
| Seated or standing | ○○○ | ○○○ |
| Arm relaxed at side, elbow at 90 degrees flexion | ○○○ | ○○○ |
| **Tester placed in proper position** | **YES** | **NO** |
| Stands on involved side | ○○○ | ○○○ |
| Holds subject's arm just above elbow | ○○○ | ○○○ |
| Places other hand over involved AC joint | ○○○ | ○○○ |
| **Tester performs test according to accepted guidelines** | **YES** | **NO** |
| Applies gentle downward pressure on the arm | ○○○ | ○○○ |
| Maintains relaxation of the limb | ○○○ | ○○○ |
| Performs assessment bilaterally | ○○○ | ○○○ |

The psychomotor skill was performed completely and in the appropriate order    **0  1  2  3  4  5**

The tester had control of the subject and the situation (showed confidence)    **0  1  2  3  4  5**

Method of performing the skill allowed the tester the ability to determine:
severity, proper progression, and the *fit* in the overall picture (Oral)    **0  1  2  3  4  5**

In order for a grade of *minimum standard* to be given, the total must be ≥11    **TOTAL =**

I_____I_____I

**Not Acceptable**          **Meets Minimum Standards**          **Exceeds Minimum Standards**

**L:** Laboratory/Classroom Testing
**C:** Clinical/Field Testing
**P:** Practicum Testing
**A:** Assessment/Mock Exam Testing
**S:** Self-Reporting

**Positive Finding:** Pain; step deformity/movement of the AC joint
**Involved Structure:** AC joint; AC/coracoclavicular ligaments (sprain)
**Special Considerations:** N/A
**Reference(s):** Konin et al; Starkey et al
**Supplies Needed:** N/A

## LIGAMENTOUS STRESS TESTS
# (LST-U-Test 2)

Peer Review _____ Peer Review _____

Skill Acquisition: _____  Practice Opportunities: _____

*Please demonstrate how you would perform the orthopedic test known as the* **Acromioclavicular Shear Test (AC Joint Compression Test)** *for the shoulder. You have 2 minutes to complete this task.*

| | YES | NO |
|---|---|---|
| **Tester places athlete and limb in appropriate position** | YES | NO |
| Seated or standing | ooo | ooo |
| Arm relaxed at side (hanging naturally to the side) | ooo | ooo |
| **Tester placed in proper position** | YES | NO |
| Stands on involved side | ooo | ooo |
| Places one hand on the subject's clavicle | ooo | ooo |
| Places other hand on the spine of the scapula | ooo | ooo |
| **Tester performs test according to accepted guidelines** | YES | NO |
| Gently squeezes the hands together (cupping motion) | ooo | ooo |
| Maintains relaxation of the limb | ooo | ooo |
| Performs assessment bilaterally | ooo | ooo |

The psychomotor skill was performed completely and in the appropriate order  **0 1 2 3 4 5**

The tester had control of the subject and the situation (showed confidence)  **0 1 2 3 4 5**

Method of performing the skill allowed the tester the ability to determine: severity, proper progression, and the *fit* in the overall picture (Oral)  **0 1 2 3 4 5**

In order for a grade of *minimum standard* to be given, the total must be ≥11    **TOTAL =**

I_____I_____I
**Not Acceptable      Meets Minimum Standards      Exceeds Minimum Standards**

**L:** Laboratory/Classroom Testing
**C:** Clinical/Field Testing
**P:** Practicum Testing
**A:** Assessment/Mock Exam Testing
**S:** Self-Reporting

**Positive Finding:** Pain; movement of the clavicle
**Involved Structure:** AC joint; AC/coracoclavicular ligaments (sprain)
**Special Considerations:** Do not perform if obvious AC joint deformity
**Reference(s):** Konin et al; Magee; Starkey et al
**Supplies Needed:** N/A

# LIGAMENTOUS STRESS TESTS
## (LST-U-Test 3)

Peer Review _____ Peer Review _____

Skill Acquisition: _____  Practice Opportunities: _____

*Please demonstrate how you would perform the orthopedic test known as the* **Anterior Drawer Test for the Shoulder** *to help rule out joint laxity. You have 2 minutes to complete this task.*

| Tester places athlete and limb in appropriate position | YES | NO |
|---|---|---|
| Supine | ○○○ | ○○○ |
| Places arm in: | | |
|   Abduction | ○○○ | ○○○ |
|   Forward flexion (horizontal flexion); around 10 degrees | ○○○ | ○○○ |
|   Lateral rotation | ○○○ | ○○○ |

| Tester placed in proper position | YES | NO |
|---|---|---|
| Places on hand in the axilla area (holding athlete's arm) | ○○○ | ○○○ |
| Stabilizes the athlete's scapula with the opposite hand | ○○○ | ○○○ |
| Applies counterpressure to the athlete's coracoid process with thumb | ○○○ | ○○○ |

| Tester performs test according to accepted guidelines | YES | NO |
|---|---|---|
| Instructs the athlete to relax | ○○○ | ○○○ |
| Appropriate pressure administered (direction and intensity, forward displacement of the humerus) | ○○○ | ○○○ |
| Maintains relaxation of the limb | ○○○ | ○○○ |
| Performs assessment bilaterally | ○○○ | ○○○ |

The psychomotor skill was performed completely and in the appropriate order    0 1 2 3 4 5

The tester had control of the subject and the situation (showed confidence)    0 1 2 3 4 5

Method of performing the skill allowed the tester the ability to determine: severity, proper progression, and the *fit* in the overall picture (Oral)    0 1 2 3 4 5

In order for a grade of *minimum standard* to be given, the total must be ≥11    **TOTAL =**

I_____I_____I

**Not Acceptable**    **Meets Minimum Standards**    **Exceeds Minimum Standards**

**L:** Laboratory/Classroom Testing
**C:** Clinical/Field Testing
**P:** Practicum Testing
**A:** Assessment/Mock Exam Testing
**S:** Self-Reporting

**Positive Finding:** Anterior displacement; clicking/apprehension
**Involved Structure:** Anterior instability of the shoulder
**Special Considerations:** N/A
**Reference(s):** Konin et al; Magee
**Supplies Needed:** N/A

## LIGAMENTOUS STRESS TESTS
# (LST-U-Test 4)

Peer Review _____ Peer Review _____

Skill Acquisition: _____    Practice Opportunities: _____

*Please demonstrate how you would perform the orthopedic test known as the* **Clunk Test for the Shoulder**. *You have 2 minutes to complete this task.*

| Tester places athlete and limb in appropriate position | YES | NO |
|---|---|---|
| Supine | ○○○ | ○○○ |
| Arm in full abduction/external rotation (passive) | ○○○ | ○○○ |
| **Tester placed in proper position** | **YES** | **NO** |
| Standing behind athlete's head | ○○○ | ○○○ |
| Supports posterior humeral head with one hand | ○○○ | ○○○ |
| Grips posterior humerus just proximal to elbow with other hand | ○○○ | ○○○ |
| **Tester performs test according to accepted guidelines** | **YES** | **NO** |
| Pushes anteriorly on humeral head | ○○○ | ○○○ |
| Rotates humerus in a lateral rotation with other hand (may continue by internally rotating and circumducting the humeral head) | ○○○ | ○○○ |
| Maintains relaxation of the limb | ○○○ | ○○○ |
| Performs assessment bilaterally | ○○○ | ○○○ |

The psychomotor skill was performed completely and in the appropriate order    **0  1  2  3  4  5**

The tester had control of the subject and the situation (showed confidence)    **0  1  2  3  4  5**

Method of performing the skill allowed the tester the ability to determine:
severity, proper progression, and the *fit* in the overall picture (Oral)    **0  1  2  3  4  5**

In order for a grade of *minimum standard* to be given, the total must be ≥11    **TOTAL =**

I_____I_____I

**Not Acceptable**            **Meets Minimum Standards**        **Exceeds Minimum Standards**

**L:** Laboratory/Classroom Testing
**C:** Clinical/Field Testing
**P:** Practicum Testing
**A:** Assessment/Mock Exam Testing
**S:** Self-Reporting

**Positive Finding:** Grinding, clunking
**Involved Structure:** Glenoid labrum tear
**Special Considerations:** N/A
**Reference(s):** Konin et al; Magee
**Supplies Needed:** Table

## Ligamentous Stress Tests
# (LST-U-Test 5)

Peer Review _____    Peer Review _____

Skill Acquisition: _____    Practice Opportunities: _____

*Please demonstrate how you would perform the orthopedic test known as the* **Feagin Test for the Shoulder.** *You have 2 minutes to complete this task.*

| Tester places athlete and limb in appropriate position | YES | NO |
|---|---|---|
| Standing | OOO | OOO |
| Shoulder abducted to 90 degrees, with elbow fully extended | OOO | OOO |
| Forearm resting on examiner's shoulder | OOO | OOO |
| **Tester placed in proper position** | **YES** | **NO** |
| Stands to the side of athlete, faces the athlete | OOO | OOO |
| Hands clasped together around upper and middle third of humerus | OOO | OOO |
| **Tester performs test according to accepted guidelines** | **YES** | **NO** |
| Pushes humerus down and forward | OOO | OOO |
| Maintains relaxation of the limb | OOO | OOO |
| Performs assessment bilaterally | OOO | OOO |

The psychomotor skill was performed completely and in the appropriate order    **0  1  2  3  4  5**

The tester had control of the subject and the situation (showed confidence)    **0  1  2  3  4  5**

Method of performing the skill allowed the tester the ability to determine:
severity, proper progression, and the *fit* in the overall picture (Oral)    **0  1  2  3  4  5**

In order for a grade of *minimum standard* to be given, the total must be ≥11    **TOTAL =**

I_____I_____I

**Not Acceptable**        **Meets Minimum Standards**        **Exceeds Minimum Standards**

**L:** Laboratory/Classroom Testing
**C:** Clinical/Field Testing
**P:** Practicum Testing
**A:** Assessment/Mock Exam Testing
**S:** Self-Reporting

**Positive Finding:** Apprehension
**Involved Structure:** Anteroinferior instability
**Special Considerations:** Modification of the sulcus sign test
**Reference(s):** Magee
**Supplies Needed:** N/A

# LIGAMENTOUS STRESS TESTS
# (LST-U-Test 6)

Peer Review _____ Peer Review _____

Skill Acquisition: _____    Practice Opportunities: _____

*Please demonstrate how you would perform the orthopedic test known as the* **Sternoclavicular Joint Stress Test for the Shoulder**. *You have 2 minutes to complete this task.*

| Tester places athlete and limb in appropriate position | YES | NO |
|---|---|---|
| Seated or standing | OOO | OOO |
| Arm relaxed at side | OOO | OOO |
| **Tester placed in proper position** | **YES** | **NO** |
| Stands in front of the athlete | OOO | OOO |
| Places one hand on the proximal end of the athlete's clavicle | OOO | OOO |
| Places the other hand on the spine of the scapula | OOO | OOO |
| **Tester performs test according to accepted guidelines** | **YES** | **NO** |
| Applies gentle downward and inward pressure on the clavicle | OOO | OOO |
| Notes any movement at the sternoclavicular joint | OOO | OOO |
| Maintains relaxation of the involved limb | OOO | OOO |
| Performs assessment bilaterally | OOO | OOO |

The psychomotor skill was performed completely and in the appropriate order      0  1  2  3  4  5

The tester had control of the subject and the situation (showed confidence)      0  1  2  3  4  5

Method of performing the skill allowed the tester the ability to determine:
severity, proper progression, and the *fit* in the overall picture (Oral)      0  1  2  3  4  5

In order for a grade of *minimum standard* to be given, the total must be ≥11      TOTAL =

I_____I_____I
**Not Acceptable**      **Meets Minimum Standards**      **Exceeds Minimum Standards**

**L:** Laboratory/Classroom Testing
**C:** Clinical/Field Testing
**P:** Practicum Testing
**A:** Assessment/Mock Exam Testing
**S:** Self-Reporting

**Positive Finding:** Pain and/or movement
**Involved Structure:** Clavicle; SC ligament sprain, possibly involving the costoclavicular ligament
**Special Considerations:** N/A
**Reference(s):** Konin et al
**Supplies Needed:** N/A

# LIGAMENTOUS STRESS TESTS
## (LST-U-Test 7)

Peer Review _____ Peer Review _____

Skill Acquisition: _____     Practice Opportunities: _____

*Please demonstrate how you would perform the orthopedic test known as the* **Posterior Drawer Test for the Shoulder**. *You have 2 minutes to complete this task.*

| Tester places athlete and limb in appropriate position | YES | NO |
|---|---|---|
| Supine | ○○○ | ○○○ |
| Arm passively placed in the 90-90 position | ○○○ | ○○○ |
| **Tester placed in proper position** | **YES** | **NO** |
| Stands next to the involved shoulder | ○○○ | ○○○ |
| Places one hand on the athlete's distal humerus | ○○○ | ○○○ |
| Places the other hand posterior to shoulder capsule to stabilize the scapula (thumb on the coracoid process) | ○○○ | ○○○ |
| **Tester performs test according to accepted guidelines** | **YES** | **NO** |
| Moves the shoulder to about 30 degrees of horizontal flexion | ○○○ | ○○○ |
| Applies passive internal rotation to the shoulder | ○○○ | ○○○ |
| Applies downward pressure (forcing the head of humerus posteriorly) | ○○○ | ○○○ |
| Maintains relaxation of the limb | ○○○ | ○○○ |
| Performs assessment bilaterally | ○○○ | ○○○ |

The psychomotor skill was performed completely and in the appropriate order     **0  1  2  3  4  5**

The tester had control of the subject and the situation (showed confidence)     **0  1  2  3  4  5**

Method of performing the skill allowed the tester the ability to determine:
severity, proper progression, and the *fit* in the overall picture (Oral)     **0  1  2  3  4  5**

In order for a grade of *minimum standard* to be given, the total must be ≥11     **TOTAL =**

I_____I_____I

**Not Acceptable**          **Meets Minimum Standards**          **Exceeds Minimum Standards**

**L:** Laboratory/Classroom Testing
**C:** Clinical/Field Testing
**P:** Practicum Testing
**A:** Assessment/Mock Exam Testing
**S:** Self-Reporting

**Positive Finding:** Posterior instability of the humeral head; apprehension
**Involved Structure:** Posterior structures
**Special Considerations:** N/A
**Reference(s):** Konin et al; Magee
**Supplies Needed:** Table

## LIGAMENTOUS STRESS TESTS
# (LST-U-Test 8)

Peer Review _____ Peer Review _____

Skill Acquisition: _____     Practice Opportunities: _____

*Please demonstrate how you would perform the orthopedic test known as the* **Jobe Relocation Test (Fowler Sign/Fowler Test/Relocation Test)** *for the shoulder. You have 2 minutes to complete this task.*

| Tester places athlete and limb in appropriate position | YES | NO |
|---|---|---|
| Supine | ○○○ | ○○○ |
| Shoulder in 90 degrees abduction | ○○○ | ○○○ |
| Shoulder in full external rotation | ○○○ | ○○○ |
| **Tester placed in proper position** | **YES** | **NO** |
| Stands next the involved shoulder | ○○○ | ○○○ |
| Places distal hand on the subject's wrist | ○○○ | ○○○ |
| Places the other hand over subject's humeral head (anterior) | ○○○ | ○○○ |
| **Tester performs test according to accepted guidelines** | **YES** | **NO** |
| Applies posterior force to the humeral head | ○○○ | ○○○ |
| Applies passive external rotation to the shoulder | ○○○ | ○○○ |
| Maintains relaxation of the limb | ○○○ | ○○○ |
| Performs assessment bilaterally | ○○○ | ○○○ |

The psychomotor skill was performed completely and in the appropriate order     0 1 2 3 4 5

The tester had control of the subject and the situation (showed confidence)     0 1 2 3 4 5

Method of performing the skill allowed the tester the ability to determine:
severity, proper progression, and the *fit* in the overall picture (Oral)     0 1 2 3 4 5

In order for a grade of *minimum standard* to be given, the total must be ≥11     **TOTAL =**

I_____I_____I

    **Not Acceptable**     **Meets Minimum Standards**     **Exceeds Minimum Standards**

**L:** Laboratory/Classroom Testing
**C:** Clinical/Field Testing
**P:** Practicum Testing
**A:** Assessment/Mock Exam Testing
**S:** Self-Reporting

**Positive Finding:** Reduction of pain; apprehension
**Involved Structure:** Anterior structures of the shoulder
**Special Considerations:** Should be performed immediately following the apprehension test (anterior)
**Reference(s):** Konin et al; Magee
**Supplies Needed:** Table

# LIGAMENTOUS STRESS TESTS
## (LST-U-Test 9)

Peer Review _____ Peer Review _____

Skill Acquisition: _____     Practice Opportunities: _____

*Please demonstrate how you would perform the orthopedic test known as the* **Apprehension Test (Crank Test)** *for an anterior shoulder dislocation. You have 2 minutes to complete this task.*

| Tester places athlete and limb in appropriate position | YES | NO |
|---|---|---|
| Supine | ○○○ | ○○○ |
| Shoulder placed in 90 degrees abduction | ○○○ | ○○○ |
| Elbow placed in 90 degrees of flexion | ○○○ | ○○○ |
| **Tester placed in proper position** | **YES** | **NO** |
| Stands next to the involved shoulder | ○○○ | ○○○ |
| Places one hand on the subject's wrist | ○○○ | ○○○ |
| Post the other hand under the distal humerus | ○○○ | ○○○ |
| **Tester performs test according to accepted guidelines** | **YES** | **NO** |
| Moves the limb slowly into external rotation | ○○○ | ○○○ |
| Maintains relaxation of the limb | ○○○ | ○○○ |
| Performs assessment bilaterally | ○○○ | ○○○ |

| | |
|---|---|
| The psychomotor skill was performed completely and in the appropriate order | 0  1  2  3  4  5 |
| The tester had control of the subject and the situation (showed confidence) | 0  1  2  3  4  5 |
| Method of performing the skill allowed the tester the ability to determine: severity, proper progression, and the *fit* in the overall picture (Oral) | 0  1  2  3  4  5 |

In order for a grade of *minimum standard* to be given, the total must be ≥11      **TOTAL =**

I_____I_____I

**Not Acceptable**          **Meets Minimum Standards**          **Exceeds Minimum Standards**

**L:** Laboratory/Classroom Testing
**C:** Clinical/Field Testing
**P:** Practicum Testing
**A:** Assessment/Mock Exam Testing
**S:** Self-Reporting

**Positive Finding:** Apprehension, pain
**Involved Structure:** Anterior structures
**Special Considerations:** Do not perform when there is obvious deformity
**Reference(s):** Konin et al; Magee; Starkey et al
**Supplies Needed:** Table

## LIGAMENTOUS STRESS TESTS
# (LST-U-Test 10)

Peer Review _____ Peer Review _____

Skill Acquisition: _____     Practice Opportunities: _____

*This problem allows you the opportunity to demonstrate the* **Test for Inferior Shoulder Instability (Sulcus Sign/Sulcus Test)**. *You have 2 minutes to complete this task.*

| Tester places athlete and limb in appropriate position | YES | NO |
|---|---|---|
| Seated or standing | OOO | OOO |
| Arms relaxed by side; elbow flexed to 90 degrees (resting in lap) | OOO | OOO |
| **Tester placed in proper position** | **YES** | **NO** |
| Sits perpendicular to the athlete | OOO | OOO |
| Places one hand on the scapula | OOO | OOO |
| Places the other hand on the elbow or forearm | OOO | OOO |
| **Tester performs test according to accepted guidelines** | **YES** | **NO** |
| Inferiorly distracts the humerus (pulls distally) | OOO | OOO |
| Maintains relaxation of the limb | OOO | OOO |
| Performs assessment bilaterally | OOO | OOO |

The psychomotor skill was performed completely and in the appropriate order      0  1  2  3  4  5

The tester had control of the subject and the situation (showed confidence)      0  1  2  3  4  5

Method of performing the skill allowed the tester the ability to determine:
severity, proper progression, and the *fit* in the overall picture (Oral)      0  1  2  3  4  5

In order for a grade of *minimum standard* to be given, the total must be ≥11      TOTAL =

I_____I_____I

**Not Acceptable**          **Meets Minimum Standards**          **Exceeds Minimum Standards**

**L:** Laboratory/Classroom Testing
**C:** Clinical/Field Testing
**P:** Practicum Testing
**A:** Assessment/Mock Exam Testing
**S:** Self-Reporting

**Positive Finding:** Step-off deformity; sunken area
**Involved Structure:** Superior glenohumeral ligament
**Special Considerations:** N/A
**Reference(s):** Konin et al; Magee; Starkey et al
**Supplies Needed:** N/A

# LIGAMENTOUS STRESS TESTS
# (LST-U-Test 11)

Peer Review _____ Peer Review _____

Skill Acquisition: _____    Practice Opportunities: _____

*This problem allows you the opportunity to demonstrate the* **Posterior Apprehension Test (Posterior Stress Test) for the Shoulder.** *You have 2 minutes to complete this task.*

| Tester places athlete and limb in appropriate position | YES | NO |
|---|---|---|
| Supine | OOO | OOO |
| Shoulder positioned in 90 degrees of flexion | OOO | OOO |
| Elbow positioned in 90 degrees of flexion | OOO | OOO |
| **Tester placed in proper position** | **YES** | **NO** |
| Stands beside the athlete | OOO | OOO |
| Stabilizes the shoulder with one hand | OOO | OOO |
| Places the other hand on the elbow or forearm | OOO | OOO |
| **Tester performs test according to accepted guidelines** | **YES** | **NO** |
| Positions the shoulder in internal rotation | OOO | OOO |
| Applies a posterior force through the long axis (push down toward the floor) | OOO | OOO |
| Maintains relaxation of the limb | OOO | OOO |
| Performs assessment bilaterally | OOO | OOO |

The psychomotor skill was performed completely and in the appropriate order    0 1 2 3 4 5

The tester had control of the subject and the situation (showed confidence)    0 1 2 3 4 5

Method of performing the skill allowed the tester the ability to determine:
severity, proper progression, and the *fit* in the overall picture (Oral)    0 1 2 3 4 5

In order for a grade of *minimum standard* to be given, the total must be ≥11    **TOTAL =**

I_____I_____I

**Not Acceptable**    **Meets Minimum Standards**    **Exceeds Minimum Standards**

**L:** Laboratory/Classroom Testing
**C:** Clinical/Field Testing
**P:** Practicum Testing
**A:** Assessment/Mock Exam Testing
**S:** Self-Reporting

**Positive Finding:** Apprehension, guarding
**Involved Structure:** Posterior capsule, posterior structures
**Special Considerations:** N/A
**Reference(s):** Konin et al; Magee; Starkey et al
**Supplies Needed:** Table

## LIGAMENTOUS STRESS TESTS
# (LST-U-Test 12)

Peer Review _____ Peer Review _____

Skill Acquisition: _____    Practice Opportunities: _____

*This problem allows you the opportunity to demonstrate the orthopedic test known as the* **Valgus Stress Test for the Elbow**. *You have 2 minutes to complete this task.*

| Tester places athlete and limb in appropriate position | YES | NO |
|---|---|---|
| Stands or sits facing the examiner | OOO | OOO |
| Arms relaxed, elbow flexed to 20 to 30 degrees flexion | OOO | OOO |
| **Tester placed in proper position** | **YES** | **NO** |
| Grasps distal forearm with one hand | OOO | OOO |
| Places other hand over the lateral epicondyle of the elbow | OOO | OOO |
| **Tester performs test according to accepted guidelines** | **YES** | **NO** |
| Applies a valgus stress to the lateral epicondyle of the elbow | OOO | OOO |
| Maintains relaxation of the limb | OOO | OOO |
| Performs assessment bilaterally | OOO | OOO |

The psychomotor skill was performed completely and in the appropriate order    **0  1  2  3  4  5**

The tester had control of the subject and the situation (showed confidence)    **0  1  2  3  4  5**

Method of performing the skill allowed the tester the ability to determine:
severity, proper progression, and the *fit* in the overall picture (Oral)    **0  1  2  3  4  5**

In order for a grade of *minimum standard* to be given, the total must be ≥11    **TOTAL =**

I_____I_____I

**Not Acceptable**        **Meets Minimum Standards**    **Exceeds Minimum Standards**

**L:** Laboratory/Classroom Testing
**C:** Clinical/Field Testing ·
**P:** Practicum Testing
**A:** Assessment/Mock Exam Testing
**S:** Self-Reporting

**Positive Finding:** Pain and laxity
**Involved Structure:** Ulnar collateral ligament
**Special Considerations:** N/A
**Reference(s):** Konin et al; Starkey et al
**Supplies Needed:** N/A

# LIGAMENTOUS STRESS TESTS
# (LST-U-Test 13)

Skill Acquisition: _____     Practice Opportunities: _____

*Please demonstrate the proper technique for administering the orthopedic test known as* **Varus Stress Test for the Elbow**. *You have 2 minutes to complete this task.*

| Tester places athlete and limb in appropriate position | YES | NO |
|---|---|---|
| Stands or sits facing the examiner | OOO | OOO |
| Arms relaxed, elbow flexed to 20 to 30 degrees | OOO | OOO |
| **Tester placed in proper position** | **YES** | **NO** |
| Grasps distal forearm with one hand | OOO | OOO |
| Places other hand over the medial epicondyle of the elbow | OOO | OOO |
| **Tester performs test according to accepted guidelines** | **YES** | **NO** |
| Applies a varus stress to the medial epicondyle of the elbow | OOO | OOO |
| Maintains relaxation of the limb | OOO | OOO |
| Performs assessment bilaterally | OOO | OOO |

| | |
|---|---|
| The psychomotor skill was performed completely and in the appropriate order | 0  1  2  3  4  5 |
| The tester had control of the subject and the situation (showed confidence) | 0  1  2  3  4  5 |
| Method of performing the skill allowed the tester the ability to determine: severity, proper progression, and the *fit* in the overall picture (Oral) | 0  1  2  3  4  5 |

In order for a grade of *minimum standard* to be given, the total must be ≥11          **TOTAL =**

I_____I_____I
**Not Acceptable**          **Meets Minimum Standards**     **Exceeds Minimum Standards**

**L:** Laboratory/Classroom Testing
**C:** Clinical/Field Testing
**P:** Practicum Testing
**A:** Assessment/Mock Exam Testing
**S:** Self-Reporting

**Positive Finding:** Pain and laxity
**Involved Structure:** Radial collateral ligament
**Special Considerations:** N/A
**Reference(s):** Konin et al; Starkey et al
**Supplies Needed:** N/A

## LIGAMENTOUS STRESS TESTS
# (LST-U-Test 14)

Peer Review _____ Peer Review _____

Skill Acquisition: _____    Practice Opportunities: _____

*Please demonstrate the proper technique for administering an* **Anterior-Posterior Glide of the Radial Head.** *You have 2 minutes to complete this task.*

| Tester places athlete and limb in appropriate position | YES | NO |
|---|---|---|
| Seated | OOO | OOO |
| Elbow resting supinated on a table (table serves as support) | OOO | OOO |
| Elbow flexed between 30 to 70 degrees | OOO | OOO |
| **Tester placed in proper position** | **YES** | **NO** |
| Thumbs and index fingers are placed to control the proximal radius (radial head) | OOO | OOO |
| **Tester performs test according to accepted guidelines** | **YES** | **NO** |
| Thumb and index finger apply a mobilization force in a posterior direction | OOO | OOO |
| Oscillation of the posterior glide is performed two to three times | OOO | OOO |
| Maintains relaxation of the limb | OOO | OOO |
| Performs assessment bilaterally | OOO | OOO |

The psychomotor skill was performed completely and in the appropriate order    0 1 2 3 4 5

The tester had control of the subject and the situation (showed confidence)    0 1 2 3 4 5

Method of performing the skill allowed the tester the ability to determine:
severity, proper progression, and the *fit* in the overall picture (Oral)    0 1 2 3 4 5

In order for a grade of *minimum standard* to be given, the total must be ≥11    **TOTAL =**

I_____I_____I
**Not Acceptable**      **Meets Minimum Standards**    **Exceeds Minimum Standards**

**L:** Laboratory/Classroom Testing
**C:** Clinical/Field Testing
**P:** Practicum Testing
**A:** Assessment/Mock Exam Testing
**S:** Self-Reporting

**Positive Finding:** Increased extension
**Involved Structure:** Joint capsule
**Special Considerations:** N/A
**Reference(s):** Edmond; Prentice; Houglum
**Supplies Needed:** Table

# LIGAMENTOUS STRESS TESTS
## (LST-U-Test 15)

Peer Review _____ Peer Review _____

Skill Acquisition: _____     Practice Opportunities: _____

*Please demonstrate the proper technique for administering an* **Anterior-Posterior Glide of the Wrist (Radiocarpal Joint)**. *You have 2 minutes to complete this task.*

| Tester places athlete and limb in appropriate position | YES | NO |
|---|---|---|
| Seated | OOO | OOO |
| Forearm resting supinated on a table (table serves as support) | OOO | OOO |
| **Tester placed in proper position** | **YES** | **NO** |
| Stabilizes the (distal) radius and ulna with one hand | OOO | OOO |
| Placed the other hand around the carpal bones (proximal row) | OOO | OOO |
| **Tester performs test according to accepted guidelines** | **YES** | **NO** |
| Hand on the carpal bones applies a mobilization force in an anterior direction | OOO | OOO |
| Oscillation of the anterior glide is performed two to three times | OOO | OOO |
| Maintains relaxation of the limb | OOO | OOO |
| Performs assessment bilaterally | OOO | OOO |

The psychomotor skill was performed completely and in the appropriate order      0  1  2  3  4  5

The tester had control of the subject and the situation (showed confidence)      0  1  2  3  4  5

Method of performing the skill allowed the tester the ability to determine:
severity, proper progression, and the *fit* in the overall picture (Oral)      0  1  2  3  4  5

In order for a grade of *minimum standard* to be given, the total must be ≥11      **TOTAL =**

I_____I_____I

**Not Acceptable**          **Meets Minimum Standards**          **Exceeds Minimum Standards**

**L:** Laboratory/Classroom Testing
**C:** Clinical/Field Testing
**P:** Practicum Testing
**A:** Assessment/Mock Exam Testing
**S:** Self-Reporting

**Positive Finding:** Increase motion (wrist extension)
**Involved Structure:** Joint capsule
**Special Considerations:** N/A
**Reference(s):** Edmond; Prentice; Houglum
**Supplies Needed:** Table

## LIGAMENTOUS STRESS TESTS
# (LST-U-Test 16)

Peer Review _____ Peer Review _____

Skill Acquisition: _____    Practice Opportunities: _____

*Please demonstrate the proper technique for administering an* **Anterior-Posterior Glide of the Second Metacarpophalangeal (MCP) Joint**. *You have 2 minutes to complete this task.*

| Tester places athlete and limb in appropriate position | YES | NO |
|---|---|---|
| Seated | ○○○ | ○○○ |
| Forearm resting supinated on a table (table serves as support) | ○○○ | ○○○ |
| **Tester placed in proper position** | **YES** | **NO** |
| Stabilizes the second metacarpal with one hand | ○○○ | ○○○ |
| Other hand is placed around the proximal phalange | ○○○ | ○○○ |
| **Tester performs test according to accepted guidelines** | **YES** | **NO** |
| Hand on the proximal phalange applies a mobilization force in a posterior direction | ○○○ | ○○○ |
| Oscillation of the posterior glide is performed two to three times | ○○○ | ○○○ |
| Maintains relaxation of the limb | ○○○ | ○○○ |
| Performs assessment bilaterally | ○○○ | ○○○ |

The psychomotor skill was performed completely and in the appropriate order    **0  1  2  3  4  5**

The tester had control of the subject and the situation (showed confidence)    **0  1  2  3  4  5**

Method of performing the skill allowed the tester the ability to determine:
severity, proper progression, and the *fit* in the overall picture (Oral)    **0  1  2  3  4  5**

In order for a grade of *minimum standard* to be given, the total must be ≥11    **TOTAL =**

I_____I_____I
    **Not Acceptable**         **Meets Minimum Standards**    **Exceeds Minimum Standards**

**L:** Laboratory/Classroom Testing
**C:** Clinical/Field Testing
**P:** Practicum Testing
**A:** Assessment/Mock Exam Testing
**S:** Self-Reporting

**Positive Finding:** Increase motion (extension)
**Involved Structure:** Joint capsule
**Special Considerations:** N/A
**Reference(s):** Edmond; Prentice; Houglum
**Supplies Needed:** Table

# LIGAMENTOUS STRESS TESTS
## (LST-U-Test 17)

Peer Review _____ Peer Review _____

Skill Acquisition: _____     Practice Opportunities: _____

*This problem allows you the opportunity to demonstrate the orthopedic test known as the* **Valgus Stress Test for the Second Proximal Interphalangeal (PIP) Joint**. *You have 2 minutes to complete this task.*

| Tester places athlete and limb in appropriate position | YES | NO |
|---|---|---|
| Stands or sits facing the examiner | ○○○ | ○○○ |
| Second PIP is flexed (15 to 30 degrees) | ○○○ | ○○○ |
| **Tester placed in proper position** | **YES** | **NO** |
| Grasps the distal end of the proximal phalanx with one hand (thumb and index finger) | ○○○ | ○○○ |
| Places other hand over the middle phalanx (thumb and index finger) | ○○○ | ○○○ |
| **Tester performs test according to accepted guidelines** | **YES** | **NO** |
| Applies a valgus stress to the joint (second proximal interphalangeal joint) | ○○○ | ○○○ |
| Maintains relaxation of the limb | ○○○ | ○○○ |
| Performs assessment bilaterally | ○○○ | ○○○ |

| | | |
|---|---|---|
| The psychomotor skill was performed completely and in the appropriate order | 0 1 2 3 4 5 |
| The tester had control of the subject and the situation (showed confidence) | 0 1 2 3 4 5 |
| Method of performing the skill allowed the tester the ability to determine: severity, proper progression, and the *fit* in the overall picture (Oral) | 0 1 2 3 4 5 |

In order for a grade of *minimum standard* to be given, the total must be ≥11          **TOTAL =**

I_____I_____I

**Not Acceptable**          **Meets Minimum Standards**          **Exceeds Minimum Standards**

**L:** Laboratory/Classroom Testing
**C:** Clinical/Field Testing
**P:** Practicum Testing
**A:** Assessment/Mock Exam Testing
**S:** Self-Reporting

**Positive Finding:** Pain and laxity
**Involved Structure:** Medial collateral ligament (finger)
**Special Considerations:** N/A
**Reference(s):** Magee; Starkey et al
**Supplies Needed:** N/A

## LIGAMENTOUS STRESS TESTS
# (LST-U-Test 18)

Peer Review _____    Peer Review _____

Skill Acquisition: _____    Practice Opportunities: _____

*This problem allows you the opportunity to demonstrate the orthopedic test known as the* **Varus Stress Test for the Third Distal Interphalangeal (DIP) Joint**. *You have 2 minutes to complete this task.*

| Tester places athlete and limb in appropriate position | YES | NO |
|---|---|---|
| Stands or sits facing the examiner | OOO | OOO |
| Third DIP is flexed (15 to 30 degrees) | OOO | OOO |
| **Tester placed in proper position** | **YES** | **NO** |
| Grasps the distal end of the middle phalanx with one hand (thumb and index finger) | OOO | OOO |
| Places other hand over the distal phalanx (thumb and index finger) | OOO | OOO |
| **Tester performs test according to accepted guidelines** | **YES** | **NO** |
| Applies a varus stress to the joint (third PIP joint) | OOO | OOO |
| Maintains relaxation of the limb | OOO | OOO |
| Performs assessment bilaterally | OOO | OOO |

The psychomotor skill was performed completely and in the appropriate order    **0  1  2  3  4  5**

The tester had control of the subject and the situation (showed confidence)    **0  1  2  3  4  5**

Method of performing the skill allowed the tester the ability to determine:
severity, proper progression, and the *fit* in the overall picture (Oral)    **0  1  2  3  4  5**

In order for a grade of *minimum standard* to be given, the total must be ≥11    **TOTAL =**

I_____I_____I
**Not Acceptable**          **Meets Minimum Standards**    **Exceeds Minimum Standards**

**L:** Laboratory/Classroom Testing
**C:** Clinical/Field Testing
**P:** Practicum Testing
**A:** Assessment/Mock Exam Testing
**S:** Self-Reporting

**Positive Finding:** Pain and laxity
**Involved Structure:** Lateral collateral ligament (finger)
**Special Considerations:** N/A
**Reference(s):** Magee; Starkey et al
**Supplies Needed:** N/A

## LIGAMENTOUS STRESS TESTS
# (LST-U-Test 19)

Peer Review _____ Peer Review _____

Skill Acquisition: _____    Practice Opportunities: _____

*Please demonstrate the proper technique for administering an* **Anterior-Posterior Glide of the Glenohumeral Joint**. *You have 2 minutes to complete this task.*

| Tester places athlete and limb in appropriate position | YES | NO |
|---|---|---|
| Supine | OOO | OOO |
| Shoulder at the edge of the table | OOO | OOO |
| **Tester placed in proper position** | **YES** | **NO** |
| Tester stands to the side of the athlete | OOO | OOO |
| One hand supports the shoulder (stabilize the scapula) | OOO | OOO |
| Other hand is placed on the proximal end of the humerus (a distraction force is applied and held) | OOO | OOO |
| **Tester performs test according to accepted guidelines** | **YES** | **NO** |
| Hand on the humerus applies a mobilization force in a posterior direction | OOO | OOO |
| Oscillation of the posterior glide is performed two to three times | OOO | OOO |
| Maintains relaxation of the limb | OOO | OOO |
| Performs assessment bilaterally | OOO | OOO |

The psychomotor skill was performed completely and in the appropriate order       0  1  2  3  4  5

The tester had control of the subject and the situation (showed confidence)       0  1  2  3  4  5

Method of performing the skill allowed the tester the ability to determine:
severity, proper progression, and the *fit* in the overall picture (Oral)       0  1  2  3  4  5

In order for a grade of *minimum standard* to be given, the total must be ≥11       **TOTAL =**

I_____I_____I
**Not Acceptable**     **Meets Minimum Standards**   **Exceeds Minimum Standards**

**L:** Laboratory/Classroom Testing
**C:** Clinical/Field Testing
**P:** Practicum Testing
**A:** Assessment/Mock Exam Testing
**S:** Self-Reporting

**Positive Finding:** Increased motion
**Involved Structure:** Joint capsule
**Special Considerations:** N/A
**Reference(s):** Prentice; Houglum
**Supplies Needed:** Table

# LIGAMENTOUS STRESS TESTS
# (LST-L-Test 1)

Peer Review _____ Peer Review _____

Skill Acquisition: _____    Practice Opportunities: _____

*Please demonstrate how you would perform the ligamentous stress test for the ankle known as the **Anterior Drawer Test for the Ankle**. You have 2 minutes to complete this task.*

| Tester places athlete and limb in appropriate position | YES | NO |
|---|---|---|
| Supine or sitting with feet relaxed over edge of table | ○○○ | ○○○ |
| Knee flexed to 90 degrees | ○○○ | ○○○ |
| **Tester placed in proper position** | **YES** | **NO** |
| Stabilizes tibia and fibula with one hand | ○○○ | ○○○ |
| Holds foot in 20 degrees of plantar flexion | ○○○ | ○○○ |
| **Tester performs test according to accepted guidelines** | **YES** | **NO** |
| Maintains relaxation of the limb | ○○○ | ○○○ |
| Draws talus forward (anterior displacement) on lower leg | ○○○ | ○○○ |
| Performs assessment bilaterally | ○○○ | ○○○ |

The psychomotor skill was performed completely and in the appropriate order    0 1 2 3 4 5

The tester had control of the subject and the situation (showed confidence)    0 1 2 3 4 5

Method of performing the skill allowed the tester the ability to determine:
severity, proper progression, and the *fit* in the overall picture (Oral)    0 1 2 3 4 5

In order for a grade of *minimum standard* to be given, the total must be ≥11    **TOTAL =**

I_____I_____I
**Not Acceptable        Meets Minimum Standards        Exceeds Minimum Standards**

**L:** Laboratory/Classroom Testing
**C:** Clinical/Field Testing
**P:** Practicum Testing
**A:** Assessment/Mock Exam Testing
**S:** Self-Reporting

**Positive Finding:** Anterior translation; clunk
**Involved Structure:** Anterior talofibular ligament
**Special Considerations:** N/A
**Reference(s):** Konin et al; Magee; Starkey et al
**Supplies Needed:** Table or chair

# LIGAMENTOUS STRESS TESTS
## (LST-L-Test 2)

Peer Review _____ Peer Review _____

Skill Acquisition: _____     Practice Opportunities: _____

*This problem allows you the opportunity to demonstrate a ligamentous stress test known as the* **Talar Tilt Test (Inversion Stress Test).** *You have 2 minutes to complete this task.*

| | YES | NO |
|---|---|---|
| **Tester places athlete and limb in appropriate position** | YES | NO |
| Seated/supine (may be done side lying on the uninvolved side) | ○○○ | ○○○ |
| Foot over the edge of the table | ○○○ | ○○○ |
| Knee flexed to 90 degrees | ○○○ | ○○○ |
| **Tester placed in proper position** | YES | NO |
| Stabilizes tibia and fibula with one hand | ○○○ | ○○○ |
| Holds foot in neutral position with other hand | ○○○ | ○○○ |
| **Tester performs test according to accepted guidelines** | YES | NO |
| Maintains relaxation of the limb | ○○○ | ○○○ |
| Passively inverts the calcaneus | ○○○ | ○○○ |
| Performs assessment bilaterally | ○○○ | ○○○ |

The psychomotor skill was performed completely and in the appropriate order          **0  1  2  3  4  5**

The tester had control of the subject and the situation (showed confidence)          **0  1  2  3  4  5**

Method of performing the skill allowed the tester the ability to determine:
severity, proper progression, and the *fit* in the overall picture (Oral)          **0  1  2  3  4  5**

In order for a grade of *minimum standard* to be given, the total must be ≥11          **TOTAL =**

I_____I_____I

**Not Acceptable          Meets Minimum Standards          Exceeds Minimum Standards**

**L:** Laboratory/Classroom Testing
**C:** Clinical/Field Testing
**P:** Practicum Testing
**A:** Assessment/Mock Exam Testing
**S:** Self-Reporting

**Positive Finding:** Inversion greater than the uninvolved limb; pain, laxity
**Involved Structure:** Calcaneofibular ligament
**Special Considerations:** N/A
**Reference(s):** Konin; Magee; Starkey
**Supplies Needed:** Table or chair

# LIGAMENTOUS STRESS TESTS
# (LST-L-Test 3)

Peer Review _____ Peer Review _____

Skill Acquisition: _____     Practice Opportunities: _____

*Please demonstrate how you would do the ligamentous stress test known as the* **Kleiger Test (External Rotation Test).** *You have 2 minutes to complete this task.*

| Tester places athlete and limb in appropriate position | YES | NO |
|---|---|---|
| Seated | ○○○ | ○○○ |
| Knee flexed to 90 degrees (legs over the edge of the table) | ○○○ | ○○○ |
| Foot placed in a neutral position (0 degrees dorsiflexion) | ○○○ | ○○○ |
| **Tester placed in proper position** | **YES** | **NO** |
| Stabilizes tibia (do not compress the fibula) with one hand | ○○○ | ○○○ |
| Grasps the foot (medial aspect) with the other hand | ○○○ | ○○○ |
| **Tester performs test according to accepted guidelines** | **YES** | **NO** |
| Maintains relaxation of the limb | ○○○ | ○○○ |
| Rotates the foot laterally (calcaneus and talus) | ○○○ | ○○○ |
| Performs assessment bilaterally | ○○○ | ○○○ |

The psychomotor skill was performed completely and in the appropriate order    **0  1  2  3  4  5**

The tester had control of the subject and the situation (showed confidence)    **0  1  2  3  4  5**

Method of performing the skill allowed the tester the ability to determine:
severity, proper progression, and the *fit* in the overall picture (Oral)    **0  1  2  3  4  5**

In order for a grade of *minimum standard* to be given, the total must be ≥11    **TOTAL =**

I_____I_____I
**Not Acceptable**          **Meets Minimum Standards**    **Exceeds Minimum Standards**

**L:** Laboratory/Classroom Testing
**C:** Clinical/Field Testing
**P:** Practicum Testing
**A:** Assessment/Mock Exam Testing
**S:** Self-Reporting

**Positive Finding:** Pain
**Involved Structure:** Deltoid ligament; syndesmosis
**Special Considerations:** Pay close attention to the location of the pain
**Reference(s):** Magee; Starkey
**Supplies Needed:** Table or chair

# LIGAMENTOUS STRESS TESTS
# (LST-L-Test 4)

Peer Review _____ Peer Review _____

Skill Acquisition: _____     Practice Opportunities: _____

*This problem allows you the opportunity to demonstrate a ligamentous stress test known as the **Eversion Stress Test (Eversion Talar Tilt Test)**. You have 2 minutes to complete this task.*

| Tester places athlete and limb in appropriate position | YES | NO |
|---|---|---|
| Seated/supine | ○○○ | ○○○ |
| Foot over the edge of the table | ○○○ | ○○○ |
| Knee flexed to 90 degrees | ○○○ | ○○○ |
| **Tester placed in proper position** | **YES** | **NO** |
| Stabilizes tibia and fibula with one hand | ○○○ | ○○○ |
| Holds foot in neutral position with other hand | ○○○ | ○○○ |
| **Tester performs test according to accepted guidelines** | **YES** | **NO** |
| Maintains relaxation of the limb | ○○○ | ○○○ |
| Passively everts the calcaneus | ○○○ | ○○○ |
| Performs assessment bilaterally | ○○○ | ○○○ |

The psychomotor skill was performed completely and in the appropriate order    **0  1  2  3  4  5**

The tester had control of the subject and the situation (showed confidence)    **0  1  2  3  4  5**

Method of performing the skill allowed the tester the ability to determine:
severity, proper progression, and the *fit* in the overall picture (Oral)    **0  1  2  3  4  5**

In order for a grade of *minimum standard* to be given, the total must be ≥11    **TOTAL =**

I_____I_____I

**Not Acceptable        Meets Minimum Standards        Exceeds Minimum Standards**

**L:** Laboratory/Classroom Testing
**C:** Clinical/Field Testing
**P:** Practicum Testing
**A:** Assessment/Mock Exam Testing
**S:** Self-Reporting

**Positive Finding:** Eversion greater than the uninvolved limb
**Involved Structure:** Deltoid ligament
**Special Considerations:** N/A
**Reference(s):** Starkey et al
**Supplies Needed:** Table

## LIGAMENTOUS STRESS TESTS
# (LST-L-Test 5)

Peer Review _____ Peer Review _____

Skill Acquisition: _____    Practice Opportunities: _____

*This problem allows you the opportunity to demonstrate an orthopedic test known as the* **Valgus Stress Test for the Knee**. *You have 2 minutes to complete this task.*

| Tester places athlete and limb in appropriate position | YES | NO |
|---|---|---|
| Supine | ○○○ | ○○○ |
| Knee in 20 to 30 degrees of flexion (superficial MCL) | ○○○ | ○○○ |
| Knee in 0 degrees of extension (deep MCL) | ○○○ | ○○○ |
| **Tester placed in proper position** | **YES** | **NO** |
| Places one hand on distal, medial tibia | ○○○ | ○○○ |
| Places the other hand on distal, lateral femur | ○○○ | ○○○ |
| **Tester performs test according to accepted guidelines** | **YES** | **NO** |
| Maintains relaxation of the limb | ○○○ | ○○○ |
| Applies valgus stress to the knee joint | ○○○ | ○○○ |
| Prevents the tibia and femur from rotating during the test | ○○○ | ○○○ |
| Performs assessment bilaterally | ○○○ | ○○○ |

The psychomotor skill was performed completely and in the appropriate order    **0  1  2  3  4  5**

The tester had control of the subject and the situation (showed confidence)    **0  1  2  3  4  5**

Method of performing the skill allowed the tester the ability to determine:
severity, proper progression, and the *fit* in the overall picture (Oral)    **0  1  2  3  4  5**

In order for a grade of *minimum standard* to be given, the total must be ≥11    **TOTAL =**

I_____I_____I

**Not Acceptable**          **Meets Minimum Standards**          **Exceeds Minimum Standards**

**L:** Laboratory/Classroom Testing
**C:** Clinical/Field Testing
**P:** Practicum Testing
**A:** Assessment/Mock Exam Testing
**S:** Self-Reporting

**Positive Finding:** Laxity; pain
**Involved Structure:** Medial collateral ligament
**Special Considerations:** 0 degrees extension = deep MCL
20 to 30 degrees extension = superficial portion of the MCL
**Reference(s):** Konin et al; Starkey et al
**Supplies Needed:** Table

# LIGAMENTOUS STRESS TESTS
# (LST-L-Test 6)

Peer Review _____ Peer Review _____

Skill Acquisition: _____     Practice Opportunities: _____

*This problem allows you the opportunity to demonstrate an orthopedic test known as the **Varus Stress Test for the Knee**. You have 2 minutes to complete this task.*

| Tester places athlete and limb in appropriate position | YES | NO |
|---|---|---|
| Supine | ○○○ | ○○○ |
| Knee in 20 to 30 degrees of flexion | ○○○ | ○○○ |
| **Tester placed in proper position** | **YES** | **NO** |
| Places one hand on distal, medial tibia | ○○○ | ○○○ |
| Places the other hand on distal, lateral femur | ○○○ | ○○○ |
| **Tester performs test according to accepted guidelines** | **YES** | **NO** |
| Maintains relaxation of the limb | ○○○ | ○○○ |
| Applies varus stress to the knee joint | ○○○ | ○○○ |
| Prevents the tibia and femur from rotating during the test | ○○○ | ○○○ |
| Performs assessment bilaterally | ○○○ | ○○○ |

The psychomotor skill was performed completely and in the appropriate order    0 1 2 3 4 5

The tester had control of the subject and the situation (showed confidence)    0 1 2 3 4 5

Method of performing the skill allowed the tester the ability to determine:
severity, proper progression, and the *fit* in the overall picture (Oral)    0 1 2 3 4 5

In order for a grade of *minimum standard* to be given, the total must be ≥11    **TOTAL =**

I_____I_____I
**Not Acceptable**         **Meets Minimum Standards**    **Exceeds Minimum Standards**

**L:** Laboratory/Classroom Testing
**C:** Clinical/Field Testing
**P:** Practicum Testing
**A:** Assessment/Mock Exam Testing
**S:** Self-Reporting

**Positive Finding:** Laxity, pain
**Involved Structure:** Lateral collateral ligament
**Special Considerations:** N/A
**Reference(s):** Konin; Starkey
**Supplies Needed:** Table

## LIGAMENTOUS STRESS TESTS
# (LST-L-Test 7)

Peer Review _____ Peer Review _____

Skill Acquisition: _____ Practice Opportunities: _____

*This problem allows you the opportunity to demonstrate the* **Lachman Test (Anterior Lachman/Ritchie/Trillat/ Lachman-Trillat Test)**. *You have 2 minutes to complete this task.*

| Tester places athlete and limb in appropriate position | YES | NO |
|---|---|---|
| Supine | ○○○ | ○○○ |
| Knee in 10 to 25 degrees of flexion | ○○○ | ○○○ |
| **Tester placed in proper position** | **YES** | **NO** |
| Stabilizes posteriorly on calf with one hand | ○○○ | ○○○ |
| Stabilizes anteriorly on distal femur with other hand (just proximal to the patella) | ○○○ | ○○○ |
| **Tester performs test according to accepted guidelines** | **YES** | **NO** |
| Maintains relaxation of the limb | ○○○ | ○○○ |
| Attempts to anteriorly displace tibia on femur (draws anteriorly) | ○○○ | ○○○ |
| Performs assessment bilaterally | ○○○ | ○○○ |

The psychomotor skill was performed completely and in the appropriate order    **0 1 2 3 4 5**

The tester had control of the subject and the situation (showed confidence)    **0 1 2 3 4 5**

Method of performing the skill allowed the tester the ability to determine:
severity, proper progression, and the *fit* in the overall picture (Oral)    **0 1 2 3 4 5**

In order for a grade of *minimum standard* to be given, the total must be ≥11    **TOTAL =**

I_____I_____I
**Not Acceptable**      **Meets Minimum Standards**      **Exceeds Minimum Standards**

**L:** Laboratory/Classroom Testing
**C:** Clinical/Field Testing
**P:** Practicum Testing
**A:** Assessment/Mock Exam Testing
**S:** Self-Reporting

**Positive Finding:** Excessive anterior translation
**Involved Structure:** ACL
**Special Considerations:** Many variations to this test
**Reference(s):** Konin et al; Magee; Starkey et al
**Supplies Needed:** Table

# Ligamentous Stress Tests
## (LST-L-Test 8)

Peer Review _____ Peer Review _____

Skill Acquisition: _____     Practice Opportunities: _____

*This problem allows you the opportunity to demonstrate the **Anterior Drawer Test (Drawer Sign) for the Knee**. You have 2 minutes to complete this task.*

| Tester places athlete and limb in appropriate position | YES | NO |
|---|---|---|
| Supine | ○○○ | ○○○ |
| Hip is flexed to 45 degrees | ○○○ | ○○○ |
| Knee is flexed to 90 degrees (foot in neutral) | ○○○ | ○○○ |
| **Tester placed in proper position** | **YES** | **NO** |
| Sits on athlete's involved foot | ○○○ | ○○○ |
| Cups the hands around the proximal (posterior) aspect of the lower leg, thumbs on the tibial plateau | ○○○ | ○○○ |
| **Tester performs test according to accepted guidelines** | **YES** | **NO** |
| Applies an anterior force to the proximal aspect of the lower leg | ○○○ | ○○○ |
| Maintains relaxation of the limb | ○○○ | ○○○ |
| Performs assessment bilaterally | ○○○ | ○○○ |

The psychomotor skill was performed completely and in the appropriate order    0 1 2 3 4 5

The tester had control of the subject and the situation (showed confidence)    0 1 2 3 4 5

Method of performing the skill allowed the tester the ability to determine:
severity, proper progression, and the *fit* in the overall picture (Oral)    0 1 2 3 4 5

In order for a grade of *minimum standard* to be given, the total must be ≥11    TOTAL =

I_____I_____I

Not Acceptable        Meets Minimum Standards        Exceeds Minimum Standards

**L:** Laboratory/Classroom Testing
**C:** Clinical/Field Testing
**P:** Practicum Testing
**A:** Assessment/Mock Exam Testing
**S:** Self-Reporting

**Positive Finding:** Anterior displacement
**Involved Structure:** ACL
**Special Considerations:** Check posterior cruciate ligament first; relax hamstrings
**Reference(s):** Konin et al; Magee; Starkey et al
**Supplies Needed:** Table

## LIGAMENTOUS STRESS TESTS
# (LST-L-Test 9)

Peer Review _____ Peer Review _____

Skill Acquisition: _____    Practice Opportunities: _____

*This problem allows you the opportunity to demonstrate the* **Posterior Drawer Test for the Knee**. *You have 2 minutes to complete this task.*

| Tester places athlete and limb in appropriate position | YES | NO |
|---|---|---|
| Supine | ○○○ | ○○○ |
| Hip is flexed to 45 degrees | ○○○ | ○○○ |
| Knee is flexed to 90 degrees (foot in neutral) | ○○○ | ○○○ |
| **Tester placed in proper position** | **YES** | **NO** |
| Sits on athlete's involved foot | ○○○ | ○○○ |
| Cups the hands around the proximal (posterior) aspect of the lower leg, thumbs on the tibial plateau | ○○○ | ○○○ |
| **Tester performs test according to accepted guidelines** | **YES** | **NO** |
| Applies a posterior force to the proximal aspect of the lower leg | ○○○ | ○○○ |
| Maintains relaxation of the limb | ○○○ | ○○○ |
| Performs assessment bilaterally | ○○○ | ○○○ |

The psychomotor skill was performed completely and in the appropriate order    **0  1  2  3  4  5**

The tester had control of the subject and the situation (showed confidence)    **0  1  2  3  4  5**

Method of performing the skill allowed the tester the ability to determine:
severity, proper progression, and the *fit* in the overall picture (Oral)    **0  1  2  3  4  5**

In order for a grade of *minimum standard* to be given, the total must be ≥11    **TOTAL =**

I_____I_____I
**Not Acceptable**          **Meets Minimum Standards**          **Exceeds Minimum Standards**

**L:** Laboratory/Classroom Testing
**C:** Clinical/Field Testing
**P:** Practicum Testing
**A:** Assessment/Mock Exam Testing
**S:** Self-Reporting

**Positive Finding:** Posterior displacement
**Involved Structure:** PCL
**Special Considerations:** N/A
**Reference(s):** Konin et al; Starkey et al
**Supplies Needed:** Table

# LIGAMENTOUS STRESS TESTS
## (LST-L-Test 10)

Peer Review _____ Peer Review _____

Skill Acquisition: _____    Practice Opportunities: _____

*This problem allows you the opportunity to demonstrate the **Slocum Test (Internal Tibial Rotation) for the Knee**. You have 2 minutes to complete this task.*

| Tester places athlete and limb in appropriate position | YES | NO |
|---|---|---|
| Supine | ○○○ | ○○○ |
| Hip is flexed to 45 degrees | ○○○ | ○○○ |
| Knee is flexed to 90 degrees (foot in neutral) | ○○○ | ○○○ |
| Tibia internally rotated 15 to 30 degrees | ○○○ | ○○○ |
| **Tester placed in proper position** | YES | NO |
| Sits on athlete's involved foot | ○○○ | ○○○ |
| Cups the hands around the proximal (posterior) aspect of the lower leg, thumbs on the tibial plateau | ○○○ | ○○○ |
| **Tester performs test according to accepted guidelines** | YES | NO |
| Applies an anterior force to the proximal aspect of the lower leg | ○○○ | ○○○ |
| Maintains relaxation of the limb | ○○○ | ○○○ |
| Performs assessment bilaterally | ○○○ | ○○○ |

The psychomotor skill was performed completely and in the appropriate order    0 1 2 3 4 5

The tester had control of the subject and the situation (showed confidence)    0 1 2 3 4 5

Method of performing the skill allowed the tester the ability to determine: severity, proper progression, and the *fit* in the overall picture (Oral)    0 1 2 3 4 5

In order for a grade of *minimum standard* to be given, the total must be ≥11    **TOTAL =**

I_____I_____I
**Not Acceptable**    **Meets Minimum Standards**    **Exceeds Minimum Standards**

**L:** Laboratory/Classroom Testing
**C:** Clinical/Field Testing
**P:** Practicum Testing
**A:** Assessment/Mock Exam Testing
**S:** Self-Reporting

**Positive Finding:** Anterior displacement
**Involved Structure:** ACL; posterolateral capsule
**Special Considerations:** Hamstring guarding
**Reference(s):** Konin et al; Magee
**Supplies Needed:** Table

## LIGAMENTOUS STRESS TESTS
# (LST-L-Test 11)

Peer Review _____ Peer Review _____

Skill Acquisition: _____    Practice Opportunities: _____

*This problem allows you the opportunity to demonstrate the* **Slocum Test (External Tibial Rotation) for the Knee**. *You have 2 minutes to complete this task.*

| Tester places athlete and limb in appropriate position | YES | NO |
|---|---|---|
| Supine | OOO | OOO |
| Hip is flexed to 45 degrees | OOO | OOO |
| Knee is flexed to 90 degrees (foot in neutral) | OOO | OOO |
| Tibia externally rotated 15 to 20 degrees | OOO | OOO |
| **Tester placed in proper position** | **YES** | **NO** |
| Sits on athlete's involved foot | OOO | OOO |
| Cups the hands around the proximal (posterior) aspect of the lower leg, thumbs on the tibial plateau | OOO | OOO |
| **Tester performs test according to accepted guidelines** | **YES** | **NO** |
| Applies an anterior force to the proximal aspect of the lower leg | OOO | OOO |
| Maintains relaxation of the limb | OOO | OOO |
| Performs assessment bilaterally | OOO | OOO |

The psychomotor skill was performed completely and in the appropriate order    **0  1  2  3  4  5**

The tester had control of the subject and the situation (showed confidence)    **0  1  2  3  4  5**

Method of performing the skill allowed the tester the ability to determine:
severity, proper progression, and the *fit* in the overall picture (Oral)    **0  1  2  3  4  5**

In order for a grade of *minimum standard* to be given, the total must be ≥11    **TOTAL =**

I_____I_____I

**Not Acceptable**        **Meets Minimum Standards**    **Exceeds Minimum Standards**

**L:** Laboratory/Classroom Testing
**C:** Clinical/Field Testing
**P:** Practicum Testing
**A:** Assessment/Mock Exam Testing
**S:** Self-Reporting

**Positive Finding:** Anterior displacement
**Involved Structure:** ACL; posteromedial capsule
**Special Considerations:** Hamstring guarding
**Reference(s):** Konin; Magee
**Supplies Needed:** Table

## LIGAMENTOUS STRESS TESTS
# (LST-L-Test 12)

Peer Review _____ Peer Review _____

Skill Acquisition: _____    Practice Opportunities: _____

*This problem allows you the opportunity to demonstrate the* **Hughston Posteromedial Drawer Test for the Knee**. *You have 2 minutes to complete this task.*

| Tester places athlete and limb in appropriate position | YES | NO |
|---|---|---|
| Supine | ○○○ | ○○○ |
| Hip is flexed to 45 degrees | ○○○ | ○○○ |
| Knee is flexed to 90 degrees (foot in neutral) | ○○○ | ○○○ |
| Tibia internally rotated 15 to 30 degrees | ○○○ | ○○○ |
| **Tester placed in proper position** | **YES** | **NO** |
| Sits on athlete's involved foot | ○○○ | ○○○ |
| Cups the hands around the proximal (posterior) aspect of the lower leg, thumbs on the tibial plateau | ○○○ | ○○○ |
| **Tester performs test according to accepted guidelines** | **YES** | **NO** |
| Applies an anterior force to the proximal aspect of the lower leg | ○○○ | ○○○ |
| Maintains relaxation of the limb | ○○○ | ○○○ |
| Performs assessment bilaterally | ○○○ | ○○○ |

The psychomotor skill was performed completely and in the appropriate order    0 1 2 3 4 5

The tester had control of the subject and the situation (showed confidence)    0 1 2 3 4 5

Method of performing the skill allowed the tester the ability to determine:
severity, proper progression, and the *fit* in the overall picture (Oral)    0 1 2 3 4 5

In order for a grade of *minimum standard* to be given, the total must be ≥11    **TOTAL =**

I_____I_____I
**Not Acceptable**          **Meets Minimum Standards**      **Exceeds Minimum Standards**

**L:** Laboratory/Classroom Testing
**C:** Clinical/Field Testing
**P:** Practicum Testing
**A:** Assessment/Mock Exam Testing
**S:** Self-Reporting

**Positive Finding:** Posterior displacement
**Involved Structure:** PCL; posteromedial capsule
**Special Considerations:** N/A
**Reference(s):** Konin et al; Magee
**Supplies Needed:** Table

## LIGAMENTOUS STRESS TESTS
# (LST-L-Test 13)

Peer Review _____    Peer Review _____

Skill Acquisition: _____    Practice Opportunities: _____

*This problem allows you the opportunity to demonstrate the* **Hughston Posterolateral Drawer Test for the Knee.**
*You have 2 minutes to complete this task.*

| Tester places athlete and limb in appropriate position | YES | NO |
|---|---|---|
| Supine | OOO | OOO |
| Hip is flexed to 45 degrees | OOO | OOO |
| Knee is flexed to 90 degrees (foot in neutral) | OOO | OOO |
| Tibia externally rotated 15 to 20 degrees | OOO | OOO |
| **Tester placed in proper position** | **YES** | **NO** |
| Sits on athlete's involved foot | OOO | OOO |
| Cups the hands around the proximal (posterior) aspect of the lower leg, thumbs on the tibial plateau | OOO | OOO |
| **Tester performs test according to accepted guidelines** | **YES** | **NO** |
| Applies an anterior force to the proximal aspect of the lower leg | OOO | OOO |
| Maintains relaxation of the limb | OOO | OOO |
| Performs assessment bilaterally | OOO | OOO |

The psychomotor skill was performed completely and in the appropriate order     **0  1  2  3  4  5**

The tester had control of the subject and the situation (showed confidence)     **0  1  2  3  4  5**

Method of performing the skill allowed the tester the ability to determine:
severity, proper progression, and the *fit* in the overall picture (Oral)     **0  1  2  3  4  5**

In order for a grade of *minimum standard* to be given, the total must be ≥11     **TOTAL =**

I_____I_____I
**Not Acceptable**          **Meets Minimum Standards**          **Exceeds Minimum Standards**

**L:** Laboratory/Classroom Testing
**C:** Clinical/Field Testing
**P:** Practicum Testing
**A:** Assessment/Mock Exam Testing
**S:** Self-Reporting

**Positive Finding:** Posterior displacement
**Involved Structure:** PCL; posterolateral capsule
**Special Considerations:** N/A
**Reference(s):** Konin et al; Magee
**Supplies Needed:** Table

# LIGAMENTOUS STRESS TESTS
## (LST-L-Test 14)

Peer Review _____ Peer Review _____

Skill Acquisition: _____    Practice Opportunities: _____

This problem allows you the opportunity to demonstrate the **Posterior Sag Test (Gravity Drawer Test) for the Knee**. You have 2 minutes to complete this task.

| Tester places athlete and limb in appropriate position | YES | NO |
|---|---|---|
| Supine | ○○○ | ○○○ |
| Hips flexed to 45 degrees | ○○○ | ○○○ |
| Knee is flexed to 90 degrees (foot in neutral) | ○○○ | ○○○ |
| **Tester placed in proper position** | **YES** | **NO** |
| Stands to the side of the athlete | ○○○ | ○○○ |
| **Tester performs test according to accepted guidelines** | **YES** | **NO** |
| Observes tibial tubercles for posterior displacement of the tibia on the femur | ○○○ | ○○○ |
| Maintains relaxation of the limb | ○○○ | ○○○ |
| Observes bilaterally | ○○○ | ○○○ |

The psychomotor skill was performed completely and in the appropriate order    **0  1  2  3  4  5**

The tester had control of the subject and the situation (showed confidence)    **0  1  2  3  4  5**

Method of performing the skill allowed the tester the ability to determine:
severity, proper progression, and the *fit* in the overall picture (Oral)    **0  1  2  3  4  5**

In order for a grade of *minimum standard* to be given, the total must be ≥11    **TOTAL =**

I_____I_____I

**Not Acceptable**　　　**Meets Minimum Standards**　　　**Exceeds Minimum Standards**

**L:** Laboratory/Classroom Testing
**C:** Clinical/Field Testing
**P:** Practicum Testing
**A:** Assessment/Mock Exam Testing
**S:** Self-Reporting

**Positive Finding:** Posterior displacement (looking for a "sag")
**Involved Structure:** PCL
**Special Considerations:** Adding active contraction of the quad is the voluntary anterior draw sign
**Reference(s):** Konin et al; Magee
**Supplies Needed:** Table

## LIGAMENTOUS STRESS TESTS
# (LST-L-Test 15)

Skill Acquisition: _____    Practice Opportunities: _____

*This problem allows you the opportunity to demonstrate the* **Godfrey Test (Godfrey 90/90/Godfrey Gravity Test) for the Knee**. *You have 2 minutes to complete this task.*

| Tester places athlete and limb in appropriate position | YES | NO |
|---|---|---|
| Supine | OOO | OOO |
| Passively flexes the athlete's hips and knee to 90 degrees (90/90 position) | OOO | OOO |
| **Tester placed in proper position** | **YES** | **NO** |
| Stands to the side of the athlete | OOO | OOO |
| Places both hands under the distal aspect of both lower legs (stabilizes the femur) | OOO | OOO |
| **Tester performs test according to accepted guidelines** | **YES** | **NO** |
| Observes tibial tubercles for posterior displacement of the tibia on the femur | OOO | OOO |
| Maintains relaxation of the limb | OOO | OOO |
| Observes bilaterally | OOO | OOO |

The psychomotor skill was performed completely and in the appropriate order    **0  1  2  3  4  5**

The tester had control of the subject and the situation (showed confidence)    **0  1  2  3  4  5**

Method of performing the skill allowed the tester the ability to determine:
severity, proper progression, and the *fit* in the overall picture (Oral)    **0  1  2  3  4  5**

In order for a grade of *minimum standard* to be given, the total must be ≥11    **TOTAL =**

I_____I_____I
**Not Acceptable**         **Meets Minimum Standards**    **Exceeds Minimum Standards**

**L:** Laboratory/Classroom Testing
**C:** Clinical/Field Testing
**P:** Practicum Testing
**A:** Assessment/Mock Exam Testing
**S:** Self-Reporting

**Positive Finding:** Downward displacement of the involved tibia
**Involved Structure:** PCL
**Special Considerations:** N/A
**Reference(s):** Konin et al; Magee; Starkey et al
**Supplies Needed:** Table

# LIGAMENTOUS STRESS TESTS
# (LST-L-Test 16)

Peer Review _____ Peer Review _____

Skill Acquisition: _____     Practice Opportunities: _____

*This problem allows you the opportunity to demonstrate the* **Lateral Pivot-Shift (MacIntosh Test/Lamaire Test) for the Knee.** *You have 2 minutes to complete this task.*

| Tester places athlete and limb in appropriate position | YES | NO |
|---|---|---|
| Supine | OOO | OOO |
| Hips flexed to 20 to 40 degrees | OOO | OOO |
| Knee in full extension (bounce home reinforces full extension) | OOO | OOO |
| **Tester placed in proper position** | **YES** | **NO** |
| Stands to the side of the athlete | OOO | OOO |
| Grasps the distal aspect of the lower leg with one hand | OOO | OOO |
| Places the other hand laterally over the fibular head | OOO | OOO |
| **Tester performs test according to accepted guidelines** | **YES** | **NO** |
| Applies a valgus stress over the knee | OOO | OOO |
| Maintains internal rotation of the tibia | OOO | OOO |
| Passively flexes the athlete's knee through 90 degrees, slowly | OOO | OOO |
| Palpates for a backward shift of the tibia | OOO | OOO |
| Maintains relaxation of the limb | OOO | OOO |
| Performs assessment bilaterally | OOO | OOO |

The psychomotor skill was performed completely and in the appropriate order    **0  1  2  3  4  5**

The tester had control of the subject and the situation (showed confidence)    **0  1  2  3  4  5**

Method of performing the skill allowed the tester the ability to determine:
severity, proper progression, and the *fit* in the overall picture (Oral)    **0  1  2  3  4  5**

In order for a grade of *minimum standard* to be given, the total must be ≥11    **TOTAL =**

I_____I_____I
**Not Acceptable**     **Meets Minimum Standards**     **Exceeds Minimum Standards**

**Positive Finding:** "Clunk"; posterior displacement of the tibia; slight external rotation of the tibia

**L:** Laboratory/Classroom Testing
**C:** Clinical/Field Testing
**P:** Practicum Testing
**A:** Assessment/Mock Exam Testing
**S:** Self-Reporting

**Involved Structure:** ACL; posterolateral capsule
**Special Considerations:** Positive sign occurs around 25 degrees
**Reference(s):** Magee; Starkey et al
**Supplies Needed:** Table

## Ligamentous Stress Tests
# (LST-L-Test 17)

Peer Review _____ Peer Review _____

Skill Acquisition: _____     Practice Opportunities: _____

*This problem allows you the opportunity to demonstrate the* **Jerk Test (Jerk Test of Hughston) for the Knee.** *You have 2 minutes to complete this task.*

| Tester places athlete and limb in appropriate position | YES | NO |
|---|---|---|
| Supine | OOO | OOO |
| Hip flexed to 45 degrees | OOO | OOO |
| Knee in full flexion | OOO | OOO |
| **Tester placed in proper position** | **YES** | **NO** |
| Stands to the side of the athlete | OOO | OOO |
| Grasps the distal aspect of the lower leg with one hand | OOO | OOO |
| Places the other hand laterally over the fibular head | OOO | OOO |
| **Tester performs test according to accepted guidelines** | **YES** | **NO** |
| Applies a valgus stress over the knee | OOO | OOO |
| Maintains internal rotation of the tibia | OOO | OOO |
| Passively extends the athlete's knee from 90 degrees to full extension, slowly | OOO | OOO |
| Maintains relaxation of the limb | OOO | OOO |
| Performs assessment bilaterally | OOO | OOO |

The psychomotor skill was performed completely and in the appropriate order    **0  1  2  3  4  5**

The tester had control of the subject and the situation (showed confidence)    **0  1  2  3  4  5**

Method of performing the skill allowed the tester the ability to determine:
severity, proper progression, and the *fit* in the overall picture (Oral)    **0  1  2  3  4  5**

In order for a grade of *minimum standard* to be given, the total must be ≥11         **TOTAL =**

I_____I_____I

**Not Acceptable**       **Meets Minimum Standards**    **Exceeds Minimum Standards**

**Positive Finding:** "Clunk/jerk"; anterior subluxation or displacement of the tibia; slight internal rotation of the tibia

**L:** Laboratory/Classroom Testing
**C:** Clinical/Field Testing
**P:** Practicum Testing
**A:** Assessment/Mock Exam Testing
**S:** Self-Reporting

**Involved Structure:** ACL; posterolateral capsule
**Special Considerations:** Positive sign occurs around 25 degrees
**Reference(s):** Konin et al; Magee
**Supplies Needed:** Table

# LIGAMENTOUS STRESS TESTS
# (LST-L-Test 18)

Skill Acquisition: _____      Practice Opportunities: _____

*Please demonstrate the proper technique for administering an* **Anterior-Posterior Glide of the Tibiofemoral Joint.** *You have 2 minutes to complete this task.*

| Tester places athlete and limb in appropriate position | YES | NO |
|---|---|---|
| Seated | ○○○ | ○○○ |
| Legs hanging off the table (table supporting distal femur) | ○○○ | ○○○ |
| Knee in slight flexion (30 to 40 degrees) | ○○○ | ○○○ |
| **Tester placed in proper position** | **YES** | **NO** |
| Stands/sits in front of the involved side | ○○○ | ○○○ |
| Applies distraction force to the tibia and holds with both hands | ○○○ | ○○○ |
| **Tester performs test according to accepted guidelines** | **YES** | **NO** |
| Applies a mobilization force in a posterior direction in and around the tibial plateau | ○○○ | ○○○ |
| Oscillation of the posterior glide is performed two to three times | ○○○ | ○○○ |
| Maintains relaxation of the limb | ○○○ | ○○○ |
| Performs assessment bilaterally | ○○○ | ○○○ |

| | |
|---|---|
| The psychomotor skill was performed completely and in the appropriate order | 0  1  2  3  4  5 |
| The tester had control of the subject and the situation (showed confidence) | 0  1  2  3  4  5 |
| Method of performing the skill allowed the tester the ability to determine: severity, proper progression, and the *fit* in the overall picture (Oral) | 0  1  2  3  4  5 |

In order for a grade of *minimum standard* to be given, the total must be ≥11        **TOTAL =**

I_____I_____I
**Not Acceptable**        **Meets Minimum Standards**        **Exceeds Minimum Standards**

**L:** Laboratory/Classroom Testing
**C:** Clinical/Field Testing
**P:** Practicum Testing
**A:** Assessment/Mock Exam Testing
**S:** Self-Reporting

**Positive Finding:** Increased joint motion (flexion)
**Involved Structure:** Joint capsule
**Special Considerations:** May be done supine with towel roll under the knee joint
**Reference(s):** Prentice; Houglum
**Supplies Needed:** Table

*Chapter*

# MANUAL MUSCLE TESTING

# MANUAL MUSCLE TESTING
# (MMT-U-Test 1)

Peer Review _____ Peer Review _____

Skill Acquisition: _____    Practice Opportunities: _____

*This problem allows you the opportunity to demonstrate a manual muscle test for the* **pectoralis minor** *muscle. You have 2 minutes to complete this task.*

| | YES | NO |
|---|---|---|
| **Tester places athlete and limb in appropriate position** | **YES** | **NO** |
| Supine (head at the end of the table) | OOO | OOO |
| Arm at the side | OOO | OOO |
| **Tester placed in proper position** | **YES** | **NO** |
| Stands to the side, facing the athlete | OOO | OOO |
| Places one hand on the anterior aspect of the shoulder | OOO | OOO |
| **Tester performs test according to accepted guidelines** | **YES** | **NO** |
| Has the athlete actively thrust the shoulder forward (lift off the table) | OOO | OOO |
| Applies downward resistance against anterior shoulder (toward the table) | OOO | OOO |
| Holds resistance for 5 seconds | OOO | OOO |
| Performs assessment bilaterally | OOO | OOO |

The psychomotor skill was performed completely and in the appropriate order    **0  1  2  3  4  5**

The tester had control of the subject and the situation (showed confidence)    **0  1  2  3  4  5**

Method of performing the skill allowed the tester the ability to determine:
severity, proper progression, and the *fit* in the overall picture (Oral)    **0  1  2  3  4  5**

In order for a grade of *minimum standard* to be given, the total must be ≥11    **TOTAL =**

I_____I_____I
**Not Acceptable**        **Meets Minimum Standards**        **Exceeds Minimum Standards**

**L:** Laboratory/Classroom Testing
**C:** Clinical/Field Testing
**P:** Practicum Testing
**A:** Assessment/Mock Exam Testing
**S:** Self-Reporting

**Positive Finding:** Decreased ability to hold con-
traction
**Involved Structure:** Pectoralis minor
**Special Considerations:** N/A
**Reference(s):** Kendall et al
**Supplies Needed:** Table

## Manual Muscle Testing
# (MMT-U-Test 2)

Peer Review _____ Peer Review _____

Skill Acquisition: _____     Practice Opportunities: _____

*This problem allows you the opportunity to demonstrate a manual muscle test for the* **extensor pollicis longus** *muscle. You have 2 minutes to complete this task.*

| Tester places athlete and limb in appropriate position | YES | NO |
|---|---|---|
| Seated or standing | ○○○ | ○○○ |
| **Tester placed in proper position** | **YES** | **NO** |
| Stands to the side, facing the athlete | ○○○ | ○○○ |
| Places one hand on the under side of the hand and wrist | ○○○ | ○○○ |
| Places the other hand against the dorsal surface of the distal phalanx of the thumb | ○○○ | ○○○ |
| **Tester performs test according to accepted guidelines** | **YES** | **NO** |
| Has the athlete actively extend the thumb | ○○○ | ○○○ |
| Applies resistance against the thumb (distal phalanx) in the direction of flexion | ○○○ | ○○○ |
| Holds resistance for 5 seconds | ○○○ | ○○○ |
| Performs assessment bilaterally | ○○○ | ○○○ |

The psychomotor skill was performed completely and in the appropriate order    0 1 2 3 4 5

The tester had control of the subject and the situation (showed confidence)    0 1 2 3 4 5

Method of performing the skill allowed the tester the ability to determine:
severity, proper progression, and the *fit* in the overall picture (Oral)    0 1 2 3 4 5

In order for a grade of *minimum standard* to be given, the total must be ≥11    **TOTAL =**

I_____I_____I

**Not Acceptable          Meets Minimum Standards     Exceeds Minimum Standards**

**L:** Laboratory/Classroom Testing
**C:** Clinical/Field Testing
**P:** Practicum Testing
**A:** Assessment/Mock Exam Testing
**S:** Self-Reporting

**Positive Finding:** Decreased ability to hold contraction
**Involved Structure:** Extensor pollicis longus
**Special Considerations:** N/A
**Reference(s):** Kendall et al
**Supplies Needed:** N/A

# MANUAL MUSCLE TESTING
## (MMT-U-Test 3)

Peer Review _____ Peer Review _____

Skill Acquisition: _____     Practice Opportunities: _____

*This problem allows you the opportunity to demonstrate a manual muscle test for the* **extensor pollicis brevis** *muscle. You have 2 minutes to complete this task.*

| | YES | NO |
|---|---|---|
| **Tester places athlete and limb in appropriate position** | YES | NO |
| Seated or standing | OOO | OOO |
| **Tester placed in proper position** | YES | NO |
| Stands to the side, facing the athlete | OOO | OOO |
| Places one hand on the underside of the hand and wrist | OOO | OOO |
| Places the other hand against the dorsal surface of the proximal phalanx of the thumb | OOO | OOO |
| **Tester performs test according to accepted guidelines** | YES | NO |
| Has the athlete actively extend the thumb | OOO | OOO |
| Applies resistance against the thumb (proximal phalanx) in the direction of flexion | OOO | OOO |
| Holds resistance for 5 seconds | OOO | OOO |
| Performs assessment bilaterally | OOO | OOO |

| | |
|---|---|
| The psychomotor skill was performed completely and in the appropriate order | **0  1  2  3  4  5** |
| The tester had control of the subject and the situation (showed confidence) | **0  1  2  3  4  5** |
| Method of performing the skill allowed the tester the ability to determine: severity, proper progression, and the *fit* in the overall picture (Oral) | **0  1  2  3  4  5** |

In order for a grade of *minimum standard* to be given, the total must be ≥11        **TOTAL =**

I_____I_____I
**Not Acceptable        Meets Minimum Standards    Exceeds Minimum Standards**

**L:** Laboratory/Classroom Testing
**C:** Clinical/Field Testing
**P:** Practicum Testing
**A:** Assessment/Mock Exam Testing
**S:** Self-Reporting

**Positive Finding:** Decreased ability to hold contraction
**Involved Structure:** Extensor pollicis brevis
**Special Considerations:** N/A
**Reference(s):** Kendall et al
**Supplies Needed:** N/A

## MANUAL MUSCLE TESTING
# (MMT-U-Test 4)

Peer Review _____ Peer Review _____

Skill Acquisition: _____          Practice Opportunities: _____

*This problem allows you the opportunity to demonstrate a manual muscle test for the* **abductor pollicis brevis** *muscle. You have 2 minutes to complete this task.*

| Tester places athlete and limb in appropriate position | YES | NO |
|---|---|---|
| Seated or standing | OOO | OOO |
| **Tester placed in proper position** | **YES** | **NO** |
| Stands to the side, facing the athlete | OOO | OOO |
| Places one hand on the underside of the hand and wrist | OOO | OOO |
| Places the other hand against the dorsal surface of the proximal phalanx of the thumb | OOO | OOO |
| **Tester performs test according to accepted guidelines** | **YES** | **NO** |
| Has the athlete actively abduct the thumb | OOO | OOO |
| Applies resistance against thumb (proximal phalanx) in the direction of adduction (toward the palm) | OOO | OOO |
| Holds resistance for 5 seconds | OOO | OOO |
| Performs assessment bilaterally | OOO | OOO |

The psychomotor skill was performed completely and in the appropriate order          0  1  2  3  4  5

The tester had control of the subject and the situation (showed confidence)          0  1  2  3  4  5

Method of performing the skill allowed the tester the ability to determine:
severity, proper progression, and the *fit* in the overall picture (Oral)          0  1  2  3  4  5

In order for a grade of *minimum standard* to be given, the total must be ≥11          **TOTAL =**

I_____I_____I

**Not Acceptable          Meets Minimum Standards          Exceeds Minimum Standards**

**L:** Laboratory/Classroom Testing
**C:** Clinical/Field Testing
**P:** Practicum Testing
**A:** Assessment/Mock Exam Testing
**S:** Self-Reporting

**Positive Finding:** Decreased ability to hold contraction
**Involved Structure:** Abductor pollicis brevis
**Special Considerations:** N/A
**Reference(s):** Kendall et al
**Supplies Needed:** N/A

# MANUAL MUSCLE TESTING
# (MMT-U-Test 5)

Peer Review _____  Peer Review _____

Skill Acquisition: _____    Practice Opportunities: _____

*This problem allows you the opportunity to demonstrate a manual muscle test for the* **flexor pollicis longus** *muscle. You have 2 minutes to complete this task.*

| | YES | NO |
|---|---|---|
| **Tester places athlete and limb in appropriate position** | YES | NO |
| Seated or supine | OOO | OOO |
| **Tester placed in proper position** | YES | NO |
| Stands to the side, facing the athlete | OOO | OOO |
| Places one hand on the underside of the hand and wrist (stabilizing the metacarpal and proximal phalanx) | OOO | OOO |
| Places the other hand against the palmar surface of the distal phalanx of the thumb | OOO | OOO |
| **Tester performs test according to accepted guidelines** | YES | NO |
| Has the athlete actively flex the thumb | OOO | OOO |
| Applies resistance against the thumb (distal phalanx) in the direction of flexion | OOO | OOO |
| Holds resistance for 5 seconds | OOO | OOO |
| Performs assessment bilaterally | OOO | OOO |

| | |
|---|---|
| The psychomotor skill was performed completely and in the appropriate order | 0 1 2 3 4 5 |
| The tester had control of the subject and the situation (showed confidence) | 0 1 2 3 4 5 |
| Method of performing the skill allowed the tester the ability to determine: severity, proper progression, and the *fit* in the overall picture (Oral) | 0 1 2 3 4 5 |

In order for a grade of *minimum standard* to be given, the total must be ≥11        **TOTAL =**

I_____I_____I
**Not Acceptable        Meets Minimum Standards    Exceeds Minimum Standards**

**L:** Laboratory/Classroom Testing
**C:** Clinical/Field Testing
**P:** Practicum Testing
**A:** Assessment/Mock Exam Testing
**S:** Self-Reporting

**Positive Finding:** Decreased ability to hold contraction
**Involved Structure:** Flexor pollicis longus and brevis
**Special Considerations:** N/A
**Reference(s):** Kendall et al
**Supplies Needed:** N/A

# Manual Muscle Testing
# (MMT-U-Test 6A)

Peer Review _____ Peer Review _____

Skill Acquisition: _____    Practice Opportunities: _____

*This problem allows you the opportunity to demonstrate a manual muscle test for the **rhomboid/levator** muscle. You have 2 minutes to complete this task.*

| Tester places athlete and limb in appropriate position | YES | NO |
|---|---|---|
| Prone (shoulder at the edge of the table) | OOO | OOO |
| Shoulder extended (hyperextended)/slight lateral rotation/full adduction | OOO | OOO |
| Elbow flexed to 90 degrees | OOO | OOO |
| **Tester placed in proper position** | **YES** | **NO** |
| Stands to the side, facing the athlete | OOO | OOO |
| Places one hand on the shoulder/scapula | OOO | OOO |
| Places the other hand against the medial aspect of the elbow | OOO | OOO |
| **Tester performs test according to accepted guidelines** | **YES** | **NO** |
| Has the athlete actively attain the position | OOO | OOO |
| Applies resistance against the arm in the direction of abduction/lateral rotation of the inferior angle of the scapula | OOO | OOO |
| Applies a depressive force to the shoulder with the other hand | OOO | OOO |
| Holds resistance for 5 seconds | OOO | OOO |
| Performs assessment bilaterally | OOO | OOO |

The psychomotor skill was performed completely and in the appropriate order    0 1 2 3 4 5

The tester had control of the subject and the situation (showed confidence)    0 1 2 3 4 5

Method of performing the skill allowed the tester the ability to determine: severity, proper progression, and the *fit* in the overall picture (Oral)    0 1 2 3 4 5

In order for a grade of *minimum standard* to be given, the total must be ≥11    TOTAL =

I_____I_____I

**Not Acceptable**    **Meets Minimum Standards**    **Exceeds Minimum Standards**

**L:** Laboratory/Classroom Testing
**C:** Clinical/Field Testing
**P:** Practicum Testing
**A:** Assessment/Mock Exam Testing
**S:** Self-Reporting

**Positive Finding:** Decreased ability to hold contraction
**Involved Structure:** Rhomboid/levator
**Special Considerations:** N/A
**Reference(s):** Kendall et al
**Supplies Needed:** Table

# Manual Muscle Testing
# (MMT-U-Test 6B)

Peer Review _____ Peer Review _____

Skill Acquisition: _____    Practice Opportunities: _____

*This problem allows you the opportunity to demonstrate a manual muscle test for the* **rhomboid (Alternate Test)** *muscle. You have 2 minutes to complete this task.*

| Tester places athlete and limb in appropriate position | YES | NO |
|---|---|---|
| Prone | ○○○ | ○○○ |
| Shoulder abducted to 90 degrees | ○○○ | ○○○ |
| Shoulder medially rotated with thumb pointing downward | ○○○ | ○○○ |
| **Tester placed in proper position** | **YES** | **NO** |
| Stands to the side, facing the athlete | ○○○ | ○○○ |
| Places one hand on the opposite scapula | ○○○ | ○○○ |
| Places the other hand against the distal forearm (radius/ulna) | ○○○ | ○○○ |
| **Tester performs test according to accepted guidelines** | **YES** | **NO** |
| Has the athlete actively horizontally extend the shoulder | ○○○ | ○○○ |
| Applies resistance against the arm in the direction of horizontal flexion (downward direction toward the table) | ○○○ | ○○○ |
| Holds resistance for 5 seconds | ○○○ | ○○○ |
| Performs assessment bilaterally | ○○○ | ○○○ |

The psychomotor skill was performed completely and in the appropriate order    0  1  2  3  4  5

The tester had control of the subject and the situation (showed confidence)    0  1  2  3  4  5

Method of performing the skill allowed the tester the ability to determine:
severity, proper progression, and the *fit* in the overall picture (Oral)    0  1  2  3  4  5

In order for a grade of *minimum standard* to be given, the total must be ≥11    **TOTAL =**

I_____I_____I
**Not Acceptable**        **Meets Minimum Standards**    **Exceeds Minimum Standards**

**L:** Laboratory/Classroom Testing
**C:** Clinical/Field Testing
**P:** Practicum Testing
**A:** Assessment/Mock Exam Testing
**S:** Self-Reporting

**Positive Finding:** Decreased ability to hold contraction
**Involved Structure:** Rhomboid (alternate)
**Special Considerations:** N/A
**Reference(s):** Kendall et al
**Supplies Needed:** Table

## MANUAL MUSCLE TESTING
# (MMT-U-Test 7)

Peer Review _____ Peer Review _____

Skill Acquisition: _____    Practice Opportunities: _____

*This problem allows you the opportunity to demonstrate a manual muscle test for the* **biceps brachii** *muscle. You have 2 minutes to complete this task.*

| Tester places athlete and limb in appropriate position | YES | NO |
|---|---|---|
| Supine or seated | ○○○ | ○○○ |
| Places the elbow in 30 to 45 degrees flexion | ○○○ | ○○○ |
| Places forearm in a supinated position | ○○○ | ○○○ |
| **Tester placed in proper position** | **YES** | **NO** |
| Stands to the side, facing the athlete | ○○○ | ○○○ |
| Places one hand under the elbow | ○○○ | ○○○ |
| Places the other hand against the distal forearm (radius/ulna) | ○○○ | ○○○ |
| **Tester performs test according to accepted guidelines** | **YES** | **NO** |
| Instructs the athlete to maintain the flexed position | ○○○ | ○○○ |
| Applies resistance against the arm in the direction of extension | ○○○ | ○○○ |
| Holds resistance for 5 seconds | ○○○ | ○○○ |
| Performs assessment bilaterally | ○○○ | ○○○ |

The psychomotor skill was performed completely and in the appropriate order      0  1  2  3  4  5

The tester had control of the subject and the situation (showed confidence)      0  1  2  3  4  5

Method of performing the skill allowed the tester the ability to determine:
severity, proper progression, and the *fit* in the overall picture (Oral)      0  1  2  3  4  5

In order for a grade of *minimum standard* to be given, the total must be ≥11      **TOTAL =**

I_____I_____I

**Not Acceptable**        **Meets Minimum Standards**      **Exceeds Minimum Standards**

**L:** Laboratory/Classroom Testing
**C:** Clinical/Field Testing
**P:** Practicum Testing
**A:** Assessment/Mock Exam Testing
**S:** Self-Reporting

**Positive Finding:** Decreased ability to hold con-
traction
**Involved Structure:** Biceps brachii
**Special Considerations:** N/A
**Reference(s):** Kendall et al
**Supplies Needed:** N/A

# MANUAL MUSCLE TESTING
## (MMT-U-Test 8)

Peer Review _____ Peer Review _____

Skill Acquisition: _____    Practice Opportunities: _____

*This problem allows you the opportunity to demonstrate a manual muscle test for the **serratus anterior** muscle. You have 2 minutes to complete this task.*

| Tester places athlete and limb in appropriate position | YES | NO |
|---|---|---|
| Supine | OOO | OOO |
| Shoulder flexed to 90 degrees | OOO | OOO |
| Shoulder elevated off the table (abduction of the scapula/as if punching) | OOO | OOO |
| Fingers clenched in a fist | OOO | OOO |
| **Tester placed in proper position** | **YES** | **NO** |
| Stands to the side, facing the athlete (may need a stool to stand on) | OOO | OOO |
| Clasps one or both hands over the elevated fist | OOO | OOO |
| **Tester performs test according to accepted guidelines** | **YES** | **NO** |
| Instructs the athlete to maintain the elevated position | OOO | OOO |
| Applies a downward resistance against the clenched fist (axial pressure pushing shoulder back down to the table) | OOO | OOO |
| Holds resistance for 5 seconds | OOO | OOO |
| Performs assessment bilaterally | OOO | OOO |

The psychomotor skill was performed completely and in the appropriate order    0  1  2  3  4  5

The tester had control of the subject and the situation (showed confidence)    0  1  2  3  4  5

Method of performing the skill allowed the tester the ability to determine:
severity, proper progression, and the *fit* in the overall picture (Oral)    0  1  2  3  4  5

In order for a grade of *minimum standard* to be given, the total must be ≥11    **TOTAL =**

I_____I_____I

**Not Acceptable**        **Meets Minimum Standards**        **Exceeds Minimum Standards**

**L:** Laboratory/Classroom Testing
**C:** Clinical/Field Testing
**P:** Practicum Testing
**A:** Assessment/Mock Exam Testing
**S:** Self-Reporting

**Positive Finding:** Decreased ability to hold contraction
**Involved Structure:** Serratus anterior
**Special Considerations:** N/A
**Reference(s):** Kendall et al
**Supplies Needed:** Table

# MANUAL MUSCLE TESTING
## (MMT-U-Test 9)

Peer Review _____ Peer Review _____

Skill Acquisition: _____    Practice Opportunities: _____

*This problem allows you the opportunity to demonstrate a manual muscle test for the **middle trapezius** muscle. You have 2 minutes to complete this task.*

| Tester places athlete and limb in appropriate position | YES | NO |
|---|---|---|
| Prone | OOO | OOO |
| Shoulder abducted to 90 degrees | OOO | OOO |
| Shoulder laterally rotated with thumb pointing upward | OOO | OOO |
| **Tester placed in proper position** | **YES** | **NO** |
| Stands to the side, facing the athlete | OOO | OOO |
| Places one hand on the opposite scapula | OOO | OOO |
| Places the other hand against the distal forearm (radius/ulna) | OOO | OOO |
| **Tester performs test according to accepted guidelines** | **YES** | **NO** |
| Has the athlete actively horizontally extend the shoulder | OOO | OOO |
| Applies resistance against the arm in the direction of horizontal flexion (downward direction toward the table) | OOO | OOO |
| Holds resistance for 5 seconds | OOO | OOO |
| Performs assessment bilaterally | OOO | OOO |

| | |
|---|---|
| The psychomotor skill was performed completely and in the appropriate order | 0  1  2  3  4  5 |
| The tester had control of the subject and the situation (showed confidence) | 0  1  2  3  4  5 |
| Method of performing the skill allowed the tester the ability to determine: severity, proper progression, and the *fit* in the overall picture (Oral) | 0  1  2  3  4  5 |

In order for a grade of *minimum standard* to be given, the total must be ≥11          **TOTAL =**

I_____I_____I

**Not Acceptable          Meets Minimum Standards     Exceeds Minimum Standards**

**L:** Laboratory/Classroom Testing
**C:** Clinical/Field Testing
**P:** Practicum Testing
**A:** Assessment/Mock Exam Testing
**S:** Self-Reporting

**Positive Finding:** Decreased ability to hold contraction
**Involved Structure:** Middle trapezius
**Special Considerations:** N/A
**Reference(s):** Kendall et al
**Supplies Needed:** Table

# MANUAL MUSCLE TESTING
# (MMT-U-Test 10)

Peer Review _____ Peer Review _____

Skill Acquisition: _____     Practice Opportunities: _____

*This problem allows you the opportunity to demonstrate a manual muscle test for the **lower trapezius** muscle. You have 2 minutes to complete this task.*

| Tester places athlete and limb in appropriate position | YES | NO |
|---|---|---|
| Prone (shoulder at the edge of the table) | OOO | OOO |
| Shoulder abducted to 130 degrees | OOO | OOO |
| Shoulder laterally rotated with thumb pointing upward | OOO | OOO |
| **Tester placed in proper position** | **YES** | **NO** |
| Stands to the side, facing the athlete | OOO | OOO |
| Places one hand on the opposite scapula | OOO | OOO |
| Places the other hand against the distal forearm (radius/ulna) | OOO | OOO |
| **Tester performs test according to accepted guidelines** | **YES** | **NO** |
| Has the athlete actively horizontally extend the shoulder | OOO | OOO |
| Applies resistance against the arm in the direction of horizontal flexion (downward direction toward the table) | OOO | OOO |
| Holds resistance for 5 seconds | OOO | OOO |
| Performs assessment bilaterally | OOO | OOO |

| | |
|---|---|
| The psychomotor skill was performed completely and in the appropriate order | 0  1  2  3  4  5 |
| The tester had control of the subject and the situation (showed confidence) | 0  1  2  3  4  5 |
| Method of performing the skill allowed the tester the ability to determine: severity, proper progression, and the *fit* in the overall picture (Oral) | 0  1  2  3  4  5 |

In order for a grade of *minimum standard* to be given, the total must be ≥11      **TOTAL =**

I_____I_____I

**Not Acceptable**        **Meets Minimum Standards**        **Exceeds Minimum Standards**

**L:** Laboratory/Classroom Testing
**C:** Clinical/Field Testing
**P:** Practicum Testing
**A:** Assessment/Mock Exam Testing
**S:** Self-Reporting

**Positive Finding:** Decreased ability to hold contraction
**Involved Structure:** Lower trapezius
**Special Considerations:** N/A
**Reference(s):** Kendall et al
**Supplies Needed:** Table

# MANUAL MUSCLE TESTING
# (MMT-U-Test 11)

Peer Review _____ Peer Review _____

Skill Acquisition: _____     Practice Opportunities: _____

*This problem allows you the opportunity to demonstrate a manual muscle test for the **upper trapezius** muscle. You have 2 minutes to complete this task.*

| Tester places athlete and limb in appropriate position | YES | NO |
|---|---|---|
| Seated | ○○○ | ○○○ |
| Elevates acrominal end of clavicle toward the head | ○○○ | ○○○ |
| Brings the head toward the elevated clavicle (lateral flexion) | ○○○ | ○○○ |
| Laterally rotates the head toward the opposite side | ○○○ | ○○○ |
| **Tester placed in proper position** | **YES** | **NO** |
| Stands facing the back of the athlete | ○○○ | ○○○ |
| Places one hand on the side of the head | ○○○ | ○○○ |
| Places the other hand against the shoulder | ○○○ | ○○○ |
| **Tester performs test according to accepted guidelines** | **YES** | **NO** |
| Instructs the athlete to hold the position | ○○○ | ○○○ |
| Applies resistance against the head in the direction of lateral flexion to the opposite side | ○○○ | ○○○ |
| Applies resistance against the shoulder in the direction of depression (downward pressure) | ○○○ | ○○○ |
| Holds resistance for 5 seconds | ○○○ | ○○○ |
| Performs assessment bilaterally | ○○○ | ○○○ |

The psychomotor skill was performed completely and in the appropriate order    0 1 2 3 4 5

The tester had control of the subject and the situation (showed confidence)    0 1 2 3 4 5

Method of performing the skill allowed the tester the ability to determine: severity, proper progression, and the *fit* in the overall picture (Oral)    0 1 2 3 4 5

In order for a grade of *minimum standard* to be given, the total must be ≥11    **TOTAL =**

I_____I_____I

**Not Acceptable**          **Meets Minimum Standards**          **Exceeds Minimum Standards**

**L:** Laboratory/Classroom Testing
**C:** Clinical/Field Testing
**P:** Practicum Testing
**A:** Assessment/Mock Exam Testing
**S:** Self-Reporting

**Positive Finding:** Decreased ability to hold contraction
**Involved Structure:** Upper trapezius
**Special Considerations:** N/A
**Reference(s):** Kendall et al
**Supplies Needed:** Stool/chair

# MANUAL MUSCLE TESTING
# (MMT-U-Test 12)

Peer Review _____ Peer Review _____

Skill Acquisition: _____    Practice Opportunities: _____

*This problem allows you the opportunity to demonstrate a manual muscle test for the* **flexor carpi radialis** *muscle. You have 2 minutes to complete this task.*

| Tester places athlete and limb in appropriate position | YES | NO |
|---|---|---|
| Seated or supine | ooo | ooo |
| Forearm placed in slightly less than full supination | ooo | ooo |
| **Tester placed in proper position** | **YES** | **NO** |
| Stands in front, facing the athlete | ooo | ooo |
| Places one hand on the underside of the wrist | ooo | ooo |
| Places the other hand on the thenar eminence | ooo | ooo |
| **Tester performs test according to accepted guidelines** | **YES** | **NO** |
| Has the athlete actively flex the wrist | ooo | ooo |
| Applies resistance against the thenar eminence in the direction of extension (toward the ulnar side) | ooo | ooo |
| Holds resistance for 5 seconds | ooo | ooo |
| Performs assessment bilaterally | ooo | ooo |

The psychomotor skill was performed completely and in the appropriate order    0 1 2 3 4 5

The tester had control of the subject and the situation (showed confidence)    0 1 2 3 4 5

Method of performing the skill allowed the tester the ability to determine: severity, proper progression, and the *fit* in the overall picture (Oral)    0 1 2 3 4 5

In order for a grade of *minimum standard* to be given, the total must be ≥11    **TOTAL =**

I_____I_____I

**Not Acceptable**    **Meets Minimum Standards**    **Exceeds Minimum Standards**

**L:** Laboratory/Classroom Testing
**C:** Clinical/Field Testing
**P:** Practicum Testing
**A:** Assessment/Mock Exam Testing
**S:** Self-Reporting

**Positive Finding:** Decreased ability to hold contraction
**Involved Structure:** Flexor carpi radialis
**Special Considerations:** N/A
**Reference(s):** Kendall et al
**Supplies Needed:** N/A

# MANUAL MUSCLE TESTING
# (MMT-U-Test 13)

Peer Review _____ Peer Review _____

Skill Acquisition: _____    Practice Opportunities: _____

*This problem allows you the opportunity to demonstrate a manual muscle test for the* **flexor carpi ulnaris** *muscle. You have 2 minutes to complete this task.*

| Tester places athlete and limb in appropriate position | YES | NO |
|---|---|---|
| Seated or supine | ooo | ooo |
| Forearm placed in full supination | ooo | ooo |
| **Tester placed in proper position** | **YES** | **NO** |
| Stands in front, facing the athlete | ooo | ooo |
| Places one hand on the underside of the wrist | ooo | ooo |
| Places the other hand on the hypothenar eminence | ooo | ooo |
| **Tester performs test according to accepted guidelines** | **YES** | **NO** |
| Has the athlete actively flex the wrist | ooo | ooo |
| Applies resistance against the hypothenar eminence in the direction of extension (toward the radial side) | ooo | ooo |
| Holds resistance for 5 seconds | ooo | ooo |
| Performs assessment bilaterally | ooo | ooo |

The psychomotor skill was performed completely and in the appropriate order          0  1  2  3  4  5

The tester had control of the subject and the situation (showed confidence)          0  1  2  3  4  5

Method of performing the skill allowed the tester the ability to determine:
severity, proper progression, and the *fit* in the overall picture (Oral)          0  1  2  3  4  5

In order for a grade of *minimum standard* to be given, the total must be ≥11          **TOTAL =**

I_____I_____I

**Not Acceptable          Meets Minimum Standards     Exceeds Minimum Standards**

**L:** Laboratory/Classroom Testing
**C:** Clinical/Field Testing
**P:** Practicum Testing
**A:** Assessment/Mock Exam Testing
**S:** Self-Reporting

**Positive Finding:** Decreased ability to hold contraction
**Involved Structure:** Flexor carpi ulnaris
**Special Considerations:** N/A
**Reference(s):** Kendall et al
**Supplies Needed:** N/A

# MANUAL MUSCLE TESTING
# (MMT-U-Test 14)

Peer Review _____ Peer Review _____

Skill Acquisition: _____    Practice Opportunities: _____

*This problem allows you the opportunity to demonstrate a manual muscle test for the* **extensor carpi ulnaris** *muscle. You have 2 minutes to complete this task.*

| Tester places athlete and limb in appropriate position | YES | NO |
|---|---|---|
| Seated or supine | OOO | OOO |
| Forearm placed in full pronation | OOO | OOO |
| **Tester placed in proper position** | **YES** | **NO** |
| Stands in front, facing the athlete | OOO | OOO |
| Places one hand on the underside of the forearm/wrist | OOO | OOO |
| Places the other hand against the dorsum of the fifth metacarpal | OOO | OOO |
| **Tester performs test according to accepted guidelines** | **YES** | **NO** |
| Has the athlete actively extend the wrist | OOO | OOO |
| Applies resistance against the dorsum of the fifth metacarpal in the direction of flexion (toward the radial side) | OOO | OOO |
| Holds resistance for 5 seconds | OOO | OOO |
| Performs assessment bilaterally | OOO | OOO |

The psychomotor skill was performed completely and in the appropriate order      **0  1  2  3  4  5**

The tester had control of the subject and the situation (showed confidence)      **0  1  2  3  4  5**

Method of performing the skill allowed the tester the ability to determine: severity, proper progression, and the *fit* in the overall picture (Oral)      **0  1  2  3  4  5**

In order for a grade of *minimum standard* to be given, the total must be ≥11      **TOTAL =**

I_____I_____I

**Not Acceptable**          **Meets Minimum Standards**          **Exceeds Minimum Standards**

**L:** Laboratory/Classroom Testing
**C:** Clinical/Field Testing
**P:** Practicum Testing
**A:** Assessment/Mock Exam Testing
**S:** Self-Reporting

**Positive Finding:** Decreased ability to hold contraction
**Involved Structure:** Extensor carpi ulnaris
**Special Considerations:** N/A
**Reference(s):** Kendall et al
**Supplies Needed:** N/A

## Manual Muscle Testing
# (MMT-U-Test 15)

Peer Review _____ Peer Review _____

Skill Acquisition: _____     Practice Opportunities: _____

*This problem allows you the opportunity to demonstrate a manual muscle test for the **opponens digiti minimi** muscle. You have 2 minutes to complete this task.*

| Tester places athlete and limb in appropriate position | YES | NO |
|---|---|---|
| Seated or supine | ООО | ООО |
| Wrist placed in full supination | ООО | ООО |
| **Tester placed in proper position** | **YES** | **NO** |
| Stands in front, facing the athlete | ООО | ООО |
| Places one hand on the underside of the hand (first metacarpal is gripped firmly) | ООО | ООО |
| Places the other hand against the palmar surface of the fifth metacarpal | ООО | ООО |
| **Tester performs test according to accepted guidelines** | **YES** | **NO** |
| Has the athlete actively oppose the fifth metacarpal/finger (moves toward the thumb) | ООО | ООО |
| Applies resistance against palmar surface of the fifth metacarpal (attempting to flatten the hand) | ООО | ООО |
| Holds resistance for 5 seconds | ООО | ООО |
| Performs assessment bilaterally | ООО | ООО |

The psychomotor skill was performed completely and in the appropriate order     **0  1  2  3  4  5**

The tester had control of the subject and the situation (showed confidence)     **0  1  2  3  4  5**

Method of performing the skill allowed the tester the ability to determine: severity, proper progression, and the *fit* in the overall picture (Oral)     **0  1  2  3  4  5**

In order for a grade of *minimum standard* to be given, the total must be ≥11     **TOTAL =**

I_____I_____I
   **Not Acceptable**        **Meets Minimum Standards**     **Exceeds Minimum Standards**

**L:** Laboratory/Classroom Testing
**C:** Clinical/Field Testing
**P:** Practicum Testing
**A:** Assessment/Mock Exam Testing
**S:** Self-Reporting

**Positive Finding:** Decreased ability to hold contraction
**Involved Structure:** Opponens digiti minimi
**Special Considerations:** N/A
**Reference(s):** Kendall et al
**Supplies Needed:** N/A

# MANUAL MUSCLE TESTING
# (MMT-U-Test 16)

Peer Review _____ Peer Review _____

Skill Acquisition: _____    Practice Opportunities: _____

*This problem allows you the opportunity to demonstrate a manual muscle test for the* **flexor digitorum profundus** *muscle. You have 2 minutes to complete this task.*

| Tester places athlete and limb in appropriate position | YES | NO |
|---|---|---|
| Seated or supine | OOO | OOO |
| Wrist placed in full supination (slight extension) | OOO | OOO |
| **Tester placed in proper position** | **YES** | **NO** |
| Stands in front, facing the athlete | OOO | OOO |
| Stabilizes the proximal and middle phalanges with one hand | OOO | OOO |
| Places the other hand against the palmar surface of the distal phalanx (2, 3, 4, 5) | OOO | OOO |
| **Tester performs test according to accepted guidelines** | **YES** | **NO** |
| Has the athlete actively flex the DIP joints of the second to fifth phalanges | OOO | OOO |
| Applies resistance against the palmar surface of each phalange in the direction of extension | OOO | OOO |
| Isolates each phalange separately (2, 3, 4, 5) | OOO | OOO |
| Holds resistance for 5 seconds | OOO | OOO |
| Performs assessment bilaterally | OOO | OOO |

The psychomotor skill was performed completely and in the appropriate order   0 1 2 3 4 5

The tester had control of the subject and the situation (showed confidence)   0 1 2 3 4 5

Method of performing the skill allowed the tester the ability to determine:
severity, proper progression, and the *fit* in the overall picture (Oral)   0 1 2 3 4 5

In order for a grade of *minimum standard* to be given, the total must be ≥11   **TOTAL =**

I_____I_____I

**Not Acceptable**    **Meets Minimum Standards**    **Exceeds Minimum Standards**

**L:** Laboratory/Classroom Testing
**C:** Clinical/Field Testing
**P:** Practicum Testing
**A:** Assessment/Mock Exam Testing
**S:** Self-Reporting

**Positive Finding:** Decreased ability to hold contraction
**Involved Structure:** Flexor digitorum profundus
**Special Considerations:** N/A
**Reference(s):** Kendall et al
**Supplies Needed:** N/A

# MANUAL MUSCLE TESTING
# (MMT-U-Test 17)

Peer Review _____ Peer Review _____

Skill Acquisition: _____    Practice Opportunities: _____

*This problem allows you the opportunity to demonstrate a manual muscle test for the* **pronator quadratus** *muscle. You have 2 minutes to complete this task.*

| Tester places athlete and limb in appropriate position | YES | NO |
|---|---|---|
| Seated or supine | ○○○ | ○○○ |
| Elbow placed in full flexion | ○○○ | ○○○ |
| Elbow/forearm placed in full pronation | ○○○ | ○○○ |
| Elbow placed against athlete's side (avoid shoulder abduction) | ○○○ | ○○○ |
| **Tester placed in proper position** | **YES** | **NO** |
| Stands to the side, facing the athlete | ○○○ | ○○○ |
| Stabilizes the elbow against the side with one hand | ○○○ | ○○○ |
| Places the other hand around the distal forearm | ○○○ | ○○○ |
| **Tester performs test according to accepted guidelines** | **YES** | **NO** |
| Instructs the athlete to hold the position | ○○○ | ○○○ |
| Applies resistance in a rotating motion against the distal forearm in the direction of supination | ○○○ | ○○○ |
| Holds resistance for 5 seconds | ○○○ | ○○○ |
| Performs assessment bilaterally | ○○○ | ○○○ |

| | |
|---|---|
| The psychomotor skill was performed completely and in the appropriate order | 0  1  2  3  4  5 |
| The tester had control of the subject and the situation (showed confidence) | 0  1  2  3  4  5 |
| Method of performing the skill allowed the tester the ability to determine: severity, proper progression, and the *fit* in the overall picture (Oral) | 0  1  2  3  4  5 |

In order for a grade of *minimum standard* to be given, the total must be ≥11          TOTAL =

I_____I_____I
Not Acceptable          Meets Minimum Standards          Exceeds Minimum Standards

**L:** Laboratory/Classroom Testing
**C:** Clinical/Field Testing
**P:** Practicum Testing
**A:** Assessment/Mock Exam Testing
**S:** Self-Reporting

**Positive Finding:** Decreased ability to hold contraction
**Involved Structure:** Pronator quadratus
**Special Considerations:** N/A
**Reference(s):** Kendall et al
**Supplies Needed:** Table

# MANUAL MUSCLE TESTING
## (MMT-U-Test 18)

Skill Acquisition: _____    Practice Opportunities: _____

*This problem allows you the opportunity to demonstrate a manual muscle test for the* **supinator (biceps elongated)** *muscle. You have 2 minutes to complete this task.*

| Tester places athlete and limb in appropriate position | YES | NO |
|---|---|---|
| Seated or standing | OOO | OOO |
| Shoulder placed in extension | OOO | OOO |
| Elbow placed in full extension | OOO | OOO |
| **Tester placed in proper position** | **YES** | **NO** |
| Stands behind the athlete | OOO | OOO |
| Stabilizes the elbow with one hand | OOO | OOO |
| Places the other hand around the distal forearm | OOO | OOO |
| **Tester performs test according to accepted guidelines** | **YES** | **NO** |
| Instructs the athlete to hold the position | OOO | OOO |
| Applies resistance in a rotating motion against the distal forearm in the direction of pronation | OOO | OOO |
| Holds resistance for 5 seconds | OOO | OOO |
| Performs assessment bilaterally | OOO | OOO |

The psychomotor skill was performed completely and in the appropriate order    **0 1 2 3 4 5**

The tester had control of the subject and the situation (showed confidence)    **0 1 2 3 4 5**

Method of performing the skill allowed the tester the ability to determine:
severity, proper progression, and the *fit* in the overall picture (Oral)    **0 1 2 3 4 5**

In order for a grade of *minimum standard* to be given, the total must be ≥11    **TOTAL =**

I_____I_____I

**Not Acceptable**    **Meets Minimum Standards**    **Exceeds Minimum Standards**

**L:** Laboratory/Classroom Testing
**C:** Clinical/Field Testing
**P:** Practicum Testing
**A:** Assessment/Mock Exam Testing
**S:** Self-Reporting

**Positive Finding:** Decreased ability to hold contraction
**Involved Structure:** Supinator (biceps elongated)
**Special Considerations:** N/A
**Reference(s):** Kendall et al
**Supplies Needed:** Stool/chair

## MANUAL MUSCLE TESTING
# (MMT-U-Test 19)

Peer Review _____ Peer Review _____

Skill Acquisition: _____     Practice Opportunities: _____

*This problem allows you the opportunity to demonstrate a manual muscle test for the* **supraspinatus** *muscle. You have 2 minutes to complete this task.*

| Tester places athlete and limb in appropriate position | YES | NO |
|---|---|---|
| Seated or standing | ○○○ | ○○○ |
| Arm placed at the side (palm flat against the side) | ○○○ | ○○○ |
| Head and neck extended and laterally flexed | ○○○ | ○○○ |
| Neck/face laterally rotated to the opposite side | ○○○ | ○○○ |
| **Tester placed in proper position** | **YES** | **NO** |
| Stands facing the athlete | ○○○ | ○○○ |
| Stabilizes the opposite shoulder with one hand | ○○○ | ○○○ |
| Places the other hand against the distal forearm | ○○○ | ○○○ |
| **Tester performs test according to accepted guidelines** | **YES** | **NO** |
| Instructs the athlete to initiate abduction of the shoulder | ○○○ | ○○○ |
| Applies resistance in the direction of adduction | ○○○ | ○○○ |
| Holds resistance for 5 seconds | ○○○ | ○○○ |
| Performs assessment bilaterally | ○○○ | ○○○ |

The psychomotor skill was performed completely and in the appropriate order     **0  1  2  3  4  5**

The tester had control of the subject and the situation (showed confidence)     **0  1  2  3  4  5**

Method of performing the skill allowed the tester the ability to determine:
severity, proper progression, and the *fit* in the overall picture (Oral)     **0  1  2  3  4  5**

In order for a grade of *minimum standard* to be given, the total must be ≥11     **TOTAL =**

I_____I_____I
**Not Acceptable**          **Meets Minimum Standards**     **Exceeds Minimum Standards**

**L:** Laboratory/Classroom Testing
**C:** Clinical/Field Testing
**P:** Practicum Testing
**A:** Assessment/Mock Exam Testing
**S:** Self-Reporting

**Positive Finding:** Decreased ability to hold contraction
**Involved Structure:** Supraspinatus
**Special Considerations:** N/A
**Reference(s):** Kendall et al
**Supplies Needed:** N/A

# MANUAL MUSCLE TESTING
## (MMT-U-Test 20A)

Peer Review _____ Peer Review _____

Skill Acquisition: _____    Practice Opportunities: _____

*This problem allows you the opportunity to demonstrate a manual muscle test for the* **triceps brachii (supine)** *muscle. You have 2 minutes to complete this task.*

| Tester places athlete and limb in appropriate position | YES | NO |
|---|---|---|
| Supine | ○○○ | ○○○ |
| Shoulder flexed to 90 degrees (arm perpendicular to the table) | ○○○ | ○○○ |
| Elbow extended to about 10 degrees (slightly less than full extension) | ○○○ | ○○○ |
| **Tester placed in proper position** | **YES** | **NO** |
| Stands to the side, facing the athlete | ○○○ | ○○○ |
| Places one hand on the biceps to stabilize the humerus | ○○○ | ○○○ |
| Places the other hand around the distal forearm | ○○○ | ○○○ |
| **Tester performs test according to accepted guidelines** | **YES** | **NO** |
| Instructs the athlete to hold this position | ○○○ | ○○○ |
| Applies resistance in the direction of flexion | ○○○ | ○○○ |
| Holds resistance for 5 seconds | ○○○ | ○○○ |
| Performs assessment bilaterally | ○○○ | ○○○ |

The psychomotor skill was performed completely and in the appropriate order    **0  1  2  3  4  5**

The tester had control of the subject and the situation (showed confidence)    **0  1  2  3  4  5**

Method of performing the skill allowed the tester the ability to determine:
severity, proper progression, and the *fit* in the overall picture (Oral)    **0  1  2  3  4  5**

In order for a grade of *minimum standard* to be given, the total must be ≥11    **TOTAL =**

I_____I_____I

**Not Acceptable          Meets Minimum Standards     Exceeds Minimum Standards**

**L:** Laboratory/Classroom Testing
**C:** Clinical/Field Testing
**P:** Practicum Testing
**A:** Assessment/Mock Exam Testing
**S:** Self-Reporting

**Positive Finding:** Decreased ability to hold contraction
**Involved Structure:** Triceps brachii
**Special Considerations:** N/A
**Reference(s):** Kendall et al
**Supplies Needed:** Table

## Manual Muscle Testing
# (MMT-U-Test 20B)

Skill Acquisition: _____     Practice Opportunities: _____

*This problem allows you the opportunity to demonstrate a manual muscle test for the* **triceps brachii (prone)** *muscle. You have 2 minutes to complete this task.*

| Tester places athlete and limb in appropriate position | YES | NO |
|---|---|---|
| Prone | ○○○ | ○○○ |
| Shoulder abducted to 90 degrees (arm supported by the table) | ○○○ | ○○○ |
| Elbow placed in a slightly flexed position | ○○○ | ○○○ |
| **Tester placed in proper position** | **YES** | **NO** |
| Stands to the side, facing the athlete | ○○○ | ○○○ |
| Places one hand under the arm near the elbow | ○○○ | ○○○ |
| Places the other hand around the distal forearm | ○○○ | ○○○ |
| **Tester performs test according to accepted guidelines** | **YES** | **NO** |
| Instructs the athlete to hold this position | ○○○ | ○○○ |
| Applies resistance in the direction of flexion | ○○○ | ○○○ |
| Holds resistance for 5 seconds | ○○○ | ○○○ |
| Performs assessment bilaterally | ○○○ | ○○○ |

The psychomotor skill was performed completely and in the appropriate order    **0  1  2  3  4  5**

The tester had control of the subject and the situation (showed confidence)    **0  1  2  3  4  5**

Method of performing the skill allowed the tester the ability to determine:
severity, proper progression, and the *fit* in the overall picture (Oral)    **0  1  2  3  4  5**

In order for a grade of *minimum standard* to be given, the total must be ≥11    **TOTAL =**

I_____I_____I

**Not Acceptable**        **Meets Minimum Standards**    **Exceeds Minimum Standards**

**L:** Laboratory/Classroom Testing
**C:** Clinical/Field Testing
**P:** Practicum Testing
**A:** Assessment/Mock Exam Testing
**S:** Self-Reporting

**Positive Finding:** Decreased ability to hold con-
traction
**Involved Structure:** Triceps brachii/anconeus
**Special Considerations:** N/A
**Reference(s):** Kendall et al
**Supplies Needed:** Table

# MANUAL MUSCLE TESTING
## (MMT-U-Test 21)

Peer Review _____ Peer Review _____

Skill Acquisition: _____    Practice Opportunities: _____

*This problem allows you the opportunity to demonstrate a* **Myotome Assessment** *in order to rule out damage to nerve root* **C5**. *You have 2 minutes to complete this task.*

| Tester places athlete and limb in appropriate position | YES | NO |
|---|---|---|
| Seated or standing | ○○○ | ○○○ |
| **Tester performs test according to accepted guidelines** | **YES** | **NO** |
| Instructs the athlete to abduct the shoulder against resistance (deltoid) *and/or* | ○○○ | ○○○ |
| Instructs the athlete to flex the elbow against resistance (biceps) | ○○○ | ○○○ |
| Performs a break test at some point in the range of motion | ○○○ | ○○○ |
| Holds resistance for 5 seconds | ○○○ | ○○○ |
| Performs assessment bilaterally | ○○○ | ○○○ |

The psychomotor skill was performed completely and in the appropriate order      0  1  2  3  4  5

The tester had control of the subject and the situation (showed confidence)      0  1  2  3  4  5

Method of performing the skill allowed the tester the ability to determine:
severity, proper progression, and the *fit* in the overall picture (Oral)      0  1  2  3  4  5

In order for a grade of *minimum standard* to be given, the total must be ≥11      **TOTAL =**

I_____I_____I
**Not Acceptable**          **Meets Minimum Standards**      **Exceeds Minimum Standards**

**L:** Laboratory/Classroom Testing
**C:** Clinical/Field Testing
**P:** Practicum Testing
**A:** Assessment/Mock Exam Testing
**S:** Self-Reporting

**Positive Finding:** Unable to maintain position against resistance
**Involved Structure:** Nerve root C5
**Special Considerations:** Rule out muscle damage
**Reference(s):** Hoppenfeld
**Supplies Needed:** N/A

## MANUAL MUSCLE TESTING
# (MMT-U-Test 22)

Peer Review _____ Peer Review _____

Skill Acquisition: _____    Practice Opportunities: _____

*This problem allows you the opportunity to demonstrate a* **Myotome Assessment** *in order to rule out damage to nerve root* **C6**. *You have 2 minutes to complete this task.*

| Tester places athlete and limb in appropriate position | YES | NO |
|---|---|---|
| Seated or standing | ○○○ | ○○○ |
| **Tester performs test according to accepted guidelines** | **YES** | **NO** |
| Instructs the athlete to extend the wrist against resistance (exterior carpi radialis longus and brevis) *and/or* | ○○○ | ○○○ |
| Instructs the athlete to flex the elbow against resistance (biceps) | ○○○ | ○○○ |
| Performs a break test at some point in the range of motion | ○○○ | ○○○ |
| Holds resistance for 5 seconds | ○○○ | ○○○ |
| Performs assessment bilaterally | ○○○ | ○○○ |

The psychomotor skill was performed completely and in the appropriate order    **0  1  2  3  4  5**

The tester had control of the subject and the situation (showed confidence)    **0  1  2  3  4  5**

Method of performing the skill allowed the tester the ability to determine:
severity, proper progression, and the *fit* in the overall picture (Oral)    **0  1  2  3  4  5**

In order for a grade of *minimum standard* to be given, the total must be ≥11    **TOTAL =**

I_____I_____I
**Not Acceptable          Meets Minimum Standards     Exceeds Minimum Standards**

**L:** Laboratory/Classroom Testing
**C:** Clinical/Field Testing
**P:** Practicum Testing
**A:** Assessment/Mock Exam Testing
**S:** Self-Reporting

**Positive Finding:** Unable to maintain position against resistance
**Involved Structure:** Nerve root C6
**Special Considerations:** Rule out muscle damage
**Reference(s):** Hoppenfeld
**Supplies Needed:** N/A

# MANUAL MUSCLE TESTING
# (MMT-U-Test 23)

Peer Review _____ Peer Review _____

Skill Acquisition: _____    Practice Opportunities: _____

*This problem allows you the opportunity to demonstrate a **Myotome Assessment** in order to rule out damage to nerve root **C7**. You have 2 minutes to complete this task.*

| Tester places athlete and limb in appropriate position | YES | NO |
|---|---|---|
| Seated or standing | ○○○ | ○○○ |
| **Tester performs test according to accepted guidelines** | **YES** | **NO** |
| Instructs the athlete to flex the wrist against resistance *and/or* | ○○○ | ○○○ |
| Instructs the athlete to extend the elbow against resistance | ○○○ | ○○○ |
| Performs a break test at some point in the range of motion | ○○○ | ○○○ |
| Holds resistance for 5 seconds | ○○○ | ○○○ |
| Performs assessment bilaterally | ○○○ | ○○○ |

| | |
|---|---|
| The psychomotor skill was performed completely and in the appropriate order | 0  1  2  3  4  5 |
| The tester had control of the subject and the situation (showed confidence) | 0  1  2  3  4  5 |
| Method of performing the skill allowed the tester the ability to determine: severity, proper progression, and the *fit* in the overall picture (Oral) | 0  1  2  3  4  5 |

In order for a grade of *minimum standard* to be given, the total must be ≥11          TOTAL =

I_____I_____I
**Not Acceptable**          **Meets Minimum Standards**          **Exceeds Minimum Standards**

**L:** Laboratory/Classroom Testing
**C:** Clinical/Field Testing
**P:** Practicum Testing
**A:** Assessment/Mock Exam Testing
**S:** Self-Reporting

**Positive Finding:** Unable to maintain position against resistance
**Involved Structure:** Nerve root C7
**Special Considerations:** Rule out muscle damage
**Reference(s):** Hoppenfeld
**Supplies Needed:** N/A

## Manual Muscle Testing
# (MMT-U-Test 24)

Peer Review _____    Peer Review _____

Skill Acquisition: _____    Practice Opportunities: _____

*This problem allows you the opportunity to demonstrate a* **Myotome Assessment** *in order to rule out damage to nerve root* **C8***. You have 2 minutes to complete this task.*

| Tester places athlete and limb in appropriate position | YES | NO |
|---|---|---|
| Seated or standing | ○○○ | ○○○ |
| **Tester performs test according to accepted guidelines** | **YES** | **NO** |
| Instructs the athlete to flex the fingers against resistance *and/or* | ○○○ | ○○○ |
| Instructs the athlete to abduct the fingers against resistance | ○○○ | ○○○ |
| Performs a break test at some point in the range of motion | ○○○ | ○○○ |
| Holds resistance for 5 seconds | ○○○ | ○○○ |
| Performs assessment bilaterally | ○○○ | ○○○ |

| | |
|---|---|
| The psychomotor skill was performed completely and in the appropriate order | **0  1  2  3  4  5** |
| The tester had control of the subject and the situation (showed confidence) | **0  1  2  3  4  5** |
| Method of performing the skill allowed the tester the ability to determine: severity, proper progression, and the *fit* in the overall picture (Oral) | **0  1  2  3  4  5** |

In order for a grade of *minimum standard* to be given, the total must be ≥11          **TOTAL =**

I_____I_____I
**Not Acceptable          Meets Minimum Standards    Exceeds Minimum Standards**

**L:** Laboratory/Classroom Testing
**C:** Clinical/Field Testing
**P:** Practicum Testing
**A:** Assessment/Mock Exam Testing
**S:** Self-Reporting

**Positive Finding:** Unable to maintain position against resistance
**Involved Structure:** Nerve root C8
**Special Considerations:** Rule out muscle damage
**Reference(s):** Hoppenfeld; Magee
**Supplies Needed:** N/A

# MANUAL MUSCLE TESTING
## (MMT-U-Test 25)

Peer Review _____ Peer Review _____

Skill Acquisition: _____    Practice Opportunities: _____

*This problem allows you the opportunity to demonstrate a* **Myotome Assessment** *in order to rule out damage to nerve root* **T1**. *You have 2 minutes to complete this task.*

| Tester places athlete and limb in appropriate position | YES | NO |
|---|---|---|
| Seated or standing | ○○○ | ○○○ |
| **Tester performs test according to accepted guidelines** | **YES** | **NO** |
| Instructs the athlete to abduct the fingers against resistance (interossei muscles) | ○○○ | ○○○ |
| Performs a break test at some point in the range of motion | ○○○ | ○○○ |
| Holds resistance for 5 seconds | ○○○ | ○○○ |
| Performs assessment bilaterally | ○○○ | ○○○ |

The psychomotor skill was performed completely and in the appropriate order    0 1 2 3 4 5

The tester had control of the subject and the situation (showed confidence)    0 1 2 3 4 5

Method of performing the skill allowed the tester the ability to determine:
severity, proper progression, and the *fit* in the overall picture (Oral)    0 1 2 3 4 5

In order for a grade of *minimum standard* to be given, the total must be ≥11    **TOTAL =**

I_____I_____I
**Not Acceptable**        **Meets Minimum Standards**    **Exceeds Minimum Standards**

**L:** Laboratory/Classroom Testing
**C:** Clinical/Field Testing
**P:** Practicum Testing
**A:** Assessment/Mock Exam Testing
**S:** Self-Reporting

**Positive Finding:** Unable to maintain position against resistance
**Involved Structure:** Nerve root T1
**Special Considerations:** Rule out muscle damage
**Reference(s):** Hoppenfeld
**Supplies Needed:** N/A

# MANUAL MUSCLE TESTING
# (MMT-U-Test 26)

Peer Review _____ Peer Review _____

Skill Acquisition: _____    Practice Opportunities: _____

*This problem allows you the opportunity to demonstrate a manual muscle test for the **latissimus dorsi** muscle. You have 2 minutes to complete this task.*

| Tester places athlete and limb in appropriate position | YES | NO |
|---|---|---|
| Prone | ○○○ | ○○○ |
| Shoulder placed in slight extension and adduction (palm facing body) | ○○○ | ○○○ |
| **Tester placed in proper position** | **YES** | **NO** |
| Stands to the side of the athlete | ○○○ | ○○○ |
| Places one hand on the medial forearm | ○○○ | ○○○ |
| **Tester performs test according to accepted guidelines** | **YES** | **NO** |
| Instructs the athlete to hold this position | ○○○ | ○○○ |
| Applies resistance in the direction of extension and adduction | ○○○ | ○○○ |
| Holds resistance for 5 seconds | ○○○ | ○○○ |
| Performs assessment bilaterally | ○○○ | ○○○ |

The psychomotor skill was performed completely and in the appropriate order    **0  1  2  3  4  5**

The tester had control of the subject and the situation (showed confidence)    **0  1  2  3  4  5**

Method of performing the skill allowed the tester the ability to determine:
severity, proper progression, and the *fit* in the overall picture (Oral)    **0  1  2  3  4  5**

In order for a grade of *minimum standard* to be given, the total must be ≥11    **TOTAL =**

I_____I_____I
**Not Acceptable**          **Meets Minimum Standards**     **Exceeds Minimum Standards**

**L:** Laboratory/Classroom Testing
**C:** Clinical/Field Testing
**P:** Practicum Testing
**A:** Assessment/Mock Exam Testing
**S:** Self-Reporting

**Positive Finding:** Decreased ability to hold contraction
**Involved Structure:** Latissimus dorsi
**Special Considerations:** N/A
**Reference(s):** Kendall
**Supplies Needed:** Table

# MANUAL MUSCLE TESTING
# (MMT-U-Test 27A)

Peer Review _____ Peer Review _____

Skill Acquisition: _____    Practice Opportunities: _____

*This problem allows you the opportunity to demonstrate a manual muscle test for the* **pectoralis major (upper portion)** *muscle. You have 2 minutes to complete this task.*

| Tester places athlete and limb in appropriate position | YES | NO |
|---|---|---|
| Supine | OOO | OOO |
| Shoulder placed in 90 degrees of flexion with slight medial rotation | OOO | OOO |
| Elbow placed in full extension | OOO | OOO |
| **Tester placed in proper position** | **YES** | **NO** |
| Stands at the end of table, above the athlete's head | OOO | OOO |
| Places one hand on the medial forearm | OOO | OOO |
| Places other hand on the athlete's opposite shoulder (stabilizes body) | OOO | OOO |
| **Tester performs test according to accepted guidelines** | **YES** | **NO** |
| Instructs the athlete to hold this position | OOO | OOO |
| Applies resistance in the direction of horizontal abduction (horizontal extension) | OOO | OOO |
| Holds resistance for 5 seconds | OOO | OOO |
| Performs assessment bilaterally | OOO | OOO |

The psychomotor skill was performed completely and in the appropriate order    0 1 2 3 4 5

The tester had control of the subject and the situation (showed confidence)    0 1 2 3 4 5

Method of performing the skill allowed the tester the ability to determine:
severity, proper progression, and the *fit* in the overall picture (Oral)    0 1 2 3 4 5

In order for a grade of *minimum standard* to be given, the total must be ≥11    **TOTAL =**

I_____I_____I
Not Acceptable     Meets Minimum Standards     Exceeds Minimum Standards

**L:** Laboratory/Classroom Testing
**C:** Clinical/Field Testing
**P:** Practicum Testing
**A:** Assessment/Mock Exam Testing
**S:** Self-Reporting

**Positive Finding:** Decreased ability to hold contraction
**Involved Structure:** Pectoralis major (upper portion)
**Special Considerations:** N/A
**Reference(s):** Kendall
**Supplies Needed:** Table

## MANUAL MUSCLE TESTING
## (MMT-U-Test 27B)

Peer Review _____ Peer Review _____

Skill Acquisition: _____    Practice Opportunities: _____

*This problem allows you the opportunity to demonstrate a manual muscle test for the* **pectoralis major (lower portion)** *muscle. You have 2 minutes to complete this task.*

| Tester places athlete and limb in appropriate position | YES | NO |
|---|---|---|
| Supine | OOO | OOO |
| Shoulder placed in 90 degrees of flexion, slight medial rotation (moves the shoulder obliquely toward the opposite iliac crest) | OOO | OOO |
| Elbow placed in full extension | OOO | OOO |
| **Tester placed in proper position** | **YES** | **NO** |
| Stands at the end of table, above the athlete's head | OOO | OOO |
| Places one hand on the medial forearm | OOO | OOO |
| Places other hand on the athlete's opposite iliac crest (stabilizes body) | OOO | OOO |
| **Tester performs test according to accepted guidelines** | **YES** | **NO** |
| Instructs the athlete to hold this position | OOO | OOO |
| Applies resistance obliquely in the direction of horizontal abduction (horizontal extension) | OOO | OOO |
| Holds resistance for 5 seconds | OOO | OOO |
| Performs assessment bilaterally | OOO | OOO |

The psychomotor skill was performed completely and in the appropriate order      0  1  2  3  4  5

The tester had control of the subject and the situation (showed confidence)      0  1  2  3  4  5

Method of performing the skill allowed the tester the ability to determine:
severity, proper progression, and the *fit* in the overall picture (Oral)      0  1  2  3  4  5

In order for a grade of *minimum standard* to be given, the total must be ≥11      TOTAL =

I_____I_____I
**Not Acceptable      Meets Minimum Standards      Exceeds Minimum Standards**

**L:** Laboratory/Classroom Testing
**C:** Clinical/Field Testing
**P:** Practicum Testing
**A:** Assessment/Mock Exam Testing
**S:** Self-Reporting

**Positive Finding:** Decreased ability to hold contraction
**Involved Structure:** Pectoralis major (lower portion)
**Special Considerations:** N/A
**Reference(s):** Kendall
**Supplies Needed:** Table

# MANUAL MUSCLE TESTING
## (MMT-U-Test 28)

Peer Review _____ Peer Review _____

Skill Acquisition: _____    Practice Opportunities: _____

*This problem allows you the opportunity to demonstrate a manual muscle test for the* **brachioradialis** *muscle. You have 2 minutes to complete this task.*

| Tester places athlete and limb in appropriate position | YES | NO |
|---|---|---|
| Supine or seated | ○○○ | ○○○ |
| Elbow placed in slight flexion (resting on the table) | ○○○ | ○○○ |
| Forearm placed in a neutral position (between supination and pronation) | ○○○ | ○○○ |
| **Tester placed in proper position** | **YES** | **NO** |
| Places one hand under the elbow (to cushion from table pressure) | ○○○ | ○○○ |
| Places other hand around the distal forearm | ○○○ | ○○○ |
| **Tester performs test according to accepted guidelines** | **YES** | **NO** |
| Instructs the athlete to hold this position | ○○○ | ○○○ |
| Applies resistance in the direction of extension | ○○○ | ○○○ |
| Holds resistance for 5 seconds | ○○○ | ○○○ |
| Performs assessment bilaterally | ○○○ | ○○○ |

The psychomotor skill was performed completely and in the appropriate order    **0  1  2  3  4  5**

The tester had control of the subject and the situation (showed confidence)    **0  1  2  3  4  5**

Method of performing the skill allowed the tester the ability to determine:
severity, proper progression, and the *fit* in the overall picture (Oral)    **0  1  2  3  4  5**

In order for a grade of *minimum standard* to be given, the total must be ≥11    **TOTAL =**

I_____I_____I

**Not Acceptable**        **Meets Minimum Standards**        **Exceeds Minimum Standards**

**L:** Laboratory/Classroom Testing
**C:** Clinical/Field Testing
**P:** Practicum Testing
**A:** Assessment/Mock Exam Testing
**S:** Self-Reporting

**Positive Finding:** Decreased ability to hold contraction
**Involved Structure:** Brachioradialis
**Special Considerations:** N/A
**Reference(s):** Kendall
**Supplies Needed:** Chair, table

## MANUAL MUSCLE TESTING
# (MMT-U-Test 29A)

Peer Review _____ Peer Review _____

Skill Acquisition: _____    Practice Opportunities: _____

*This problem allows you the opportunity to demonstrate a manual muscle test for the **middle deltoid** muscle. You have 2 minutes to complete this task.*

| Tester places athlete and limb in appropriate position | YES | NO |
|---|---|---|
| Seated | OOO | OOO |
| Shoulder abducted to 90 degrees | OOO | OOO |
| Elbow flexed to 90 degrees (palm facing downward) | OOO | OOO |
| **Tester placed in proper position** | YES | NO |
| Stands behind or to the side of the athlete | OOO | OOO |
| Places one hand around the distal humerus | OOO | OOO |
| **Tester performs test according to accepted guidelines** | YES | NO |
| Instructs the athlete to hold this position | OOO | OOO |
| Applies resistance downward in the direction of adduction | OOO | OOO |
| Holds resistance for 5 seconds | OOO | OOO |
| Performs assessment bilaterally | OOO | OOO |

The psychomotor skill was performed completely and in the appropriate order    **0  1  2  3  4  5**

The tester had control of the subject and the situation (showed confidence)    **0  1  2  3  4  5**

Method of performing the skill allowed the tester the ability to determine:
severity, proper progression, and the *fit* in the overall picture (Oral)    **0  1  2  3  4  5**

In order for a grade of *minimum standard* to be given, the total must be ≥11    **TOTAL =**

I_____I_____I
**Not Acceptable**        **Meets Minimum Standards**    **Exceeds Minimum Standards**

**L:** Laboratory/Classroom Testing
**C:** Clinical/Field Testing
**P:** Practicum Testing
**A:** Assessment/Mock Exam Testing
**S:** Self-Reporting

**Positive Finding:** Decreased ability to hold contraction
**Involved Structure:** Middle deltoid
**Special Considerations:** Elbow may be placed into an extended position for greater leverage
**Reference(s):** Kendall
**Supplies Needed:** Chair

# MANUAL MUSCLE TESTING
# (MMT-U-Test 29B)

Peer Review _____  Peer Review _____

Skill Acquisition: _____  Practice Opportunities: _____

*This problem allows you the opportunity to demonstrate a manual muscle test in a seated position for the **anterior deltoid** muscle. You have 2 minutes to complete this task.*

| Tester places athlete and limb in appropriate position | YES | NO |
|---|---|---|
| Seated | ○○○ | ○○○ |
| Shoulder abducted to 90 degrees (slight flexion) | ○○○ | ○○○ |
| Shoulder placed in slight external rotation | ○○○ | ○○○ |
| Elbow flexed to 90 degrees (palm facing downward) | ○○○ | ○○○ |
| **Tester placed in proper position** | **YES** | **NO** |
| Stands facing the athlete | ○○○ | ○○○ |
| Places one hand around the distal humerus | ○○○ | ○○○ |
| Applies counterpressure posteriorly to the shoulder girdle with the other hand | ○○○ | ○○○ |
| **Tester performs test according to accepted guidelines** | **YES** | **NO** |
| Instructs the athlete to hold this position | ○○○ | ○○○ |
| Applies resistance downward in the direction of adduction and slight extension | ○○○ | ○○○ |
| Holds resistance for 5 seconds | ○○○ | ○○○ |
| Performs assessment bilaterally | ○○○ | ○○○ |

| | |
|---|---|
| The psychomotor skill was performed completely and in the appropriate order | 0  1  2  3  4  5 |
| The tester had control of the subject and the situation (showed confidence) | 0  1  2  3  4  5 |
| Method of performing the skill allowed the tester the ability to determine: severity, proper progression, and the *fit* in the overall picture (Oral) | 0  1  2  3  4  5 |

In order for a grade of *minimum standard* to be given, the total must be ≥11        **TOTAL =**

I_____I_____I

**Not Acceptable          Meets Minimum Standards          Exceeds Minimum Standards**

**L:** Laboratory/Classroom Testing
**C:** Clinical/Field Testing
**P:** Practicum Testing
**A:** Assessment/Mock Exam Testing
**S:** Self-Reporting

**Positive Finding:** Decreased ability to hold contraction
**Involved Structure:** Anterior deltoid
**Special Considerations:** Elbow may be placed into an extended position for greater leverage
**Reference(s):** Kendall
**Supplies Needed:** Chair

## Manual Muscle Testing
# (MMT-U-Test 29C)

Peer Review _____ Peer Review _____

Skill Acquisition: _____    Practice Opportunities: _____

*This problem allows you the opportunity to demonstrate a manual muscle test in a seated position for the* **posterior deltoid** *muscle. You have 2 minutes to complete this task.*

| Tester places athlete and limb in appropriate position | YES | NO |
|---|---|---|
| Seated | ○○○ | ○○○ |
| Shoulder abducted to 90 degrees (slight extension) | ○○○ | ○○○ |
| Shoulder placed in slight medial rotation | ○○○ | ○○○ |
| Elbow flexed to 90 degrees (palm facing downward) | ○○○ | ○○○ |
| **Tester placed in proper position** | **YES** | **NO** |
| Stands behind the athlete | ○○○ | ○○○ |
| Places one hand on the posterolateral surface of the distal humerus | ○○○ | ○○○ |
| Applies counter pressure anteriorly to the shoulder girdle with the other hand | ○○○ | ○○○ |
| **Tester performs test according to accepted guidelines** | **YES** | **NO** |
| Instructs the athlete to hold his position | ○○○ | ○○○ |
| Applies resistance downward in the direction of adduction and slight flexion | ○○○ | ○○○ |
| Holds resistance for 5 seconds | ○○○ | ○○○ |
| Performs assessment bilaterally | ○○○ | ○○○ |

| | |
|---|---|
| The psychomotor skill was performed completely and in the appropriate order | 0  1  2  3  4  5 |
| The tester had control of the subject and the situation (showed confidence) | 0  1  2  3  4  5 |
| Method of performing the skill allowed the tester the ability to determine: severity, proper progression, and the *fit* in the overall picture (Oral) | 0  1  2  3  4  5 |

In order for a grade of *minimum standard* to be given, the total must be ≥11          **TOTAL =**

I_____I_____I

**Not Acceptable**          **Meets Minimum Standards**          **Exceeds Minimum Standards**

**L:** Laboratory/Classroom Testing
**C:** Clinical/Field Testing
**P:** Practicum Testing
**A:** Assessment/Mock Exam Testing
**S:** Self-Reporting

**Positive Finding:** Decreased ability to hold contraction
**Involved Structure:** Posterior deltoid
**Special Considerations:** Elbow may be placed into an extended position for greater leverage
**Reference(s):** Kendall
**Supplies Needed:** Chair

# Manual Muscle Testing
## (MMT-U-Test 30)

Peer Review _____   Peer Review _____

Skill Acquisition: _____   Practice Opportunities: _____

*This problem allows you the opportunity to demonstrate a manual muscle test for the* **teres major** *muscle. You have 2 minutes to complete this task.*

| Tester places athlete and limb in appropriate position | YES | NO |
|---|---|---|
| Prone (head facing the test arm) | ○○○ | ○○○ |
| Shoulder extended, adducted, and medially rotated (hand on the posterior iliac crest) | ○○○ | ○○○ |
| **Tester placed in proper position** | **YES** | **NO** |
| Stands on the side of the test arm | ○○○ | ○○○ |
| Places hand on the distal humerus just above the elbow | ○○○ | ○○○ |
| **Tester performs test according to accepted guidelines** | **YES** | **NO** |
| Instructs the athlete to hold this position | ○○○ | ○○○ |
| Applies resistance downward in the direction of abduction and flexion | ○○○ | ○○○ |
| Holds resistance for 5 seconds | ○○○ | ○○○ |
| Performs assessment bilaterally | ○○○ | ○○○ |

| | |
|---|---|
| The psychomotor skill was performed completely and in the appropriate order | 0  1  2  3  4  5 |
| The tester had control of the subject and the situation (showed confidence) | 0  1  2  3  4  5 |
| Method of performing the skill allowed the tester the ability to determine: severity, proper progression, and the *fit* in the overall picture (Oral) | 0  1  2  3  4  5 |

In order for a grade of *minimum standard* to be given, the total must be ≥11          TOTAL = 

I_____I_____I

**Not Acceptable**          **Meets Minimum Standards**          **Exceeds Minimum Standards**

**L:** Laboratory/Classroom Testing
**C:** Clinical/Field Testing
**P:** Practicum Testing
**A:** Assessment/Mock Exam Testing
**S:** Self-Reporting

**Positive Finding:** Decreased ability to hold contraction
**Involved Structure:** Teres major
**Special Considerations:** NA
**Reference(s):** Kendall
**Supplies Needed:** Table

## MANUAL MUSCLE TESTING
# (MMT-U-Test 31)

Peer Review _____ Peer Review _____

Skill Acquisition: _____    Practice Opportunities: _____

*This problem allows you the opportunity to demonstrate a manual muscle test for the* **coracobrachialis** *muscle. You have 2 minutes to complete this task.*

| Tester places athlete and limb in appropriate position | YES | NO |
|---|---|---|
| Seated or supine | ООО | ООО |
| Shoulder flexed to approximately 75 degrees | ООО | ООО |
| Shoulder placed in lateral rotation | ООО | ООО |
| Elbow flexed to 90 degrees and supinated | ООО | ООО |
| **Tester placed in proper position** | **YES** | **NO** |
| Stands to the side of the athlete | ООО | ООО |
| Places one hand on the anteromedial surface of the distal humerus | ООО | ООО |
| **Tester performs test according to accepted guidelines** | **YES** | **NO** |
| Instructs the athlete to hold this position | ООО | ООО |
| Applies resistance downward in the direction of extension | ООО | ООО |
| Holds resistance for 5 seconds | ООО | ООО |
| Performs assessment bilaterally | ОО | ОО |

The psychomotor skill was performed completely and in the appropriate order    **0 1 2 3 4 5**

The tester had control of the subject and the situation (showed confidence)    **0 1 2 3 4 5**

Method of performing the skill allowed the tester the ability to determine:
severity, proper progression, and the *fit* in the overall picture (Oral)    **0 1 2 3 4 5**

In order for a grade of *minimum standard* to be given, the total must be ≥11    **TOTAL =**

I_____I_____I

**Not Acceptable**        **Meets Minimum Standards**    **Exceeds Minimum Standards**

**L:** Laboratory/Classroom Testing
**C:** Clinical/Field Testing
**P:** Practicum Testing
**A:** Assessment/Mock Exam Testing
**S:** Self-Reporting

**Positive Finding:** Decreased ability to hold contraction
**Involved Structure:** Coracobrachialis
**Special Considerations:** NA
**Reference(s):** Kendall
**Supplies Needed:** Chair

# MANUAL MUSCLE TESTING
## (MMT-U-Test 32)

Peer Review _____ Peer Review _____

Skill Acquisition: _____ Practice Opportunities: _____

*This problem allows you the opportunity to demonstrate a manual muscle test in a prone position for the **infraspinatus** muscle. You have 2 minutes to complete this task.*

| Tester places athlete and limb in appropriate position | YES | NO |
|---|---|---|
| Prone (head facing away from the test arm) | ○○○ | ○○○ |
| Shoulder flexed to 90 degrees and externally rotated to approximately 90 degrees | ○○○ | ○○○ |
| Elbow flexed to 90 degrees (elbow off the edge of table) | ○○○ | ○○○ |
| **Tester placed in proper position** | **YES** | **NO** |
| Stands on the side of the test arm | ○○○ | ○○○ |
| Places one hand under the arm near the elbow to stabilize the humerus | ○○○ | ○○○ |
| Places the other hand on the distal forearm | ○○○ | ○○○ |
| **Tester performs test according to accepted guidelines** | **YES** | **NO** |
| Instructs the athlete to hold this position | ○○○ | ○○○ |
| Applies resistance downward in the direction of medial rotation | ○○○ | ○○○ |
| Holds resistance for 5 seconds | ○○○ | ○○○ |
| Performs assessment bilaterally | ○○○ | ○○○ |

| | |
|---|---|
| The psychomotor skill was performed completely and in the appropriate order | 0 1 2 3 4 5 |
| The tester had control of the subject and the situation (showed confidence) | 0 1 2 3 4 5 |
| Method of performing the skill allowed the tester the ability to determine: severity, proper progression, and the *fit* in the overall picture (Oral) | 0 1 2 3 4 5 |

In order for a grade of *minimum standard* to be given, the total must be ≥11          **TOTAL =**

I_____I_____I
**Not Acceptable**     **Meets Minimum Standards**   **Exceeds Minimum Standards**

**L:** Laboratory/Classroom Testing
**C:** Clinical/Field Testing
**P:** Practicum Testing
**A:** Assessment/Mock Exam Testing
**S:** Self-Reporting

**Positive Finding:** Decreased ability to hold contraction
**Involved Structure:** Infraspinatus
**Special Considerations:** Same as for teres minor
**Reference(s):** Kendall
**Supplies Needed:** Table

## Manual Muscle Testing
# (MMT-U-Test 33)

Peer Review _____ Peer Review _____

Skill Acquisition: _____     Practice Opportunities: _____

*This problem allows you the opportunity to demonstrate a manual muscle test in a prone position for the* **teres minor** *muscle. You have 2 minutes to complete this task.*

| Tester places athlete and limb in appropriate position | YES | NO |
|---|---|---|
| Prone (head facing away from the test arm) | OOO | OOO |
| Shoulder flexed to 90 degrees and externally rotated to approximately 90 degrees | OOO | OOO |
| Elbow flexed to 90 degrees (elbow off the edge of the table) | OOO | OOO |
| **Tester placed in proper position** | **YES** | **NO** |
| Stands on the side of the test arm | OOO | OOO |
| Places one hand under the arm near the elbow to stabilize the humerus | OOO | OOO |
| Places the other hand on the distal forearm | OOO | OOO |
| **Tester performs test according to accepted guidelines** | **YES** | **NO** |
| Instructs the athlete to hold this position | OOO | OOO |
| Applies resistance downward in the direction of medial rotation | OOO | OOO |
| Holds resistance for 5 seconds | OOO | OOO |
| Performs assessment bilaterally | OOO | OOO |

The psychomotor skill was performed completely and in the appropriate order       0 1 2 3 4 5

The tester had control of the subject and the situation (showed confidence)       0 1 2 3 4 5

Method of performing the skill allowed the tester the ability to determine:
severity, proper progression, and the *fit* in the overall picture (Oral)       0 1 2 3 4 5

In order for a grade of *minimum standard* to be given, the total must be ≥11       **TOTAL =**

I_____I_____I

**Not Acceptable**       **Meets Minimum Standards**       **Exceeds Minimum Standards**

**L:** Laboratory/Classroom Testing
**C:** Clinical/Field Testing
**P:** Practicum Testing
**A:** Assessment/Mock Exam Testing
**S:** Self-Reporting

**Positive Finding:** Decreased ability to hold contraction
**Involved Structure:** Teres minor
**Special Considerations:** Same as for Infraspinatus
**Reference(s):** Kendall
**Supplies Needed:** Table

# MANUAL MUSCLE TESTING
# (MMT-U-Test 34)

Peer Review _____ Peer Review _____

Skill Acquisition: _____    Practice Opportunities: _____

*This problem allows you the opportunity to demonstrate a manual muscle test in a prone position for the **subscapularis** muscle. You have 2 minutes to complete this task.*

| Tester places athlete and limb in appropriate position | YES | NO |
|---|---|---|
| Prone (head facing away from the test arm) | OOO | OOO |
| Shoulder flexed to 90 degrees and internally rotated to approximately 45 degrees | OOO | OOO |
| Elbow flexed to 90 degrees (elbow off the edge of the table) | OOO | OOO |
| **Tester placed in proper position** | YES | NO |
| Stands on the side of the test arm | OOO | OOO |
| Places one hand under the arm near the elbow to stabilize the humerus | OOO | OOO |
| Places other hand at the distal forearm | OOO | OOO |
| **Tester performs test according to accepted guidelines** | YES | NO |
| Instructs the athlete to hold this position | OOO | OOO |
| Applies resistance downward in the direction of lateral rotation | OOO | OOO |
| Holds resistance for 5 seconds | OOO | OOO |
| Performs assessment bilaterally | OOO | OOO |

| | |
|---|---|
| The psychomotor skill was performed completely and in the appropriate order | 0 1 2 3 4 5 |
| The tester had control of the subject and the situation (showed confidence) | 0 1 2 3 4 5 |
| Method of performing the skill allowed the tester the ability to determine: severity, proper progression, and the *fit* in the overall picture (Oral) | 0 1 2 3 4 5 |

In order for a grade of *minimum standard* to be given, the total must be ≥11        TOTAL =

I_____I_____I
Not Acceptable    Meets Minimum Standards    Exceeds Minimum Standards

**L:** Laboratory/Classroom Testing
**C:** Clinical/Field Testing
**P:** Practicum Testing
**A:** Assessment/Mock Exam Testing
**S:** Self-Reporting

**Positive Finding:** Decreased ability to hold contraction
**Involved Structure:** Subscapularis
**Special Considerations:** N/A
**Reference(s):** Kendall
**Supplies Needed:** Table

## Manual Muscle Testing
# (MMT-L-Test 1)

Peer Review _____ Peer Review _____

Skill Acquisition: _____     Practice Opportunities: _____

*Please demonstrate a manual muscle test for the* **tibialis anterior** *muscle. You have 2 minutes to complete this task response.*

| Tester places athlete and limb in appropriate position | YES | NO |
|---|---|---|
| Supine or seated | ○○○ | ○○○ |
| **Tester placed in proper position** | **YES** | **NO** |
| Supports the leg just above the ankle joint (stabilizes) | ○○○ | ○○○ |
| **Tester performs test according to accepted guidelines** | **YES** | **NO** |
| Has athlete actively dorsiflex the ankle joint and invert the foot (without extension of the great toe) | ○○○ | ○○○ |
| Applies resistance to the medial side, dorsal surface of the foot (direction of plantar flexion of the ankle joint and eversion of the foot) | ○○○ | ○○○ |
| Holds resistance for 5 seconds | ○○○ | ○○○ |
| Performs assessment bilaterally | ○○○ | ○○○ |

| | |
|---|---|
| The psychomotor skill was performed completely and in the appropriate order | 0 1 2 3 4 5 |
| The tester had control of the subject and the situation (showed confidence) | 0 1 2 3 4 5 |
| Method of performing the skill allowed the tester the ability to determine: severity, proper progression, and the *fit* in the overall picture (Oral) | 0 1 2 3 4 5 |

In order for a grade of *minimum standard* to be given, the total must be ≥11          **TOTAL =**

I_____I_____I
**Not Acceptable**          **Meets Minimum Standards**          **Exceeds Minimum Standards**

**L:** Laboratory/Classroom Testing
**C:** Clinical/Field Testing
**P:** Practicum Testing
**A:** Assessment/Mock Exam Testing
**S:** Self-Reporting

**Positive Finding:** Decreased ability to hold contraction; may be seen as a partial "drop foot"
**Involved Structure:** Tibialis anterior
**Special Considerations:** N/A
**Reference(s):** Kendall et al
**Supplies Needed:** Table

# MANUAL MUSCLE TESTING
## (MMT-L-Test 2)

Peer Review _____ Peer Review _____

Skill Acquisition: _____    Practice Opportunities: _____

*Please demonstrate a manual muscle test for the* **flexor hallucis longus** *muscle. You have 2 minutes to complete this task response.*

| | YES | NO |
|---|---|---|
| **Tester places athlete and limb in appropriate position** | YES | NO |
| Supine or seated | ○○○ | ○○○ |
| **Tester placed in proper position** | YES | NO |
| Stabilizes the metatarsophalangeal joint in neutral position (0 degrees) | ○○○ | ○○○ |
| Maintains the ankle joint approximately midway between dorsal and plantar flexion (25 degrees) | ○○○ | ○○○ |
| **Tester performs test according to accepted guidelines** | YES | NO |
| Has athlete actively flex the interphalangeal joint of the great toe | ○○○ | ○○○ |
| Applies resistance to the plantar surface of the distal phalanx in the direction of extension | ○○○ | ○○○ |
| Holds resistance for 5 seconds | ○○○ | ○○○ |
| Performs assessment bilaterally | ○○○ | ○○○ |

| | |
|---|---|
| The psychomotor skill was performed completely and in the appropriate order | 0  1  2  3  4  5 |
| The tester had control of the subject and the situation (showed confidence) | 0  1  2  3  4  5 |
| Method of performing the skill allowed the tester the ability to determine: severity, proper progression, and the *fit* in the overall picture (Oral) | 0  1  2  3  4  5 |

In order for a grade of *minimum standard* to be given, the total must be ≥11    **TOTAL =**

I_____I_____I

**Not Acceptable**        **Meets Minimum Standards**    **Exceeds Minimum Standards**

**L:** Laboratory/Classroom Testing
**C:** Clinical/Field Testing
**P:** Practicum Testing
**A:** Assessment/Mock Exam Testing
**S:** Self-Reporting

**Positive Finding:** Decreased ability to hold contraction
**Involved Structure:** Flexor hallucis longus
**Special Considerations:** N/A
**Reference(s):** Kendall et al
**Supplies Needed:** Table

# MANUAL MUSCLE TESTING
## (MMT-L-Test 3)

Peer Review _____ Peer Review _____

Skill Acquisition: _____    Practice Opportunities: _____

*Please demonstrate a manual muscle test for the* **soleus** *muscle. You have 2 minutes to complete this task response.*

| Tester places athlete and limb in appropriate position | YES | NO |
|---|---|---|
| Prone | ○○○ | ○○○ |
| Knee flexed to 90 degrees | ○○○ | ○○○ |
| **Tester placed in proper position** | **YES** | **NO** |
| Supports the leg proximal to the ankle | ○○○ | ○○○ |
| Places the other hand on the calcaneus | ○○○ | ○○○ |
| **Tester performs test according to accepted guidelines** | **YES** | **NO** |
| Has the athlete actively plantar flex the ankle joint (without inversion and/or eversion) | ○○○ | ○○○ |
| Applies resistance to the calcaneus, pulling the heel in the direction of dorsiflexion | ○○○ | ○○○ |
| Holds resistance for 5 seconds | ○○○ | ○○○ |
| Performs assessment bilaterally | ○○○ | ○○○ |

| | |
|---|---|
| The psychomotor skill was performed completely and in the appropriate order | 0  1  2  3  4  5 |
| The tester had control of the subject and the situation (showed confidence) | 0  1  2  3  4  5 |
| Method of performing the skill allowed the tester the ability to determine: severity, proper progression, and the *fit* in the overall picture (Oral) | 0  1  2  3  4  5 |

In order for a grade of *minimum standard* to be given, the total must be ≥11        **TOTAL =**

I_____I_____I
**Not Acceptable**        **Meets Minimum Standards**    **Exceeds Minimum Standards**

**L:** Laboratory/Classroom Testing
**C:** Clinical/Field Testing
**P:** Practicum Testing
**A:** Assessment/Mock Exam Testing
**S:** Self-Reporting

**Positive Finding:** Inability to point the toes
**Involved Structure:** Soleus
**Special Considerations:** N/A
**Reference(s):** Kendall et al
**Supplies Needed:** Table

# MANUAL MUSCLE TESTING
## (MMT-L-Test 4)

Peer Review _____ Peer Review _____

Skill Acquisition: _____     Practice Opportunities: _____

*Please demonstrate a manual muscle test for the* **semitendinosus/semimembranosus** *muscle. You have 2 minutes to complete this task response.*

| | YES | NO |
|---|---|---|
| **Tester places athlete and limb in appropriate position** | | |
| Prone | ○○○ | ○○○ |
| **Tester placed in proper position** | YES | NO |
| Holds the thigh firmly against the table | ○○○ | ○○○ |
| Places the other hand against the distal tibia/fibula (posterior aspect) | ○○○ | ○○○ |
| **Tester performs test according to accepted guidelines** | YES | NO |
| Has athlete actively flex the knee between 50 and 70 degrees | ○○○ | ○○○ |
| Thigh and leg placed in medial rotation | ○○○ | ○○○ |
| Applies resistance to the leg proximal to the ankle, in the direction of knee extension | ○○○ | ○○○ |
| Holds resistance for 5 seconds | ○○○ | ○○○ |
| Performs assessment bilaterally | ○○○ | ○○○ |

| | |
|---|---|
| The psychomotor skill was performed completely and in the appropriate order | **0  1  2  3  4  5** |
| The tester had control of the subject and the situation (showed confidence) | **0  1  2  3  4  5** |
| Method of performing the skill allowed the tester the ability to determine: severity, proper progression, and the *fit* in the overall picture (Oral) | **0  1  2  3  4  5** |

In order for a grade of *minimum standard* to be given, the total must be ≥11     **TOTAL =**

I_____I_____I

**Not Acceptable**          **Meets Minimum Standards**          **Exceeds Minimum Standards**

**L:** Laboratory/Classroom Testing
**C:** Clinical/Field Testing
**P:** Practicum Testing
**A:** Assessment/Mock Exam Testing
**S:** Self-Reporting

**Positive Finding:** Decreased ability to hold contraction
**Involved Structure:** Semitendinosus, semimembranosus
**Special Considerations:** N/A
**Reference(s):** Kendall et al
**Supplies Needed:** Table

# MANUAL MUSCLE TESTING
# (MMT-L-Test 5)

Peer Review _____ Peer Review _____

Skill Acquisition: _____    Practice Opportunities: _____

*Please demonstrate a manual muscle test for the **biceps femoris** muscle. You have 2 minutes to complete this task response.*

| Tester places athlete and limb in appropriate position | YES | NO |
|---|---|---|
| Prone | ○○○ | ○○○ |
| **Tester placed in proper position** | **YES** | **NO** |
| Holds the thigh firmly against the table | ○○○ | ○○○ |
| Places the other hand against the distal tibia/fibula (posterior aspect) | ○○○ | ○○○ |
| **Tester performs test according to accepted guidelines** | **YES** | **NO** |
| Has athlete actively flex the knee between 50 and 70 degrees | ○○○ | ○○○ |
| Thigh and leg are placed in lateral rotation | ○○○ | ○○○ |
| Applies resistance to] the leg proximal to the ankle, in the direction of knee extension | ○○○ | ○○○ |
| Holds resistance for 5 seconds | ○○○ | ○○○ |
| Performs assessment bilaterally | ○○○ | ○○○ |

The psychomotor skill was performed completely and in the appropriate order     0  1  2  3  4  5

The tester had control of the subject and the situation (showed confidence)     0  1  2  3  4  5

Method of performing the skill allowed the tester the ability to determine:
severity, proper progression, and the *fit* in the overall picture (Oral)     0  1  2  3  4  5

In order for a grade of *minimum standard* to be given, the total must be ≥11     TOTAL =

I_____I_____I
**Not Acceptable**        **Meets Minimum Standards**    **Exceeds Minimum Standards**

**L:** Laboratory/Classroom Testing
**C:** Clinical/Field Testing
**P:** Practicum Testing
**A:** Assessment/Mock Exam Testing
**S:** Self-Reporting

**Positive Finding:** Decreased ability to hold contraction
**Involved Structure:** Biceps femoris
**Special Considerations:** N/A
**Reference(s):** Kendall et al
**Supplies Needed:** Table

# MANUAL MUSCLE TESTING
# (MMT-L-Test 6)

Peer Review _____ Peer Review _____

Skill Acquisition: _____    Practice Opportunities: _____

*Please demonstrate a manual muscle test for the* **quadriceps femoris** *muscle. You have 2 minutes to complete this task response.*

| Tester places athlete and limb in appropriate position | YES | NO |
|---|---|---|
| Seated | ○○○ | ○○○ |
| Knees over the side of the table (holding onto the table) | ○○○ | ○○○ |
| **Tester placed in proper position** | **YES** | **NO** |
| Holds the thigh firmly down on the table | ○○○ | ○○○ |
| Places the other hand against the distal tibia/fibula (anterior aspect) | ○○○ | ○○○ |
| **Tester performs test according to accepted guidelines** | **YES** | **NO** |
| Has the athlete actively extend the knee joint (without rotation of the thigh) | ○○○ | ○○○ |
| Applies resistance to the leg above the ankle, in the direction of flexion | ○○○ | ○○○ |
| Holds resistance for 5 seconds | ○○○ | ○○○ |
| Performs assessment bilaterally | ○○○ | ○○○ |

The psychomotor skill was performed completely and in the appropriate order    **0  1  2  3  4  5**

The tester had control of the subject and the situation (showed confidence)    **0  1  2  3  4  5**

Method of performing the skill allowed the tester the ability to determine:
severity, proper progression, and the *fit* in the overall picture (Oral)    **0  1  2  3  4  5**

In order for a grade of *minimum standard* to be given, the total must be ≥11    **TOTAL =**

I_____I_____I

**Not Acceptable**      **Meets Minimum Standards**    **Exceeds Minimum Standards**

**Positive Finding:** Decreased ability to hold contraction

**L:** Laboratory/Classroom Testing
**C:** Clinical/Field Testing
**P:** Practicum Testing
**A:** Assessment/Mock Exam Testing
**S:** Self-Reporting

**Involved Structure:** Rectus femoris, vastus lateralis, vastus intermedius, vastus medialis
**Special Considerations:** N/A
**Reference(s):** Kendall et al
**Supplies Needed:** Table

# MANUAL MUSCLE TESTING
## (MMT-L-Test 7)

Peer Review _____ Peer Review _____

Skill Acquisition: _____    Practice Opportunities: _____

*Please demonstrate a manual muscle test for the **gastrocnemius** muscle. You have 2 minutes to complete this task response.*

| Tester places athlete and limb in appropriate position | YES | NO |
|---|---|---|
| Prone | ○○○ | ○○○ |
| Knee extended with foot over the edge of the table | ○○○ | ○○○ |
| **Tester placed in proper position** | **YES** | **NO** |
| *No fixation/stabilization needed* | | |
| Places one hand on the calcaneus (heel) | ○○○ | ○○○ |
| Places other hand on the plantar surface of the forefoot | ○○○ | ○○○ |
| **Tester performs test according to accepted guidelines** | **YES** | **NO** |
| Had athlete actively plantar flex the foot | ○○○ | ○○○ |
| Applies resistance to the forefoot and calcaneus | ○○○ | ○○○ |
| Holds resistance for 5 seconds | ○○○ | ○○○ |
| Performs assessment bilaterally | ○○○ | ○○○ |

The psychomotor skill was performed completely and in the appropriate order    0 1 2 3 4 5

The tester had control of the subject and the situation (showed confidence)    0 1 2 3 4 5

Method of performing the skill allowed the tester the ability to determine:
severity, proper progression, and the *fit* in the overall picture (Oral)    0 1 2 3 4 5

In order for a grade of *minimum standard* to be given, the total must be ≥11    TOTAL =

I_____I_____I
**Not Acceptable**        **Meets Minimum Standards**    **Exceeds Minimum Standards**

**L:** Laboratory/Classroom Testing
**C:** Clinical/Field Testing
**P:** Practicum Testing
**A:** Assessment/Mock Exam Testing
**S:** Self-Reporting

**Positive Finding:** Decreased ability to hold contraction
**Involved Structure:** Gastrocnemius, plantaris
**Special Considerations:** May be done standing on one leg (rise on toes, heel off the ground)
**Reference(s):** Kendall et al
**Supplies Needed:** Table

## MANUAL MUSCLE TESTING
# (MMT-L-Test 8)

Peer Review _____  Peer Review _____

Skill Acquisition: _____    Practice Opportunities: _____

*Please demonstrate a manual muscle test for the* **iliopsoas (with emphasis on the psoas minor)** *muscle. You have 2 minutes to complete this task response.*

| | YES | NO |
|---|---|---|
| **Tester places athlete and limb in appropriate position** | YES | NO |
| Supine | OOO | OOO |
| **Tester placed in proper position** | YES | NO |
| Stabilizes the opposite iliac crest | OOO | OOO |
| Places the other hand on the distal tibia/fibula | OOO | OOO |
| **Tester performs test according to accepted guidelines** | YES | NO |
| Has the athlete actively flex the hip (slight abduction and lateral rotation) | OOO | OOO |
| Applies resistance to the anteromedial aspect of the leg (direction of extension and slight abduction) | OOO | OOO |
| Holds resistance for 5 seconds | OOO | OOO |
| Performs assessment bilaterally | OOO | OOO |

The psychomotor skill was performed completely and in the appropriate order          0  1  2  3  4  5

The tester had control of the subject and the situation (showed confidence)          0  1  2  3  4  5

Method of performing the skill allowed the tester the ability to determine: severity, proper progression, and the *fit* in the overall picture (Oral)          0  1  2  3  4  5

In order for a grade of *minimum standard* to be given, the total must be ≥11          TOTAL =

I_____I_____I
**Not Acceptable**          **Meets Minimum Standards**          **Exceeds Minimum Standards**

**L:** Laboratory/Classroom Testing
**C:** Clinical/Field Testing
**P:** Practicum Testing
**A:** Assessment/Mock Exam Testing
**S:** Self-Reporting

**Positive Finding:** Decreased ability to hold contraction
**Involved Structure:** Iliopsoas, psoas minor
**Special Considerations:** Seated hip flexion (knee flexed) isolates the iliopsoas
**Reference(s):** Kendall et al
**Supplies Needed:** Table

## MANUAL MUSCLE TESTING
# (MMT-L-Test 9)

Peer Review _____ Peer Review _____

Skill Acquisition: _____     Practice Opportunities: _____

*Please demonstrate a manual muscle test for the **tensor fasciae latae** muscle. You have 2 minutes to complete this task response.*

| Tester places athlete and limb in appropriate position | YES | NO |
|---|---|---|
| Supine | ○○○ | ○○○ |
| **Tester placed in proper position** | **YES** | **NO** |
| Stabilizes the opposite iliac crest (if needed) | ○○○ | ○○○ |
| Places the other hand on the distal tibia/fibula | ○○○ | ○○○ |
| **Tester performs test according to accepted guidelines** | **YES** | **NO** |
| Has athlete actively abduct/flex hip (medially rotate the hip with the knee extended) | ○○○ | ○○○ |
| Applies resistance to the leg in the direction of extension and adduction | ○○○ | ○○○ |
| Holds resistance for 5 seconds | ○○○ | ○○○ |
| Performs assessment bilaterally | ○○○ | ○○○ |

The psychomotor skill was performed completely and in the appropriate order     0 1 2 3 4 5

The tester had control of the subject and the situation (showed confidence)     0 1 2 3 4 5

Method of performing the skill allowed the tester the ability to determine:
severity, proper progression, and the *fit* in the overall picture (Oral)     0 1 2 3 4 5

In order for a grade of *minimum standard* to be given, the total must be ≥11     **TOTAL =**

I_____I_____I

**Not Acceptable**          **Meets Minimum Standards**          **Exceeds Minimum Standards**

**L:** Laboratory/Classroom Testing
**C:** Clinical/Field Testing
**P:** Practicum Testing
**A:** Assessment/Mock Exam Testing
**S:** Self-Reporting

**Positive Finding:** Decreased ability to hold contraction
**Involved Structure:** Tensor fasciae latae
**Special Considerations:** N/A
**Reference(s):** Kendall et al
**Supplies Needed:** Table

## MANUAL MUSCLE TESTING
# (MMT-L-Test 10)

Peer Review _____ Peer Review _____

Skill Acquisition: _____    Practice Opportunities: _____

*Please demonstrate a manual muscle test for the* **sartorius** *muscle. You have 2 minutes to complete this task response.*

| Tester places athlete and limb in appropriate position | YES | NO |
|---|---|---|
| Supine | ○○○ | ○○○ |
| Places thigh in lateral rotation, abduction, and flexion | ○○○ | ○○○ |
| Places knee in a flexed position | ○○○ | ○○○ |
| **Tester placed in proper position** | **YES** | **NO** |
| Stands in front and to the side of the athlete | ○○○ | ○○○ |
| Places hand on the anterolateral surface of the lower thigh | ○○○ | ○○○ |
| Places other hand at the distal end of the tibia/fibula | ○○○ | ○○○ |
| **Tester performs test according to accepted guidelines** | **YES** | **NO** |
| Applies resistance to hip flexion/abduction and lateral rotation | ○○○ | ○○○ |
| Applies resistance to knee flexion | ○○○ | ○○○ |
| Holds resistance for 5 seconds | ○○○ | ○○○ |
| Performs assessment bilaterally | ○○○ | ○○○ |

The psychomotor skill was performed completely and in the appropriate order    **0 1 2 3 4 5**

The tester had control of the subject and the situation (showed confidence)    **0 1 2 3 4 5**

Method of performing the skill allowed the tester the ability to determine:
severity, proper progression, and the *fit* in the overall picture (Oral)    **0 1 2 3 4 5**

In order for a grade of *minimum standard* to be given, the total must be ≥11    **TOTAL =**

I_____I_____I
**Not Acceptable**    **Meets Minimum Standards**    **Exceeds Minimum Standards**

**L:** Laboratory/Classroom Testing
**C:** Clinical/Field Testing
**P:** Practicum Testing
**A:** Assessment/Mock Exam Testing
**S:** Self-Reporting

**Positive Finding:** Decreased ability to hold contraction
**Involved Structure:** Sartorius
**Special Considerations:** Must resist multiple actions
**Reference(s):** Kendall
**Supplies Needed:** Table

## MANUAL MUSCLE TESTING
# (MMT-L-Test 11)

*Please demonstrate a manual muscle test for the* **gluteus medius** *muscle. You have 2 minutes to complete this task response.*

| Tester places athlete and limb in appropriate position | YES | NO |
|---|---|---|
| Side lying (bottom leg flexed at the hip and knee) | ooo | ooo |
| Pelvis slightly rotated forward | ooo | ooo |
| **Tester placed in proper position** | **YES** | **NO** |
| Stands behind the athlete halfway between the hips and knees | ooo | ooo |
| Stabilizes the pelvis (iliac crest) with one hand | ooo | ooo |
| Places other hand on the distal tibia/fibula | ooo | ooo |
| **Tester performs test according to accepted guidelines** | **YES** | **NO** |
| Has athlete actively abduct the hip (slight extension and external rotation) | ooo | ooo |
| Applies resistance against the lower leg in the direction of adduction and flexion | ooo | ooo |
| Holds resistance for 5 seconds | ooo | ooo |
| Performs assessment bilaterally | ooo | ooo |

The psychomotor skill was performed completely and in the appropriate order    **0  1  2  3  4  5**

The tester had control of the subject and the situation (showed confidence)    **0  1  2  3  4  5**

Method of performing the skill allowed the tester the ability to determine: severity, proper progression, and the *fit* in the overall picture (Oral)    **0  1  2  3  4  5**

In order for a grade of *minimum standard* to be given, the total must be ≥11    **TOTAL =**

I_____I_____I

**Not Acceptable**        **Meets Minimum Standards**    **Exceeds Minimum Standards**

**L:** Laboratory/Classroom Testing
**C:** Clinical/Field Testing
**P:** Practicum Testing
**A:** Assessment/Mock Exam Testing
**S:** Self-Reporting

**Positive Finding:** Decreased ability to hold contraction
**Involved Structure:** Gluteus medius
**Special Considerations:** N/A
**Reference(s):** Kendall et al
**Supplies Needed:** Table

# MANUAL MUSCLE TESTING
## (MMT-L-Test 12)

Peer Review _____ Peer Review _____

Skill Acquisition: _____     Practice Opportunities: _____

*Please demonstrate a manual muscle test for the* **gluteus minimus** *muscle. You have 2 minutes to complete this task response.*

| Tester places athlete and limb in appropriate position | YES | NO |
|---|---|---|
| Side lying (bottom leg flexed at the hip and knee) | ○○○ | ○○○ |
| **Tester placed in proper position** | **YES** | **NO** |
| Stands behind the athlete halfway between the hips and knees | ○○○ | ○○○ |
| Stabilizes the pelvis (iliac crest) with one hand | ○○○ | ○○○ |
| Places the other hand on the distal tibia/fibula | ○○○ | ○○○ |
| **Tester performs test according to accepted guidelines** | **YES** | **NO** |
| Has athlete actively abduct hip (neutral, no external rotation) | ○○○ | ○○○ |
| Applies resistance to the lower leg in the direction of adduction and extension | ○○○ | ○○○ |
| Holds resistance for 5 seconds | ○○○ | ○○○ |
| Performs assessment bilaterally | ○○○ | ○○○ |

The psychomotor skill was performed completely and in the appropriate order    0 1 2 3 4 5

The tester had control of the subject and the situation (showed confidence)    0 1 2 3 4 5

Method of performing the skill allowed the tester the ability to determine:
severity, proper progression, and the *fit* in the overall picture (Oral)    0 1 2 3 4 5

In order for a grade of *minimum standard* to be given, the total must be ≥11    **TOTAL =**

I_____I_____I

**Not Acceptable**     **Meets Minimum Standards**     **Exceeds Minimum Standards**

**L:** Laboratory/Classroom Testing
**C:** Clinical/Field Testing
**P:** Practicum Testing
**A:** Assessment/Mock Exam Testing
**S:** Self-Reporting

**Positive Finding:** Decreased ability to hold con-
traction
**Involved Structure:** Gluteus minimus
**Special Considerations:** N/A
**Reference(s):** Kendall et al
**Supplies Needed:** Table

# MANUAL MUSCLE TESTING
## (MMT-L-Test 13)

Peer Review _____ Peer Review _____

Skill Acquisition: _____    Practice Opportunities: _____

*Please demonstrate a manual muscle test for the* **gluteus maximus** *muscle. You have 2 minutes to complete this task response.*

| Tester places athlete and limb in appropriate position | YES | NO |
|---|---|---|
| Prone | ○○○ | ○○○ |
| Knee flexed at or greater than 90 degrees | ○○○ | ○○○ |
| **Tester placed in proper position** | **YES** | **NO** |
| Stands near the affected side | ○○○ | ○○○ |
| Stabilizes the pelvis with one hand | ○○○ | ○○○ |
| Places the other hand on the posterior aspect of the thigh (distal hamstrings) | ○○○ | ○○○ |
| **Tester performs test according to accepted guidelines** | **YES** | **NO** |
| Has athlete actively extend the hip | ○○○ | ○○○ |
| Applies resistance to the leg in the direction of flexion | ○○○ | ○○○ |
| Holds resistance for 5 seconds | ○○○ | ○○○ |
| Performs assessment bilaterally | ○○○ | ○○○ |

The psychomotor skill was performed completely and in the appropriate order    **0  1  2  3  4  5**

The tester had control of the subject and the situation (showed confidence)    **0  1  2  3  4  5**

Method of performing the skill allowed the tester the ability to determine:
severity, proper progression, and the *fit* in the overall picture (Oral)    **0  1  2  3  4  5**

In order for a grade of *minimum standard* to be given, the total must be ≥11    **TOTAL =**

I_____I_____I
**Not Acceptable**         **Meets Minimum Standards**    **Exceeds Minimum Standards**

**L:** Laboratory/Classroom Testing
**C:** Clinical/Field Testing
**P:** Practicum Testing
**A:** Assessment/Mock Exam Testing
**S:** Self-Reporting

**Positive Finding:** Decreased ability to hold contraction
**Involved Structure:** Gluteus maximus
**Special Considerations:** N/A
**Reference(s):** Kendall et al
**Supplies Needed:** Table

## MANUAL MUSCLE TESTING
# (MMT-L-Test 14)

Peer Review _____ Peer Review _____

Skill Acquisition: _____    Practice Opportunities: _____

*Please demonstrate a manual muscle test for the* **peroneus longus** *muscle. You have 2 minutes to complete this task response.*

| Tester places athlete and limb in appropriate position | YES | NO |
|---|---|---|
| Supine (lower leg internally rotated) or side lying | ○○○ | ○○○ |
| Places foot in inverted position | ○○○ | ○○○ |
| **Tester placed in proper position** | **YES** | **NO** |
| Stands at the end of the table facing the athlete | ○○○ | ○○○ |
| Stabilizes the lower leg with one hand | ○○○ | ○○○ |
| Places the other hand on the lateral aspect of the metatarsals | ○○○ | ○○○ |
| **Tester performs test according to accepted guidelines** | **YES** | **NO** |
| Has athlete actively evert the foot | ○○○ | ○○○ |
| Applies resistance to the foot in the direction of inversion and dorsiflexion | ○○○ | ○○○ |
| Holds resistance for 5 seconds | ○○○ | ○○○ |
| Performs assessment bilaterally | ○○○ | ○○○ |

The psychomotor skill was performed completely and in the appropriate order     0  1  2  3  4  5

The tester had control of the subject and the situation (showed confidence)     0  1  2  3  4  5

Method of performing the skill allowed the tester the ability to determine:
severity, proper progression, and the *fit* in the overall picture (Oral)     0  1  2  3  4  5

In order for a grade of *minimum standard* to be given, the total must be ≥11          **TOTAL =**

I_____I_____I
**Not Acceptable**          **Meets Minimum Standards**     **Exceeds Minimum Standards**

**L:** Laboratory/Classroom Testing
**C:** Clinical/Field Testing
**P:** Practicum Testing
**A:** Assessment/Mock Exam Testing
**S:** Self-Reporting

**Positive Finding:** Decreased ability to hold contraction
**Involved Structure:** Peroneus longus, peroneus brevis
**Special Considerations:** Assists in plantar flexion
**Reference(s):** Kendall et al
**Supplies Needed:** Table

## MANUAL MUSCLE TESTING
# (MMT-L-Test 15)

Peer Review _____ Peer Review _____

Skill Acquisition: _____    Practice Opportunities: _____

*This problem allows you the opportunity to demonstrate a* **Myotome Assessment** *in order to rule out damage to nerve root* **L3**. *You have 2 minutes to complete this task.*

| Tester places athlete and limb in appropriate position | YES | NO |
|---|---|---|
| Seated | OOO | OOO |
| **Tester performs test according to accepted guidelines** | **YES** | **NO** |
| Instructs the athlete to flex the hip against resistance (iliopsoas) | OOO | OOO |
| Performs a break test at some point in the range of motion | OOO | OOO |
| Holds resistance for 5 seconds | OOO | OOO |
| Performs assessment bilaterally | OOO | OOO |

| | |
|---|---|
| The psychomotor skill was performed completely and in the appropriate order | **0  1  2  3  4  5** |
| The tester had control of the subject and the situation (showed confidence) | **0  1  2  3  4  5** |
| Method of performing the skill allowed the tester the ability to determine: severity, proper progression, and the *fit* in the overall picture (Oral) | **0  1  2  3  4  5** |

In order for a grade of *minimum standard* to be given, the total must be ≥11          **TOTAL =**

I_____I_____I
**Not Acceptable**          **Meets Minimum Standards**          **Exceeds Minimum Standards**

**L:** Laboratory/Classroom Testing
**C:** Clinical/Field Testing
**P:** Practicum Testing
**A:** Assessment/Mock Exam Testing
**S:** Self-Reporting

**Positive Finding:** Unable to maintain proper position against resistance
**Involved Structure:** Nerve root L3
**Special Considerations:** Rule out muscle damage
**Reference(s):** Magee
**Supplies Needed:** N/A

# MANUAL MUSCLE TESTING
## (MMT-L-Test 16)

Peer Review _____ Peer Review _____

Skill Acquisition: _____        Practice Opportunities: _____

*This problem allows you the opportunity to demonstrate a* **Myotome Assessment** *in order to rule out damage to nerve root* **L4**. *You have 2 minutes to complete this task.*

| Tester places athlete and limb in appropriate position | YES | NO |
|---|---|---|
| Seated or standing | ○○○ | ○○○ |
| **Tester performs test according to accepted guidelines** | **YES** | **NO** |
| Instructs the athlete to invert the ankle against resistance (tibialis anterior) | ○○○ | ○○○ |
| Performs a break test at some point in the range of motion | ○○○ | ○○○ |
| Holds resistance for 5 seconds | ○○○ | ○○○ |
| Performs assessment bilaterally | ○○○ | ○○○ |

The psychomotor skill was performed completely and in the appropriate order    0  1  2  3  4  5

The tester had control of the subject and the situation (showed confidence)    0  1  2  3  4  5

Method of performing the skill allowed the tester the ability to determine:
severity, proper progression, and the *fit* in the overall picture (Oral)    0  1  2  3  4  5

In order for a grade of *minimum standard* to be given, the total must be ≥11    **TOTAL =**

I_____I_____I

**Not Acceptable**          **Meets Minimum Standards**          **Exceeds Minimum Standards**

**L:** Laboratory/Classroom Testing
**C:** Clinical/Field Testing
**P:** Practicum Testing
**A:** Assessment/Mock Exam Testing
**S:** Self-Reporting

**Positive Finding:** Unable to maintain proper position against resistance
**Involved Structure:** Nerve root L4
**Special Considerations:** Rule out muscle damage
**Reference(s):** Hoppenfeld
**Supplies Needed:** N/A

## Manual Muscle Testing
# (MMT-L-Test 17)

Peer Review _____ Peer Review _____

Skill Acquisition: _____    Practice Opportunities: _____

*This problem allows you the opportunity to demonstrate a* **Myotome Assessment** *in order to rule out damage to nerve root* **L5**. *You have 2 minutes to complete this task.*

| Tester places athlete and limb in appropriate position | YES | NO |
|---|---|---|
| Seated or standing | ○○○ | ○○○ |
| **Tester performs test according to accepted guidelines** | **YES** | **NO** |
| Instructs the athlete to extend the great toe against resistance (interossei muscles) | ○○○ | ○○○ |
| Performs a break test at some point in the range of motion | ○○○ | ○○○ |
| Holds resistance for 5 seconds | ○○○ | ○○○ |
| Performs assessment bilaterally | ○○○ | ○○○ |

The psychomotor skill was performed completely and in the appropriate order    **0  1  2  3  4  5**

The tester had control of the subject and the situation (showed confidence)    **0  1  2  3  4  5**

Method of performing the skill allowed the tester the ability to determine:
severity, proper progression, and the *fit* in the overall picture (Oral)    **0  1  2  3  4  5**

In order for a grade of *minimum standard* to be given, the total must be ≥11    **TOTAL =**

I_____I_____I

**Not Acceptable**      **Meets Minimum Standards**    **Exceeds Minimum Standards**

**L:** Laboratory/Classroom Testing
**C:** Clinical/Field Testing
**P:** Practicum Testing
**A:** Assessment/Mock Exam Testing
**S:** Self-Reporting

**Positive Finding:** Unable to maintain proper position against resistance
**Involved Structure:** Nerve root L5
**Special Considerations:** Rule out muscle damage
**Reference(s):** Hoppenfeld
**Supplies Needed:** N/A

# MANUAL MUSCLE TESTING
# (MMT-L-Test 18)

Peer Review _____    Peer Review _____

Skill Acquisition: _____    Practice Opportunities: _____

*This problem allows you the opportunity to demonstrate a* **Myotome Assessment** *in order to rule out damage to nerve root* **S1**. *You have 2 minutes to complete this task.*

| Tester places athlete and limb in appropriate position | YES | NO |
|---|---|---|
| Seated | ООО | ООО |
| **Tester performs test according to accepted guidelines** | **YES** | **NO** |
| Instructs the athlete to evert the ankle against resistance (peroneus longus and brevis) | ООО | ООО |
| Performs a break test at some point in the range of motion | ООО | ООО |
| Holds resistance for 5 seconds | ООО | ООО |
| Performs assessment bilaterally | ООО | ООО |

The psychomotor skill was performed completely and in the appropriate order    **0  1  2  3  4  5**

The tester had control of the subject and the situation (showed confidence)    **0  1  2  3  4  5**

Method of performing the skill allowed the tester the ability to determine:
severity, proper progression, and the *fit* in the overall picture (Oral)    **0  1  2  3  4  5**

In order for a grade of *minimum standard* to be given, the total must be ≥11    **TOTAL =**

I_____I_____I

**Not Acceptable**          **Meets Minimum Standards**          **Exceeds Minimum Standards**

**L:** Laboratory/Classroom Testing
**C:** Clinical/Field Testing
**P:** Practicum Testing
**A:** Assessment/Mock Exam Testing
**S:** Self-Reporting

**Positive Finding:** Unable to maintain proper position against resistance
**Involved Structure:** Nerve root S1
**Special Considerations:** Rule out muscle damage
**Reference(s):** Hoppenfeld
**Supplies Needed:** N/A

# MANUAL MUSCLE TESTING
## (MMT-L-Test 19)

*This problem allows you the opportunity to demonstrate a* **Myotome Assessment** *in order to rule out damage to nerve root* **S2**. *You have 2 minutes to complete this task.*

| Tester places athlete and limb in appropriate position | YES | NO |
|---|---|---|
| Seated | ○○○ | ○○○ |
| **Tester performs test according to accepted guidelines** | **YES** | **NO** |
| Instructs the athlete to flex the knee against resistance (hamstring) | ○○○ | ○○○ |
| Performs a break test at some point in the range of motion | ○○○ | ○○○ |
| Holds resistance for 5 seconds | ○○○ | ○○○ |
| Performs assessment bilaterally | ○○○ | ○○○ |

| | |
|---|---|
| The psychomotor skill was performed completely and in the appropriate order | 0  1  2  3  4  5 |
| The tester had control of the subject and the situation (showed confidence) | 0  1  2  3  4  5 |
| Method of performing the skill allowed the tester the ability to determine: severity, proper progression, and the *fit* in the overall picture (Oral) | 0  1  2  3  4  5 |

In order for a grade of *minimum standard* to be given, the total must be ≥11          TOTAL = _____

I_____I_____I
**Not Acceptable**       **Meets Minimum Standards**       **Exceeds Minimum Standards**

**L:** Laboratory/Classroom Testing
**C:** Clinical/Field Testing
**P:** Practicum Testing
**A:** Assessment/Mock Exam Testing
**S:** Self-Reporting

**Positive Finding:** Unable to maintain proper position against resistance
**Involved Structure:** Nerve root S2
**Special Considerations:** Rule out muscle damage
**Reference(s):** Magee
**Supplies Needed:** N/A

Chapter

6

# REFLEX TESTING

# REFLEX TESTING
# (RT-U-Test 1)

Peer Review _____ Peer Review _____

Skill Acquisition: _____    Practice Opportunities: _____

*Please demonstrate how you would perform a test to check the **C5 reflex (biceps)**. You have 2 minutes to complete this task.*

| Tester places athlete and limb in appropriate position | YES | NO |
|---|---|---|
| Seated or standing | OOO | OOO |
| Places the athlete's arm over the tester's opposite arm (support under the medial elbow) | OOO | OOO |
| Elbow resting at approximately a 90 degree angle | OOO | OOO |
| **Tester performs test according to accepted guidelines** | **YES** | **NO** |
| Places thumb over the biceps tendon (in the cubital fossa) | OOO | OOO |
| Maintains relaxation of the limb | OOO | OOO |
| Strikes the thumbnail over the biceps tendon | OOO | OOO |
| Uses the pointed end of the neurological hammer | OOO | OOO |
| Elicits reflex | OOO | OOO |
| Performs assessment bilaterally | OOO | OOO |

| | |
|---|---|
| The psychomotor skill was performed completely and in the appropriate order | **0  1  2  3  4  5** |
| The tester had control of the subject and the situation (showed confidence) | **0  1  2  3  4  5** |
| Method of performing the skill allowed the tester the ability to determine: severity, proper progression, and the *fit* in the overall picture (Oral) | **0  1  2  3  4  5** |

In order for a grade of *minimum standard* to be given, the total must be ≥11          **TOTAL =**

I_____I_____I

**Not Acceptable**          **Meets Minimum Standards**          **Exceeds Minimum Standards**

**L:** Laboratory/Classroom Testing
**C:** Clinical/Field Testing
**P:** Practicum Testing
**A:** Assessment/Mock Exam Testing
**S:** Self-Reporting

**Positive Finding:** No reflex or abnormal movement (hyper/hypo)
**Involved Structure:** Nerve root coming off C5
**Special Considerations:** C6 may be involved
**Reference(s):** Hoppenfeld
**Supplies Needed:** Table/chair, reflex hammer

## REFLEX TESTING
# (RT-U-Test 2)

Peer Review _____ Peer Review _____

Skill Acquisition: _____     Practice Opportunities: _____

*Please demonstrate how you would perform a test to check the **C6 reflex (brachioradialis)**. You have 2 minutes to complete this task.*

| Tester places athlete and limb in appropriate position | YES | NO |
|---|---|---|
| Seated | ○○○ | ○○○ |
| Places the athlete's arm over the tester's opposite arm (support under the medial elbow) | ○○○ | ○○○ |
| Elbow resting at approximately 90 degree angle | ○○○ | ○○○ |
| **Tester performs test according to accepted guidelines** | **YES** | **NO** |
| Maintains relaxation of the limb | ○○○ | ○○○ |
| Strikes the brachioradialis tendon at the distal end of the radius | ○○○ | ○○○ |
| Uses the flat end of the neurological hammer | ○○○ | ○○○ |
| Elicits reflex | ○○○ | ○○○ |
| Performs assessment bilaterally | ○○○ | ○○○ |

The psychomotor skill was performed completely and in the appropriate order    0 1 2 3 4 5

The tester had control of the subject and the situation (showed confidence)    0 1 2 3 4 5

Method of performing the skill allowed the tester the ability to determine: severity, proper progression, and the *fit* in the overall picture (Oral)    0 1 2 3 4 5

In order for a grade of *minimum standard* to be given, the total must be ≥11    TOTAL =

I_____I_____I
**Not Acceptable**    **Meets Minimum Standards**    **Exceeds Minimum Standards**

**L:** Laboratory/Classroom Testing
**C:** Clinical/Field Testing
**P:** Practicum Testing
**A:** Assessment/Mock Exam Testing
**S:** Self-Reporting

**Positive Finding:** No reflex or abnormal movement (hyper/hypo)
**Involved Structure:** Nerve root coming off C6
**Special Considerations:** C5 may be involved
**Reference(s):** Hoppenfeld
**Supplies Needed:** Table/chair, reflex hammer

# REFLEX TESTING
# (RT-U-Test 3)

Peer Review _____ Peer Review _____

Skill Acquisition: _____    Practice Opportunities: _____

*Please demonstrate how you would perform a test to check the* **C7 reflex (triceps)**. *You have 2 minutes to complete this task.*

| Tester places athlete and limb in appropriate position | YES | NO |
|---|---|---|
| Seated | OOO | OOO |
| Places the athlete's arm over the tester's opposite arm (support under the medial elbow) | OOO | OOO |
| Elbow resting at approximately 90 degree angle | OOO | OOO |
| **Tester performs test according to accepted guidelines** | **YES** | **NO** |
| Maintains relaxation of the limb | OOO | OOO |
| Strikes the triceps tendon where it crosses the olecranon fossa | OOO | OOO |
| Uses the pointed end of the neurological hammer | OOO | OOO |
| Elicits reflex | OOO | OOO |
| Performs assessment bilaterally | OOO | OOO |

The psychomotor skill was performed completely and in the appropriate order    **0  1  2  3  4  5**

The tester had control of the subject and the situation (showed confidence)    **0  1  2  3  4  5**

Method of performing the skill allowed the tester the ability to determine:
severity, proper progression, and the *fit* in the overall picture (Oral)    **0  1  2  3  4  5**

In order for a grade of *minimum standard* to be given, the total must be ≥11    **TOTAL =**

I_____I_____I

**Not Acceptable**        **Meets Minimum Standards**        **Exceeds Minimum Standards**

**L:** Laboratory/Classroom Testing
**C:** Clinical/Field Testing
**P:** Practicum Testing
**A:** Assessment/Mock Exam Testing
**S:** Self-Reporting

**Positive Finding:** No reflex or abnormal movement (hyper/hypo)
**Involved Structure:** Nerve root coming off C7
**Special Considerations:** C8 may be involved
**Reference(s):** Hoppenfeld
**Supplies Needed:** Table/chair, reflex hammer

## REFLEX TESTING
# (RT-L-Test 1)

Peer Review _____ Peer Review _____

Skill Acquisition: _____    Practice Opportunities: _____

*Please demonstrate how you would perform a test to check the* **S1 reflex (Achilles' tendon)**. *You have 2 minutes to complete this task.*

| Tester places athlete and limb in appropriate position | YES | NO |
|---|---|---|
| Prone or seated | ○○○ | ○○○ |
| Foot hanging over the edge of the table (prone) *or* | ○○○ | ○○○ |
| Foot dangling off the edge of the table (seated) | ○○○ | ○○○ |
| **Tester performs test according to accepted guidelines** | **YES** | **NO** |
| Applies slight stretch (gently dorsiflex the foot) | ○○○ | ○○○ |
| Maintains relaxation of the limb | ○○○ | ○○○ |
| Strikes the Achilles' tendon | ○○○ | ○○○ |
| Uses the flat end of the neurological hammer (some texts use pointed end) | ○○○ | ○○○ |
| Elicits reflex | ○○○ | ○○○ |
| Performs assessment bilaterally | ○○○ | ○○○ |

The psychomotor skill was performed completely and in the appropriate order    **0  1  2  3  4  5**

The tester had control of the subject and the situation (showed confidence)    **0  1  2  3  4  5**

Method of performing the skill allowed the tester the ability to determine:
severity, proper progression, and the *fit* in the overall picture (Oral)    **0  1  2  3  4  5**

In order for a grade of *minimum standard* to be given, the total must be ≥11    **TOTAL =**

I_____I_____I

**Not Acceptable**        **Meets Minimum Standards**        **Exceeds Minimum Standards**

**L:** Laboratory/Classroom Testing
**C:** Clinical/Field Testing
**P:** Practicum Testing
**A:** Assessment/Mock Exam Testing
**S:** Self-Reporting

**Positive Finding:** No reflex or abnormal movement (hyper/hypo)
**Involved Structure:** Nerve Root coming off S1
**Special Considerations:** S2 may be involved
**Reference(s):** Hoppenfeld
**Supplies Needed:** Table/chair, reflex hammer

# REFLEX TESTING
## (RT-L-Test 2)

Peer Review _____ Peer Review _____

Skill Acquisition: _____    Practice Opportunities: _____

*Please demonstrate how you would perform a test to check the **L4 reflex (patellar)**. You have 2 minutes to complete this task.*

| Tester places athlete and limb in appropriate position | YES | NO |
|---|---|---|
| Seated | ○○○ | ○○○ |
| Legs hanging over the edge of the table (knees at 90 degrees) | ○○○ | ○○○ |
| **Tester performs test according to accepted guidelines** | **YES** | **NO** |
| Maintains relaxation of the limb | ○○○ | ○○○ |
| Strikes the patella tendon | ○○○ | ○○○ |
| Uses the pointed end of the neurological hammer (some texts use flat end) | ○○○ | ○○○ |
| Elicits reflex | ○○○ | ○○○ |
| Performs assessment bilaterally | ○○○ | ○○○ |

The psychomotor skill was performed completely and in the appropriate order    **0  1  2  3  4  5**

The tester had control of the subject and the situation (showed confidence)    **0  1  2  3  4  5**

Method of performing the skill allowed the tester the ability to determine:
severity, proper progression, and the *fit* in the overall picture (Oral)    **0  1  2  3  4  5**

In order for a grade of *minimum standard* to be given, the total must be ≥11    **TOTAL =**

I_____I_____I

**Not Acceptable**        **Meets Minimum Standards**        **Exceeds Minimum Standards**

**L:** Laboratory/Classroom Testing
**C:** Clinical/Field Testing
**P:** Practicum Testing
**A:** Assessment/Mock Exam Testing
**S:** Self-Reporting

**Positive Finding:** No reflex or abnormal movement (hyper/hypo)
**Involved Structure:** Nerve root coming off L4
**Special Considerations:** L2/L3 may be involved
**Reference(s):** Hoppenfeld
**Supplies Needed:** Table/chair, reflex hammer

# REFLEX TESTING
## (RT-L-Test 3)

Peer Review _____ Peer Review _____

Skill Acquisition: _____     Practice Opportunities: _____

*Please demonstrate how you would perform a test for the pathological reflex known as* **Babinski's Reflex** *to rule out an upper motor neuron lesion. You have 2 minutes to complete this task.*

| Tester places athlete and limb in appropriate position | YES | NO |
|---|---|---|
| Supine | ○○○ | ○○○ |

| Tester performs test according to accepted guidelines | YES | NO |
|---|---|---|
| Maintains relaxation of the limb | ○○○ | ○○○ |
| Uses a pointed object to stroke the plantar surface of the foot: | | |
|   Lateral border | ○○○ | ○○○ |
|   Proximal to distal | ○○○ | ○○○ |
|   Even/appropriate pressure | ○○○ | ○○○ |
| Performs assessment bilaterally | ○○○ | ○○○ |

The psychomotor skill was performed completely and in the appropriate order    0 1 2 3 4 5

The tester had control of the subject and the situation (showed confidence)    0 1 2 3 4 5

Method of performing the skill allowed the tester the ability to determine: severity, proper progression, and the *fit* in the overall picture (Oral)    0 1 2 3 4 5

In order for a grade of *minimum standard* to be given, the total must be ≥11    **TOTAL =**

I_____I_____I

**Not Acceptable**     **Meets Minimum Standards**     **Exceeds Minimum Standards**

**L:** Laboratory/Classroom Testing
**C:** Clinical/Field Testing
**P:** Practicum Testing
**A:** Assessment/Mock Exam Testing
**S:** Self-Reporting

**Positive Finding:** Splaying of the toes
**Involved Structure:** Upper motor neuron lesion
**Special Considerations:** N/A
**Reference(s):** Magee
**Supplies Needed:** Table, pointed object

# REFLEX TESTING
# (RT-L-Test 4)

Peer Review _____ Peer Review _____

Skill Acquisition: _____     Practice Opportunities: _____

*This problem allows you the opportunity to demonstrate a superficial reflex known as the **superficial abdominal reflex** in order to rule out an upper motor neuron lesion. You have 2 minutes to complete this task.*

| Tester places athlete and limb in appropriate position | YES | NO |
|---|---|---|
| Supine | ○○○ | ○○○ |
| **Tester performs test according to accepted guidelines** | **YES** | **NO** |
| Maintains relaxation of the abdominal region | ○○○ | ○○○ |
| Uses a pointed object to stroke each of the four quadrants of the abdomen | ○○○ | ○○○ |
| Strokes in a triangular motion around the umbilicus | ○○○ | ○○○ |

The psychomotor skill was performed completely and in the appropriate order    0 1 2 3 4 5

The tester had control of the subject and the situation (showed confidence)    0 1 2 3 4 5

Method of performing the skill allowed the tester the ability to determine:
severity, proper progression, and the *fit* in the overall picture (Oral)    0 1 2 3 4 5

In order for a grade of *minimum standard* to be given, the total must be ≥11    **TOTAL =**

I_____I_____I
**Not Acceptable**        **Meets Minimum Standards**   **Exceeds Minimum Standards**

**L:** Laboratory/Classroom Testing
**C:** Clinical/Field Testing
**P:** Practicum Testing
**A:** Assessment/Mock Exam Testing
**S:** Self-Reporting

**Positive Finding:** No movement of the skin
**Involved Structure:** Upper motor neuron lesion—unilateral absence indicates a lower motor neuron lesion (T7-L2)
**Special Considerations:** N/A
**Reference(s):** Magee
**Supplies Needed:** Table, pointed object

## REFLEX TESTING
# (RT-L-Test 5)

Peer Review _____ Peer Review _____

Skill Acquisition: _____    Practice Opportunities: _____

*Please demonstrate how you would perform a test to check the **deep tendon reflex of L5 (posterior tibial)**. You have 2 minutes to complete this task.*

| Tester places athlete and limb in appropriate position | YES | NO |
|---|---|---|
| Prone | ○○○ | ○○○ |
| Foot hanging over the edge of the table | ○○○ | ○○○ |
| **Tester performs test according to accepted guidelines** | **YES** | **NO** |
| Applies slight stretch (plantar flexion) | ○○○ | ○○○ |
| Maintains relaxation of the limb | ○○○ | ○○○ |
| Strikes the posterior tibial tendon (just behind the medial malleolus) | ○○○ | ○○○ |
| Uses the pointed end of the neurological hammer | ○○○ | ○○○ |
| Elicits reflex | ○○○ | ○○○ |
| Performs assessment bilaterally | ○○○ | ○○○ |

The psychomotor skill was performed completely and in the appropriate order    0 1 2 3 4 5

The tester had control of the subject and the situation (showed confidence)    0 1 2 3 4 5

Method of performing the skill allowed the tester the ability to determine:
severity, proper progression, and the *fit* in the overall picture (Oral)    0 1 2 3 4 5

In order for a grade of *minimum standard* to be given, the total must be ≥11    **TOTAL =**

I_____I_____I
**Not Acceptable**      **Meets Minimum Standards**   **Exceeds Minimum Standards**

**L:** Laboratory/Classroom Testing
**C:** Clinical/Field Testing
**P:** Practicum Testing
**A:** Assessment/Mock Exam Testing
**S:** Self-Reporting

**Positive Finding:** No reflex or abnormal movement (hyper/hypo)
**Involved Structure:** Nerve root coming off L4/L5
**Special Considerations:** N/A
**Reference(s):** Magee
**Supplies Needed:** Table, reflex hammer

# REFLEX TESTING
# (RT-L-Test 6)

Peer Review _____ Peer Review _____

Skill Acquisition: _____    Practice Opportunities: _____

*Please demonstrate how you would perform a test for the pathological reflex known as the* **Oppenheim Reflex** *to rule out an upper motor neuron lesion. You have 2 minutes to complete this task.*

| Tester places athlete and limb in appropriate position | YES | NO |
|---|---|---|
| Supine | ○○○ | ○○○ |
| **Tester performs test according to accepted guidelines** | **YES** | **NO** |
| Maintains relaxation of the limb | ○○○ | ○○○ |
| Uses a pointed object along the crest of the tibia: | | |
|   Anteromedial border | ○○○ | ○○○ |
|   Even/appropriate pressure | ○○○ | ○○○ |
| Performs assessment bilaterally | ○○○ | ○○○ |

The psychomotor skill was performed completely and in the appropriate order    **0  1  2  3  4  5**

The tester had control of the subject and the situation (showed confidence)    **0  1  2  3  4  5**

Method of performing the skill allowed the tester the ability to determine:
severity, proper progression, and the *fit* in the overall picture (Oral)    **0  1  2  3  4  5**

In order for a grade of *minimum standard* to be given, the total must be ≥11    **TOTAL =**

I_____I_____I

**Not Acceptable**     **Meets Minimum Standards**     **Exceeds Minimum Standards**

**L:** Laboratory/Classroom Testing
**C:** Clinical/Field Testing
**P:** Practicum Testing
**A:** Assessment/Mock Exam Testing
**S:** Self-Reporting

**Positive Finding:** Splaying of toes
**Involved Structure:** Upper motor neuron lesion
**Special Considerations:** N/A
**Reference(s):** Magee
**Supplies Needed:** Table, pointed object

# SENSORY TESTING

# SENSORY TESTING
# (SST-U-Test 1)

Peer Review _____ Peer Review _____

Skill Acquisition: _____    Practice Opportunities: _____

*This problem allows you the opportunity to demonstrate a* **Dermatome Sensory Test** *using a in order to rule out damage to the nerve root* **C5.** *You have 2 minutes to complete this task.*

| Tester places athlete and limb in appropriate position | YES | NO |
|---|---|---|
| Seated or prone | ○○○ | ○○○ |
| **Tester performs test according to accepted guidelines** | **YES** | **NO** |
| Gives appropriate directions to the athlete | ○○○ | ○○○ |
| Explains differences in pressure | ○○○ | ○○○ |
| Demonstration given away from the injured area | ○○○ | ○○○ |
| Instructs athlete to close eyes | ○○○ | ○○○ |
| Applies varied pressure with tool or common objects: | | |
|   Sharp | ○○○ | ○○○ |
|   Dull | ○○○ | ○○○ |
|   No touch | ○○○ | ○○○ |
| Applies appropriate pressure to the lateral arm (deltoid tuberosity) | ○○○ | ○○○ |
| Performs assessment bilaterally | ○○○ | ○○○ |

The psychomotor skill was performed completely and in the appropriate order    0 1 2 3 4 5

The tester had control of the subject and the situation (showed confidence)    0 1 2 3 4 5

Method of performing the skill allowed the tester the ability to determine:
severity, proper progression, and the *fit* in the overall picture (Oral)    0 1 2 3 4 5

In order for a grade of *minimum standard* to be given, the total must be ≥11    **TOTAL =**

I_____I_____I
**Not Acceptable**        **Meets Minimum Standards**    **Exceeds Minimum Standards**

**L:** Laboratory/Classroom Testing
**C:** Clinical/Field Testing
**P:** Practicum Testing
**A:** Assessment/Mock Exam Testing
**S:** Self-Reporting

**Positive Finding:** No feeling; difficulty in distinguishing varied pressure
**Involved Structure:** Nerve root C5
**Special Considerations:** N/A
**Reference(s):** Hoppenfeld
**Supplies Needed:** Table/chair, sharp/dull object

# SENSORY TESTING
# (SST-U-Test 2)

Peer Review _____ Peer Review _____

Skill Acquisition: _____    Practice Opportunities: _____

*This problem allows you the opportunity to demonstrate a* **Dermatome Sensory Test** *in order to rule out damage to the nerve root* **C6**. *You have 2 minutes to complete this task.*

| Tester places athlete and limb in appropriate position | YES | NO |
|---|---|---|
| Seated or prone | ○○○ | ○○○ |
| **Tester performs test according to accepted guidelines** | **YES** | **NO** |
| Gives appropriate directions to the athlete | ○○○ | ○○○ |
| Explains differences in pressure | ○○○ | ○○○ |
| Demonstration given away from the injured area | ○○○ | ○○○ |
| Instructs athlete to close eyes | ○○○ | ○○○ |
| Applies varied pressure with tool or common objects: | | |
|   Sharp | ○○○ | ○○○ |
|   Dull | ○○○ | ○○○ |
|   No touch | ○○○ | ○○○ |
| Applies appropriate pressure to the lateral forearm (at web of the thumb) | ○○○ | ○○○ |
| Performs assessment bilaterally | ○○○ | ○○○ |

The psychomotor skill was performed completely and in the appropriate order    0  1  2  3  4  5

The tester had control of the subject and the situation (showed confidence)    0  1  2  3  4  5

Method of performing the skill allowed the tester the ability to determine:
severity, proper progression, and the *fit* in the overall picture (Oral)    0  1  2  3  4  5

In order for a grade of *minimum standard* to be given, the total must be ≥11    **TOTAL =**

I_____I_____I
**Not Acceptable**        **Meets Minimum Standards**    **Exceeds Minimum Standards**

**L:** Laboratory/Classroom Testing
**C:** Clinical/Field Testing
**P:** Practicum Testing
**A:** Assessment/Mock Exam Testing
**S:** Self-Reporting

**Positive Finding:** No feeling; difficulty in distinguishing varied pressure
**Involved Structure:** Nerve root C6
**Special Considerations:** N/A
**Reference(s):** Hoppenfeld
**Supplies Needed:** Table/chair, sharp/dull object

# SENSORY TESTING
# (SST-U-Test 3)

Peer Review _____ Peer Review _____

Skill Acquisition: _____     Practice Opportunities: _____

*This problem allows you the opportunity to demonstrate a* **Dermatome Sensory Test** *in order to rule out damage to the nerve root* **C7**. *You have 2 minutes to complete this task.*

| Tester places athlete and limb in appropriate position | YES | NO |
|---|---|---|
| Seated or prone | OOO | OOO |
| **Tester performs test according to accepted guidelines** | **YES** | **NO** |
| Gives appropriate directions to the athlete | OOO | OOO |
| Explains differences in pressure | OOO | OOO |
| Demonstration given away from the injured area | OOO | OOO |
| Instructs athlete to close eyes | OOO | OOO |
| Applies varied pressure with tool or common objects: | | |
| Sharp | OOO | OOO |
| Dull | OOO | OOO |
| No touch | OOO | OOO |
| Applies appropriate pressure to the middle finger (palmar surface, distal) | OOO | OOO |
| Performs assessment bilaterally | OOO | OOO |

| | |
|---|---|
| The psychomotor skill was performed completely and in the appropriate order | 0 1 2 3 4 5 |
| The tester had control of the subject and the situation (showed confidence) | 0 1 2 3 4 5 |
| Method of performing the skill allowed the tester the ability to determine: severity, proper progression, and the *fit* in the overall picture (Oral) | 0 1 2 3 4 5 |

In order for a grade of *minimum standard* to be given, the total must be ≥11     **TOTAL =**

I_____I_____I

**Not Acceptable**    **Meets Minimum Standards**    **Exceeds Minimum Standards**

**L:** Laboratory/Classroom Testing
**C:** Clinical/Field Testing
**P:** Practicum Testing
**A:** Assessment/Mock Exam Testing
**S:** Self-Reporting

**Positive Finding:** No feeling; difficulty in distinguishing varied pressure
**Involved Structure:** Nerve root C7
**Special Considerations:** N/A
**Reference(s):** Hoppenfeld
**Supplies Needed:** Table/chair, sharp/dull object

## SENSORY TESTING
# (SST-U-Test 4)

Peer Review _____  Peer Review _____

Skill Acquisition: _____    Practice Opportunities: _____

*This problem allows you the opportunity to demonstrate a* **Dermatome Sensory Test** *in order to rule out damage to the nerve root* **C8**. *You have 2 minutes to complete this task.*

| Tester places athlete and limb in appropriate position | YES | NO |
|---|---|---|
| Seated or prone | OOO | OOO |
| **Tester performs test according to accepted guidelines** | **YES** | **NO** |
| Gives appropriate directions to the athlete | OOO | OOO |
| Explains differences in pressure | OOO | OOO |
| Demonstration given away from the injured area | OOO | OOO |
| Instructs athlete to close eyes | OOO | OOO |
| Applies varied pressure with tool or common objects: | | |
|   Sharp | OOO | OOO |
|   Dull | OOO | OOO |
|   No touch | OOO | OOO |
| Applies appropriate pressureto the fourth and fifth fingers at the outside of little finger | OOO | OOO |
| Performs assessment bilaterally | OOO | OOO |

The psychomotor skill was performed completely and in the appropriate order     **0  1  2  3  4  5**

The tester had control of the subject and the situation (showed confidence)     **0  1  2  3  4  5**

Method of performing the skill allowed the tester the ability to determine:
severity, proper progression, and the *fit* in the overall picture (Oral)     **0  1  2  3  4  5**

In order for a grade of *minimum standard* to be given, the total must be ≥11     **TOTAL =**

I_____I_____I
   **Not Acceptable**        **Meets Minimum Standards**     **Exceeds Minimum Standards**

**L:** Laboratory/Classroom Testing
**C:** Clinical/Field Testing
**P:** Practicum Testing
**A:** Assessment/Mock Exam Testing
**S:** Self-Reporting

**Positive Finding:** No feeling; difficulty in distinguishing varied pressure
**Involved Structure:** Nerve root C8
**Special Considerations:** N/A
**Reference(s):** Hoppenfeld
**Supplies Needed:** Table/chair, sharp/dull objects

# SENSORY TESTING
# (SST-U-Test 5)

Skill Acquisition: _____    Practice Opportunities: _____

*This problem allows you the opportunity to demonstrate a **Dermatome Sensory Test** in order to rule out damage to the nerve root **T1**. You have 2 minutes to complete this task.*

| | YES | NO |
|---|---|---|
| **Tester places athlete and limb in appropriate position** | YES | NO |
| Seated or prone | OOO | OOO |
| **Tester performs test according to accepted guidelines** | YES | NO |
| Gives appropriate directions to the athlete | OOO | OOO |
| Explains differences in pressure | OOO | OOO |
| Demonstration given away from the injured area | OOO | OOO |
| Instructs athlete to close eyes | OOO | OOO |
| Applies varied pressure with tool or common objects: | | |
|   Sharp | OOO | OOO |
|   Dull | OOO | OOO |
|   No touch | OOO | OOO |
| Applies appropriate pressure to the upper half of the medial forearm | OOO | OOO |
| (medial epicondyle) | | |
| Performs assessment bilaterally | OOO | OOO |

| | |
|---|---|
| The psychomotor skill was performed completely and in the appropriate order | 0  1  2  3  4  5 |
| The tester had control of the subject and the situation (showed confidence) | 0  1  2  3  4  5 |
| Method of performing the skill allowed the tester the ability to determine: severity, proper progression, and the *fit* in the overall picture (Oral) | 0  1  2  3  4  5 |

In order for a grade of *minimum standard* to be given, the total must be ≥11          **TOTAL =**

I_____I_____I

**Not Acceptable**          **Meets Minimum Standards**          **Exceeds Minimum Standards**

**L:** Laboratory/Classroom Testing
**C:** Clinical/Field Testing
**P:** Practicum Testing
**A:** Assessment/Mock Exam Testing
**S:** Self-Reporting

**Positive Finding:** No feeling; difficulty in distinguishing varied pressure
**Involved Structure:** Nerve root T1
**Special Considerations:** N/A
**Reference(s):** Hoppenfeld
**Supplies Needed:** Table/chair, sharp/dull objects

## SENSORY TESTING
# (SST-U-Test 6)

*Please demonstrate how you would evaluate an athlete who is suspected of a cranial nerve injury to the **olfactory nerve (cranial nerve #1)**. You have 2 minutes to complete this task.*

| Tester places athlete and limb in appropriate position | YES | NO |
|---|---|---|
| Seated or standing | ○○○ | ○○○ |
| **Tester performs test according to accepted guidelines** | **YES** | **NO** |
| Gives appropriate directions to the athlete | ○○○ | ○○○ |
| Instructs the athlete to close eyes | ○○○ | ○○○ |
| Asks the athlete to identify a familiar odor | ○○○ | ○○○ |

| | | |
|---|---|---|
| The psychomotor skill was performed completely and in the appropriate order | | 0  1  2  3  4  5 |
| The tester had control of the subject and the situation (showed confidence) | | 0  1  2  3  4  5 |
| Method of performing the skill allowed the tester the ability to determine: severity, proper progression, and the *fit* in the overall picture (Oral) | | 0  1  2  3  4  5 |

In order for a grade of *minimum standard* to be given, the total must be ≥11          **TOTAL =**

I_____I_____I
**Not Acceptable**          **Meets Minimum Standards**          **Exceeds Minimum Standards**

**L:** Laboratory/Classroom Testing
**C:** Clinical/Field Testing
**P:** Practicum Testing
**A:** Assessment/Mock Exam Testing
**S:** Self-Reporting

**Positive Finding:** Inability to distinguish the odor
**Involved Structure:** Cranial nerve #1
**Special Considerations:** Sensory only
**Reference(s):** Magee; Starkey
**Supplies Needed:** Familiar odor (eg, tape adhesive)

# SENSORY TESTING
# (SST-U-Test 7)

Peer Review _____ Peer Review _____

Skill Acquisition: _____    Practice Opportunities: _____

*Please demonstrate how you would evaluate an athlete who is suspected of a cranial nerve injury to the* **optic nerve (cranial nerve #2)**. *You have 2 minutes to complete this task.*

| Tester places athlete and limb in appropriate position | YES | NO |
|---|---|---|
| Seated or standing | ○○○ | ○○○ |
| **Tester performs test according to accepted guidelines** | **YES** | **NO** |
| Gives appropriate directions to the athlete | ○○○ | ○○○ |
| Asks athlete to read from chart or scoreboard (visual field and distance acuity) | ○○○ | ○○○ |
| Asks the athlete to tell how many fingers he or she sees (visual field and near acuity) | ○○○ | ○○○ |

| | |
|---|---|
| The psychomotor skill was performed completely and in the appropriate order | 0  1  2  3  4  5 |
| The tester had control of the subject and the situation (showed confidence) | 0  1  2  3  4  5 |
| Method of performing the skill allowed the tester the ability to determine: severity, proper progression, and the *fit* in the overall picture (Oral) | 0  1  2  3  4  5 |

In order for a grade of *minimum standard* to be given, the total must be ≥11          **TOTAL =**

I_____I_____I

**Not Acceptable**          **Meets Minimum Standards**          **Exceeds Minimum Standards**

**L:** Laboratory/Classroom Testing
**C:** Clinical/Field Testing
**P:** Practicum Testing
**A:** Assessment/Mock Exam Testing
**S:** Self-Reporting

**Positive Finding:** Inability to see/read requested material
**Involved Structure:** Cranial nerve #2
**Special Considerations:** Sensory only
**Reference(s):** Magee; Starkey et al
**Supplies Needed:** Vision card, etc

# SENSORY TESTING
# (SST-U-Test 8)

Peer Review _____ Peer Review _____

Skill Acquisition: _____    Practice Opportunities: _____

*Please demonstrate how you would evaluate an athlete who is suspected of a cranial nerve injury to the **oculo-motor nerve (cranial nerve #3)**. You have 2 minutes to complete this task.*

| Tester places athlete and limb in appropriate position | YES | NO |
|---|---|---|
| Seated or standing | ○○○ | ○○○ |
| **Tester performs test according to accepted guidelines** | **YES** | **NO** |
| Gives appropriate directions to the athlete | ○○○ | ○○○ |
| Checks the athlete's reaction to light (pupil reaction) | ○○○ | ○○○ |
| Asks the athlete to raise the upper eyelid | ○○○ | ○○○ |
| Asks the athlete to roll the eye downward, upward, and medially | ○○○ | ○○○ |

The psychomotor skill was performed completely and in the appropriate order    0 1 2 3 4 5

The tester had control of the subject and the situation (showed confidence)    0 1 2 3 4 5

Method of performing the skill allowed the tester the ability to determine:
severity, proper progression, and the *fit* in the overall picture (Oral)    0 1 2 3 4 5

In order for a grade of *minimum standard* to be given, the total must be ≥11    **TOTAL =**

I_____I_____I
**Not Acceptable        Meets Minimum Standards    Exceeds Minimum Standards**

**L:** Laboratory/Classroom Testing
**C:** Clinical/Field Testing
**P:** Practicum Testing
**A:** Assessment/Mock Exam Testing
**S:** Self-Reporting

**Positive Finding:** Inability to complete the above tasks
**Involved Structure:** Cranial nerve #3
**Special Considerations:** Motor only
**Reference(s):** Magee; Starkey et al
**Supplies Needed:** Pen light

## SENSORY TESTING
# (SST-U-Test 9)

Peer Review _____ Peer Review _____

Skill Acquisition: _____        Practice Opportunities: _____

*Demonstrate how you would evaluate an athlete who is suspected of suffering a cranial nerve injury to the* **trigeminal nerve**. *This problem requires you to demonstrate assessment of both the sensory and motor functions of* **cranial nerve #5**. *You have 2 minutes to complete this task.*

| Tester places athlete and limb in appropriate position | YES | NO |
|---|---|---|
| Seated or standing | OOO | OOO |
| **Tester performs test according to accepted guidelines** | **YES** | **NO** |
| Gives appropriate directions to the athlete | OOO | OOO |
| Instructs the athlete to close eyes | OOO | OOO |
| Asks the athlete to recognize a light touch to the face (sensory) | OOO | OOO |
| Asks the athlete to clench teeth together (motor) | OOO | OOO |

The psychomotor skill was performed completely and in the appropriate order    0 1 2 3 4 5

The tester had control of the subject and the situation (showed confidence)    0 1 2 3 4 5

Method of performing the skill allowed the tester the ability to determine: severity, proper progression, and the *fit* in the overall picture (Oral)    0 1 2 3 4 5

In order for a grade of *minimum standard* to be given, the total must be ≥11    **TOTAL =**

I_____I_____I

**Not Acceptable**     **Meets Minimum Standards**     **Exceeds Minimum Standards**

**L:** Laboratory/Classroom Testing
**C:** Clinical/Field Testing
**P:** Practicum Testing
**A:** Assessment/Mock Exam Testing
**S:** Self-Reporting

**Positive Finding:** Inability to complete the above tasks
**Involved Structure:** Cranial nerve #5
**Special Considerations:** Motor/sensory
**Reference(s):** Magee; Starkey et al
**Supplies Needed:** N/A

## SENSORY TESTING
# (SST-U-Test 10)

Peer Review _____ Peer Review _____

Skill Acquisition: _____    Practice Opportunities: _____

*Please demonstrate how you would evaluate an athlete who is suspected of a cranial nerve injury to the* **abducens nerve (cranial nerve #6).** *You have 2 minutes to complete this task.*

| Tester places athlete and limb in appropriate position | YES | NO |
|---|---|---|
| Seated or standing | ○○○ | ○○○ |
| **Tester performs test according to accepted guidelines** | **YES** | **NO** |
| Gives appropriate directions to the athlete | ○○○ | ○○○ |
| Asks the athlete to move the eye laterally | ○○○ | ○○○ |

| | |
|---|---|
| The psychomotor skill was performed completely and in the appropriate order | **0  1  2  3  4  5** |
| The tester had control of the subject and the situation (showed confidence) | **0  1  2  3  4  5** |
| Method of performing the skill allowed the tester the ability to determine: severity, proper progression, and the *fit* in the overall picture (Oral) | **0  1  2  3  4  5** |

In order for a grade of *minimum standard* to be given, the total must be ≥11          **TOTAL =**

I_____I_____I
**Not Acceptable**          **Meets Minimum Standards**          **Exceeds Minimum Standards**

**L:** Laboratory/Classroom Testing
**C:** Clinical/Field Testing
**P:** Practicum Testing
**A:** Assessment/Mock Exam Testing
**S:** Self-Reporting

**Positive Finding:** Inability to complete the above tasks
**Involved Structure:** Cranial nerve #6
**Special Considerations:** Motor only
**Reference(s):** Magee; Starkey et al
**Supplies Needed:** Pen light

## SENSORY TESTING
# (SST-U-Test 11)

Peer Review _____ Peer Review _____

Skill Acquisition: _____    Practice Opportunities: _____

*Demonstrate how you would evaluate an athlete who is suspected of suffering a cranial nerve injury to the* **facial nerve**. *This problem requires you to demonstrate assessment of both the sensory and motor functions of* **cranial nerve #7**. *You have 2 minutes to complete this task.*

| Tester places athlete and limb in appropriate position | YES | NO |
|---|---|---|
| Seated or standing | ○○○ | ○○○ |
| **Tester performs test according to accepted guidelines** | **YES** | **NO** |
| Gives appropriate directions to the athlete | ○○○ | ○○○ |
| Instructs the athlete to close eyes | ○○○ | ○○○ |
| Asks the athlete to recognize a familiar taste on the anterior portion of the tongue (sensory) | ○○○ | ○○○ |
| Asks the athlete to smile, puff cheeks, etc to show control of facial muscles (motor) | ○○○ | ○○○ |

| | |
|---|---|
| The psychomotor skill was performed completely and in the appropriate order | 0  1  2  3  4  5 |
| The tester had control of the subject and the situation (showed confidence) | 0  1  2  3  4  5 |
| Method of performing the skill allowed the tester the ability to determine: severity, proper progression, and the *fit* in the overall picture (Oral) | 0  1  2  3  4  5 |

In order for a grade of *minimum standard* to be given, the total must be ≥11      **TOTAL =**

I_____I_____I

**Not Acceptable**       **Meets Minimum Standards**    **Exceeds Minimum Standards**

**L:** Laboratory/Classroom Testing
**C:** Clinical/Field Testing
**P:** Practicum Testing
**A:** Assessment/Mock Exam Testing
**S:** Self-Reporting

**Positive Finding:** Inability to complete the above tasks
**Involved Structure:** Cranial nerve #7
**Special Considerations:** Motor/sensory
**Reference(s):** Magee; Starkey et al
**Supplies Needed:** Sugar, etc

## SENSORY TESTING
# (SST-U-Test 12)

Skill Acquisition: _____    Practice Opportunities: _____

*Please demonstrate how you would evaluate an athlete who is suspected of a cranial nerve injury to the* **vestibu-locochlear nerve (cranial nerve #8)**. *You have 2 minutes to complete this task.*

| Tester places athlete and limb in appropriate position | YES | NO |
|---|---|---|
| Seated or standing | ○○○ | ○○○ |
| **Tester performs test according to accepted guidelines** | **YES** | **NO** |
| Gives appropriate directions to the athlete | ○○○ | ○○○ |
| Asks the athlete to listen for sounds (eg, watch ticking) | ○○○ | ○○○ |
| Moves sound further away (compared bilaterally) | ○○○ | ○○○ |
| Asks the athlete to maintain normal balance (balance/coordination test) | ○○○ | ○○○ |

The psychomotor skill was performed completely and in the appropriate order    **0  1  2  3  4  5**

The tester had control of the subject and the situation (showed confidence)    **0  1  2  3  4  5**

Method of performing the skill allowed the tester the ability to determine: severity, proper progression, and the *fit* in the overall picture (Oral)    **0  1  2  3  4  5**

In order for a grade of *minimum standard* to be given, the total must be ≥11    **TOTAL =**

I_____I_____I

**Not Acceptable**        **Meets Minimum Standards**    **Exceeds Minimum Standards**

**L:** Laboratory/Classroom Testing
**C:** Clinical/Field Testing
**P:** Practicum Testing
**A:** Assessment/Mock Exam Testing
**S:** Self-Reporting

**Positive Finding:** Inability to complete the above tasks
**Involved Structure:** Cranial nerve #8
**Special Considerations:** Sensory only (may be called acoustic nerve)
**Reference(s):** Magee; Starkey et al
**Supplies Needed:** Some type of noise

# SENSORY TESTING
# (SST-U-Test 13)

Peer Review _____ Peer Review _____

Skill Acquisition: _____    Practice Opportunities: _____

*Demonstrate how you would evaluate an athlete who is suspected of suffering a cranial nerve injury to the **glossopharyngeal nerve**. This problem requires you to demonstrate assessment of both the sensory and motor functions of **cranial nerve #9**. You have 2 minutes to complete this task.*

| Tester places athlete and limb in appropriate position | YES | NO |
|---|---|---|
| Seated or standing | OOO | OOO |
| **Tester performs test according to accepted guidelines** | **YES** | **NO** |
| Gives appropriate directions to the athlete | OOO | OOO |
| Instructs the athlete to close eyes | OOO | OOO |
| Asks the athlete to recognize a familiar taste on the posterior portion of the tongue (sensory) | OOO | OOO |
| Asks the athlete to swallow to demonstrate gag reflex (motor) | OOO | OOO |

The psychomotor skill was performed completely and in the appropriate order    0 1 2 3 4 5

The tester had control of the subject and the situation (showed confidence)    0 1 2 3 4 5

Method of performing the skill allowed the tester the ability to determine: severity, proper progression, and the *fit* in the overall picture (Oral)    0 1 2 3 4 5

In order for a grade of *minimum standard* to be given, the total must be ≥11    **TOTAL =**

I_____I_____I

**Not Acceptable**    **Meets Minimum Standards**    **Exceeds Minimum Standards**

**L:** Laboratory/Classroom Testing
**C:** Clinical/Field Testing
**P:** Practicum Testing
**A:** Assessment/Mock Exam Testing
**S:** Self-Reporting

**Positive Finding:** Inability to complete the above tasks
**Involved Structure:** Cranial nerve #9
**Special Considerations:** Motor/sensory
**Reference(s):** Magee; Konin
**Supplies Needed:** Sugar, etc

# SENSORY TESTING
# (SST-U-Test 14)

Peer Review _____ Peer Review _____

Skill Acquisition: _____    Practice Opportunities: _____

*Please demonstrate how you would evaluate an athlete who is suspected of a cranial nerve injury to the* **accessory nerve (cranial nerve #11)**. *You have 2 minutes to complete this task.*

| Tester places athlete and limb in appropriate position | YES | NO |
|---|---|---|
| Seated or standing | ○○○ | ○○○ |
| **Tester performs test according to accepted guidelines** | **YES** | **NO** |
| Gives appropriate directions to the athlete | ○○○ | ○○○ |
| Asks the athlete to shrug shoulders against resistance | ○○○ | ○○○ |
| Holds resistance for 5 seconds | ○○○ | ○○○ |

The psychomotor skill was performed completely and in the appropriate order    0  1  2  3  4  5

The tester had control of the subject and the situation (showed confidence)    0  1  2  3  4  5

Method of performing the skill allowed the tester the ability to determine:
severity, proper progression, and the *fit* in the overall picture (Oral)    0  1  2  3  4  5

In order for a grade of *minimum standard* to be given, the total must be ≥11    **TOTAL =**

I_____I_____I

**Not Acceptable**    **Meets Minimum Standards**    **Exceeds Minimum Standards**

**L:** Laboratory/Classroom Testing
**C:** Clinical/Field Testing
**P:** Practicum Testing
**A:** Assessment/Mock Exam Testing
**S:** Self-Reporting

**Positive Finding:** Inability to complete the above tasks
**Involved Structure:** Cranial nerve #11
**Special Considerations:** Motor only
**Reference(s):** Magee; Starkey et al
**Supplies Needed:** N/A

# SENSORY TESTING
# (SST-U-Test 15)

Skill Acquisition: _____    Practice Opportunities: _____

*Please demonstrate how you would evaluate an athlete who is suspected of a cranial nerve injury to the* **hypoglossal nerve (cranial nerve #12)**. *You have 2 minutes to complete this task.*

| Tester places athlete and limb in appropriate position | YES | NO |
|---|---|---|
| Seated or standing | ○○○ | ○○○ |
| **Tester performs test according to accepted guidelines** | **YES** | **NO** |
| Gives appropriate directions to the athlete | ○○○ | ○○○ |
| Asks the athlete to stick out the tongue (general tongue movements) | ○○○ | ○○○ |

The psychomotor skill was performed completely and in the appropriate order    **0  1  2  3  4  5**

The tester had control of the subject and the situation (showed confidence)    **0  1  2  3  4  5**

Method of performing the skill allowed the tester the ability to determine: severity, proper progression, and the *fit* in the overall picture (Oral)    **0  1  2  3  4  5**

In order for a grade of *minimum standard* to be given, the total must be ≥11    **TOTAL =**

I_____I_____I

**Not Acceptable**　　　　**Meets Minimum Standards**　　　**Exceeds Minimum Standards**

**L:** Laboratory/Classroom Testing
**C:** Clinical/Field Testing
**P:** Practicum Testing
**A:** Assessment/Mock Exam Testing
**S:** Self-Reporting

**Positive Finding:** Inability to complete the above tasks
**Involved Structure:** Cranial nerve #12
**Special Considerations:** Motor only
**Reference(s):** Magee; Starkey et al
**Supplies Needed:** N/A

## SENSORY TESTING
# (SST-U-Test 16)

Peer Review _____ Peer Review _____

Skill Acquisition: _____    Practice Opportunities: _____

*Please demonstrate how you would evaluate an athlete who is suspected of a cranial nerve injury to the* **trochlear nerve (cranial nerve #4)**. *You have 2 minutes to complete this task.*

| Tester places athlete and limb in appropriate position | YES | NO |
|---|---|---|
| Seated or standing | OOO | OOO |
| **Tester performs test according to accepted guidelines** | **YES** | **NO** |
| Gives appropriate directions to the athlete | OOO | OOO |
| Asks the athlete to elevate eyes (upward rolling of the eyes) | OOO | OOO |

The psychomotor skill was performed completely and in the appropriate order    **0  1  2  3  4  5**

The tester had control of the subject and the situation (showed confidence)    **0  1  2  3  4  5**

Method of performing the skill allowed the tester the ability to determine:
severity, proper progression, and the *fit* in the overall picture (Oral)    **0  1  2  3  4  5**

In order for a grade of *minimum standard* to be given, the total must be ≥11    **TOTAL =**

I_____I_____I

**Not Acceptable**        **Meets Minimum Standards**        **Exceeds Minimum Standards**

**L:** Laboratory/Classroom Testing
**C:** Clinical/Field Testing
**P:** Practicum Testing
**A:** Assessment/Mock Exam Testing
**S:** Self-Reporting

**Positive Finding:** Inability to complete the above tasks
**Involved Structure:** Cranial nerve #4
**Special Considerations:** Motor only
**Reference(s):** Konin et al; Starkey et al
**Supplies Needed:** Pen light

## SENSORY TESTING
# (SST-U-Test 17)

Peer Review _____ Peer Review _____

Skill Acquisition: _____    Practice Opportunities: _____

*Demonstrate how you would evaluate an athlete who is suspected of suffering a cranial nerve injury to the **vagus nerve**. This problem requires you to demonstrate assessment of both the sensory and motor functions of **cranial nerve #10**. You have 2 minutes to complete this task.*

| Tester places athlete and limb in appropriate position | YES | NO |
|---|---|---|
| Seated or standing | ○○○ | ○○○ |
| **Tester performs test according to accepted guidelines** | **YES** | **NO** |
| Gives appropriate directions to the athlete | ○○○ | ○○○ |
| Asks athlete to swallow (motor) | ○○○ | ○○○ |
| Asks athlete to recognize a light touch to the pharynx, larynx (sensory) | ○○○ | ○○○ |

The psychomotor skill was performed completely and in the appropriate order       0  1  2  3  4  5

The tester had control of the subject and the situation (showed confidence)       0  1  2  3  4  5

Method of performing the skill allowed the tester the ability to determine:
severity, proper progression, and the *fit* in the overall picture (Oral)       0  1  2  3  4  5

In order for a grade of *minimum standard* to be given, the total must be ≥11       **TOTAL =**

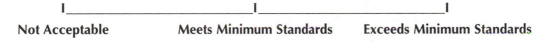

**Not Acceptable**          **Meets Minimum Standards**          **Exceeds Minimum Standards**

**L:** Laboratory/Classroom Testing
**C:** Clinical/Field Testing
**P:** Practicum Testing
**A:** Assessment/Mock Exam Testing
**S:** Self-Reporting

**Positive Finding:** Inability to complete the above tasks
**Involved Structure:** Cranial nerve #10
**Special Considerations:** Motor/sensory
**Reference(s):** Starkey et al; Konin et al
**Supplies Needed:** N/A

## SENSORY TESTING
# (SST-L-Test 1)

Peer Review _____ Peer Review _____

Skill Acquisition: _____     Practice Opportunities: _____

*This problem allows you the opportunity to demonstrate a* **Dermatome Sensory Test** *in order to rule out damage to the nerve root* **L4**. *You have 2 minutes to complete this task.*

| Tester places athlete and limb in appropriate position | YES | NO |
|---|---|---|
| Seated or prone | ○○○ | ○○○ |
| Shoes and socks off | ○○○ | ○○○ |
| **Tester performs test according to accepted guidelines** | **YES** | **NO** |
| Gives appropriate directions to the athlete | ○○○ | ○○○ |
| Explain differences in pressure | ○○○ | ○○○ |
| Demonstration given away from the injured area | ○○○ | ○○○ |
| Instructs athlete to close eyes | ○○○ | ○○○ |
| Applies varied pressure with tool or common objects: | | |
|    Sharp | ○○○ | ○○○ |
|    Dull | ○○○ | ○○○ |
|    No touch | ○○○ | ○○○ |
| Applies appropriate pressure to the medial side of the lower leg | ○○○ | ○○○ |
| Performs assessment bilaterally | ○○○ | ○○○ |

The psychomotor skill was performed completely and in the appropriate order    **0 1 2 3 4 5**

The tester had control of the subject and the situation (showed confidence)    **0 1 2 3 4 5**

Method of performing the skill allowed the tester the ability to determine:
severity, proper progression, and the *fit* in the overall picture (Oral)    **0 1 2 3 4 5**

In order for a grade of *minimum standard* to be given, the total must be ≥11     **TOTAL =**

I_____I_____I

**Not Acceptable**     **Meets Minimum Standards**     **Exceeds Minimum Standards**

**L:** Laboratory/Classroom Testing
**C:** Clinical/Field Testing
**P:** Practicum Testing
**A:** Assessment/Mock Exam Testing
**S:** Self-Reporting

**Positive Finding:** No feeling; difficulty distinguishing varied pressure
**Involved Structure:** Nerve root L4
**Special Considerations:** N/A
**Reference(s):** Hoppenfeld
**Supplies Needed:** Table/chair, sharp/dull objects

# SENSORY TESTING
## (SST-L-Test 2)

Peer Review _____ Peer Review _____

Skill Acquisition: _____    Practice Opportunities: _____

*This problem allows you the opportunity to demonstrate a **Dermatome Sensory Test** in order to rule out damage to the nerve root **L5**. You have 2 minutes to complete this task.*

| Tester places athlete and limb in appropriate position | YES | NO |
|---|---|---|
| Seated or prone | ○○○ | ○○○ |
| Shoes and socks off | ○○○ | ○○○ |
| **Tester performs test according to accepted guidelines** | **YES** | **NO** |
| Gives appropriate directions to the athlete | ○○○ | ○○○ |
| Explains differences in pressure | ○○○ | ○○○ |
| Demonstration given away from the injured area | ○○○ | ○○○ |
| Instructs athlete to close eyes | ○○○ | ○○○ |
| Applies varied pressure with tool or common objects: | | |
|   Sharp | ○○○ | ○○○ |
|   Dull | ○○○ | ○○○ |
|   No touch | ○○○ | ○○○ |
| Applies appropriate pressure to the top of the foot (and/or below the head of fibula) | ○○○ | ○○○ |
| Performs assessment bilaterally | ○○○ | ○○○ |

The psychomotor skill was performed completely and in the appropriate order    **0  1  2  3  4  5**

The tester had control of the subject and the situation (showed confidence)    **0  1  2  3  4  5**

Method of performing the skill allowed the tester the ability to determine:
severity, proper progression, and the *fit* in the overall picture (Oral)    **0  1  2  3  4  5**

In order for a grade of *minimum standard* to be given, the total must be ≥11    **TOTAL =**

I_____I_____I
**Not Acceptable**      **Meets Minimum Standards**      **Exceeds Minimum Standards**

**L:** Laboratory/Classroom Testing
**C:** Clinical/Field Testing
**P:** Practicum Testing
**A:** Assessment/Mock Exam Testing
**S:** Self-Reporting

**Positive Finding:** No feeling; difficulty distinguishing varied pressure
**Involved Structure:** Nerve root L5
**Special Considerations:** N/A
**Reference(s):** Hoppenfeld
**Supplies Needed:** Table/chair, sharp/dull objects

# SENSORY TESTING
# (SST-L-Test 3)

Peer Review _____  Peer Review _____

Skill Acquisition: _____    Practice Opportunities: _____

*This problem allows you the opportunity to demonstrate a* **Dermatome Sensory Test** *in order to rule out damage to the nerve root* **S1**. *You have 2 minutes to complete this task.*

| Tester places athlete and limb in appropriate position | YES | NO |
|---|---|---|
| Seated or prone | OOO | OOO |
| Shoes and socks off | OOO | OOO |
| **Tester performs test according to accepted guidelines** | **YES** | **NO** |
| Gives appropriate directions to the athlete | OOO | OOO |
| Explains differences in pressure | OOO | OOO |
| Demonstration given away from the injured area | OOO | OOO |
| Instructs athlete to close eyes | OOO | OOO |
| Applies varied pressure with tool or common objects: | | |
|   Sharp | OOO | OOO |
|   Dull | OOO | OOO |
|   No touch | OOO | OOO |
| Applies appropriate pressure to the lateral malleolus and/or fifth metatarsal | OOO | OOO |
| Performs assessment bilaterally | OOO | OOO |

The psychomotor skill was performed completely and in the appropriate order    **0  1  2  3  4  5**

The tester had control of the subject and the situation (showed confidence)    **0  1  2  3  4  5**

Method of performing the skill allowed the tester the ability to determine:
severity, proper progression, and the *fit* in the overall picture (Oral)    **0  1  2  3  4  5**

In order for a grade of *minimum standard* to be given, the total must be ≥11    **TOTAL =**

I_____I_____I

**Not Acceptable**          **Meets Minimum Standards**          **Exceeds Minimum Standards**

**L:** Laboratory/Classroom Testing
**C:** Clinical/Field Testing
**P:** Practicum Testing
**A:** Assessment/Mock Exam Testing
**S:** Self-Reporting

**Positive Finding:** No feeling; difficulty distinguishing varied pressure
**Involved Structure:** Nerve root S1
**Special Considerations:** N/A
**Reference(s):** Hoppenfeld
**Supplies Needed:** Table/chair, sharp/dull objects

# SENSORY TESTING
# (SST-L-Test 4)

Peer Review _____ Peer Review _____

Skill Acquisition: _____    Practice Opportunities: _____

*This problem allows you the opportunity to demonstrate a* **Dermatome Sensory Test** *in order to rule out damage to the nerve root* **L3**. *You have 2 minutes to complete this task.*

| Tester places athlete and limb in appropriate position | YES | NO |
|---|---|---|
| Seated or prone | ○○○ | ○○○ |
| **Tester performs test according to accepted guidelines** | **YES** | **NO** |
| Gives appropriate directions to the athlete | ○○○ | ○○○ |
| Explains differences in pressure | ○○○ | ○○○ |
| Demonstration given away from the injured area | ○○○ | ○○○ |
| Instructs athlete to close eyes | ○○○ | ○○○ |
| Applies varied pressure with tool or common objects: | | |
|   Sharp | ○○○ | ○○○ |
|   Dull | ○○○ | ○○○ |
|   No touch | ○○○ | ○○○ |
| Applies appropriate pressure to the area just above the superior pole of the patella | ○○○ | ○○○ |
| Performs assessment bilaterally | ○○○ | ○○○ |

The psychomotor skill was performed completely and in the appropriate order    **0  1  2  3  4  5**

The tester had control of the subject and the situation (showed confidence)    **0  1  2  3  4  5**

Method of performing the skill allowed the tester the ability to determine:
severity, proper progression, and the *fit* in the overall picture (Oral)    **0  1  2  3  4  5**

In order for a grade of *minimum standard* to be given, the total must be ≥11    **TOTAL =**

I_____I_____I
**Not Acceptable**          **Meets Minimum Standards**          **Exceeds Minimum Standards**

**L:** Laboratory/Classroom Testing
**C:** Clinical/Field Testing
**P:** Practicum Testing
**A:** Assessment/Mock Exam Testing
**S:** Self-Reporting

**Positive Finding:** No feeling; difficulty in distinguishing varied pressure
**Involved Structure:** Nerve root L3
**Special Considerations:** N/A
**Reference(s):** Magee
**Supplies Needed:** Table/chair, sharp/dull objects

## SENSORY TESTING
# (SST-L-Test 5)

Peer Review _____ Peer Review _____

Skill Acquisition: _____     Practice Opportunities: _____

*This problem allows you the opportunity to demonstrate a* **Dermatome Sensory Test** *in order to rule out damage to the nerve root* **L2**. *You have 2 minutes to complete this task.*

| Tester places athlete and limb in appropriate position | YES | NO |
|---|---|---|
| Seated or prone | ○○○ | ○○○ |
| **Tester performs test according to accepted guidelines** | **YES** | **NO** |
| Gives appropriate directions to the athlete | ○○○ | ○○○ |
| Explains differences in pressure | ○○○ | ○○○ |
| Demonstration given away from the injured area | ○○○ | ○○○ |
| Instructs athlete to close eyes | ○○○ | ○○○ |
| Applies varied pressure with tool or common objects: | | |
|   Sharp | ○○○ | ○○○ |
|   Dull | ○○○ | ○○○ |
|   No touch | ○○○ | ○○○ |
| Applies appropriate pressure to the area of the mid thigh (middle quadriceps) | ○○○ | ○○○ |
| Performs assessment bilaterally | ○○○ | ○○○ |

The psychomotor skill was performed completely and in the appropriate order    **0  1  2  3  4  5**

The tester had control of the subject and the situation (showed confidence)    **0  1  2  3  4  5**

Method of performing the skill allowed the tester the ability to determine:
severity, proper progression, and the *fit* in the overall picture (Oral)    **0  1  2  3  4  5**

In order for a grade of *minimum standard* to be given, the total must be ≥11    **TOTAL =**

I_____I_____I

**Not Acceptable**　　　　　**Meets Minimum Standards**　　　**Exceeds Minimum Standards**

**L:** Laboratory/Classroom Testing
**C:** Clinical/Field Testing
**P:** Practicum Testing
**A:** Assessment/Mock Exam Testing
**S:** Self-Reporting

**Positive Finding:** No feeling; difficulty distinguishing varied pressure
**Involved Structure:** Nerve root L2
**Special Considerations:** N/A
**Reference(s):** Magee
**Supplies Needed:** Table/chair, sharp/dull objects

# SENSORY TESTING
# (SST-L-Test 6)

Skill Acquisition: _____    Practice Opportunities: _____

*This problem allows you the opportunity to demonstrate a **Dermatome Sensory Test** in order to rule out damage to the nerve root **S2**. You have 2 minutes to complete this task.*

| Tester places athlete and limb in appropriate position | YES | NO |
|---|---|---|
| Seated or prone | ○○○ | ○○○ |
| **Tester performs test according to accepted guidelines** | **YES** | **NO** |
| Gives appropriate directions to the athlete | ○○○ | ○○○ |
| Explains differences in pressure | ○○○ | ○○○ |
| Demonstration given away from the injured area | ○○○ | ○○○ |
| Instructs athlete to close eyes | ○○○ | ○○○ |
| Applies varied pressure with tool or common objects: | | |
|   Sharp | ○○○ | ○○○ |
|   Dull | ○○○ | ○○○ |
|   No touch | ○○○ | ○○○ |
| Applies appropriate pressure to the area in and around the popliteal fossa (posterior knee) | ○○○ | ○○○ |
| Performs assessment bilaterally | ○○○ | ○○○ |

| | | |
|---|---|---|
| The psychomotor skill was performed completely and in the appropriate order | | 0  1  2  3  4  5 |
| The tester had control of the subject and the situation (showed confidence) | | 0  1  2  3  4  5 |
| Method of performing the skill allowed the tester the ability to determine: severity, proper progression, and the *fit* in the overall picture (Oral) | | 0  1  2  3  4  5 |

In order for a grade of *minimum standard* to be given, the total must be ≥11     **TOTAL =**

I_____I_____I
**Not Acceptable**        **Meets Minimum Standards**        **Exceeds Minimum Standards**

**L:** Laboratory/Classroom Testing
**C:** Clinical/Field Testing
**P:** Practicum Testing
**A:** Assessment/Mock Exam Testing
**S:** Self-Reporting

**Positive Finding:** No feeling; difficulty distinguishing varied pressure
**Involved Structure:** Nerve root S2
**Special Considerations:** N/A
**Reference(s):** Magee
**Supplies Needed:** Table/chair, sharp/dull objects

# Sensory Testing
# (SST-L-Test 7)

Peer Review _____ Peer Review _____

Skill Acquisition: _____    Practice Opportunities: _____

*This problem allows you the opportunity to demonstrate a **Dermatome Sensory Test** in order to rule out damage to the nerve root **L1**. You have 2 minutes to complete this task.*

| Tester places athlete and limb in appropriate position | YES | NO |
|---|---|---|
| Seated or prone | ○○○ | ○○○ |
| **Tester performs test according to accepted guidelines** | **YES** | **NO** |
| Gives appropriate directions to the athlete | ○○○ | ○○○ |
| Explains differences in pressure | ○○○ | ○○○ |
| Demonstration given away from the injured area | ○○○ | ○○○ |
| Instructs athlete to close eyes | ○○○ | ○○○ |
| Applies varied pressure with tool or common objects: | | |
| Sharp | ○○○ | ○○○ |
| Dull | ○○○ | ○○○ |
| No touch | ○○○ | ○○○ |
| Applies appropriate pressure to the area just below the inguinal ligament (upper anterior thigh) | ○○○ | ○○○ |
| Performs assessment bilaterally | ○○○ | ○○○ |

The psychomotor skill was performed completely and in the appropriate order    0 1 2 3 4 5

The tester had control of the subject and the situation (showed confidence)    0 1 2 3 4 5

Method of performing the skill allowed the tester the ability to determine:
severity, proper progression, and the *fit* in the overall picture (Oral)    0 1 2 3 4 5

In order for a grade of *minimum standard* to be given, the total must be ≥11    TOTAL =

I_____I_____I

**Not Acceptable**    **Meets Minimum Standards**    **Exceeds Minimum Standards**

**L:** Laboratory/Classroom Testing
**C:** Clinical/Field Testing
**P:** Practicum Testing
**A:** Assessment/Mock Exam Testing
**S:** Self-Reporting

**Positive Finding:** No feeling; difficulty distinguishing varied pressure
**Involved Structure:** Nerve root L1
**Special Considerations:** N/A
**Reference(s):** Hoppenfeld
**Supplies Needed:** Table/chair, sharp/dull objects

# SENSORY TESTING
# (SST-L-Test 8)

Skill Acquisition: _____    Practice Opportunities: _____

*This problem allows you the opportunity to demonstrate a* **Dermatome Sensory Test** *in order to rule out damage to the nerve root* **T12**. *You have 2 minutes to complete this task.*

| Tester places athlete and limb in appropriate position | YES | NO |
|---|---|---|
| Seated or prone | ○○○ | ○○○ |
| **Tester performs test according to accepted guidelines** | **YES** | **NO** |
| Gives appropriate directions to the athlete | ○○○ | ○○○ |
| Explains differences in pressure | ○○○ | ○○○ |
| Demonstration given away from the injured area | ○○○ | ○○○ |
| Instructs athlete to close eyes | ○○○ | ○○○ |
| Applies varied pressure with tool or common objects: | | |
|   Sharp | ○○○ | ○○○ |
|   Dull | ○○○ | ○○○ |
|   No touch | ○○○ | ○○○ |
| Applies appropriate pressure to the area just above the inguinal ligament | ○○○ | ○○○ |
| Performs assessment bilaterally | ○○○ | ○○○ |

The psychomotor skill was performed completely and in the appropriate order    0 1 2 3 4 5

The tester had control of the subject and the situation (showed confidence)    0 1 2 3 4 5

Method of performing the skill allowed the tester the ability to determine:
severity, proper progression, and the *fit* in the overall picture (Oral)    0 1 2 3 4 5

In order for a grade of *minimum standard* to be given, the total must be ≥11    **TOTAL =**

I_____I_____I

**Not Acceptable**　　**Meets Minimum Standards**　　**Exceeds Minimum Standards**

**L:** Laboratory/Classroom Testing
**C:** Clinical/Field Testing
**P:** Practicum Testing
**A:** Assessment/Mock Exam Testing
**S:** Self-Reporting

**Positive Finding:** No feeling; difficulty distinguishing varied pressure
**Involved Structure:** Nerve root T12
**Special Considerations:** N/A
**Reference(s):** Magee
**Supplies Needed:** Table/chair, sharp/dull objects

# SPECIAL TESTS

# SPECIAL TESTS
# (ST-U-Test 1)

Peer Review _____ Peer Review _____

Skill Acquisition: _____    Practice Opportunities: _____

*Please demonstrate how you would perform the orthopedic test known as the **Adson's Maneuver** to help rule out the condition known as thoracic outlet syndrome. You have 2 minutes to complete this task.*

| Tester places athlete and limb in appropriate position | YES | NO |
|---|---|---|
| Seated or standing | OOO | OOO |
| Arm at the side (approximately 30 degrees abduction) | OOO | OOO |
| Externally rotate the shoulder (thumb pointing upward) | OOO | OOO |
| Extend the shoulder and elbow | OOO | OOO |
| **Tester placed in proper position** | **YES** | **NO** |
| Stands behind and to the side of the athlete | OOO | OOO |
| Places two fingers over the radial pulse | OOO | OOO |
| **Tester performs test according to accepted guidelines** | **YES** | **NO** |
| Asks the athlete to extend and laterally rotate the head to the involved side | OOO | OOO |
| Asks the athlete to take a deep breath | OOO | OOO |
| Asks the athlete to hold it | OOO | OOO |
| Performs assessment bilaterally | OOO | OOO |

The psychomotor skill was performed completely and in the appropriate order    0 1 2 3 4 5

The tester had control of the subject and the situation (showed confidence)    0 1 2 3 4 5

Method of performing the skill allowed the tester the ability to determine:
severity, proper progression, and the *fit* in the overall picture (Oral)    0 1 2 3 4 5

In order for a grade of *minimum standard* to be given, the total must be ≥11    **TOTAL =**

I_____I_____I

**Not Acceptable**    **Meets Minimum Standards**    **Exceeds Minimum Standards**

**L:** Laboratory/Classroom Testing
**C:** Clinical/Field Testing
**P:** Practicum Testing
**A:** Assessment/Mock Exam Testing
**S:** Self-Reporting

**Positive Finding:** Disappearance of the radial pulse
**Involved Structure:** Subclavian artery (indicitive of thoracic outlet syndrome)
**Special Considerations:** N/A
**Reference(s):** Konin et al; Starkey et al; Magee
**Supplies Needed:** N/A

## SPECIAL TESTS
# (ST-U-Test 2)

Peer Review _____ Peer Review _____

Skill Acquisition: _____    Practice Opportunities: _____

*Please demonstrate how you would perform the orthopedic test known as the* **Empty Can Test (Supraspinatus Test)** *for the shoulder. You have 2 minutes to complete this task.*

| Tester places athlete and limb in appropriate position | YES | NO |
|---|---|---|
| Standing or seated | ○○○ | ○○○ |
| Shoulder abducted to 90 degrees | ○○○ | ○○○ |
| Horizontally flex shoulder to approximately 30 degrees | ○○○ | ○○○ |
| Internally rotate shoulder thumb pointing toward the floor (ending position is similar to draining a can) | ○○○ | ○○○ |
| **Tester placed in proper position** | **YES** | **NO** |
| Stands, facing the athlete | ○○○ | ○○○ |
| Places hand on the distal portion of the forearm | ○○○ | ○○○ |
| **Tester performs test according to accepted guidelines** | **YES** | **NO** |
| Directs athlete to hold arms in this position | ○○○ | ○○○ |
| Applies downward pressure (resist abduction) | ○○○ | ○○○ |
| Performs assessment bilaterally (both shoulders may be tested at the same time) | ○○○ | ○○○ |

The psychomotor skill was performed completely and in the appropriate order    **0  1  2  3  4  5**

The tester had control of the subject and the situation (showed confidence)    **0  1  2  3  4  5**

Method of performing the skill allowed the tester the ability to determine: severity, proper progression, and the *fit* in the overall picture (Oral)    **0  1  2  3  4  5**

In order for a grade of *minimum standard* to be given, the total must be ≥11    **TOTAL =**

I_____I_____I
**Not Acceptable**      **Meets Minimum Standards**   **Exceeds Minimum Standards**

**L:** Laboratory/Classroom Testing
**C:** Clinical/Field Testing
**P:** Practicum Testing
**A:** Assessment/Mock Exam Testing
**S:** Self-Reporting

**Positive Finding:** Pain and/or weakness
**Involved Structure:** Supraspinatus, suprascapular nerve
**Special Considerations:** N/A
**Reference(s):** Konin et al; Magee; Starkey et al
**Supplies Needed:** N/A

## SPECIAL TESTS
# (ST-U-Test 3)

Peer Review _____    Peer Review _____

Skill Acquisition: _____        Practice Opportunities: _____

*Please demonstrate how you would perform the orthopedic test known as* **Ludington's Test** *for the shoulder. You have 2 minutes to complete this task.*

| Tester places athlete and limb in appropriate position | YES | NO |
|---|---|---|
| Standing or seated | ○○○ | ○○○ |
| Athlete clasps both hands (with fingers interlocked) behind or on top of the head | ○○○ | ○○○ |
| **Tester placed in proper position** | **YES** | **NO** |
| Stands directly behind the athlete | ○○○ | ○○○ |
| Places fingers over the biceps tendon long head (bicipital groove) | ○○○ | ○○○ |
| **Tester performs test according to accepted guidelines** | **YES** | **NO** |
| Asks the athlete to alternately contract biceps (contract/relax) | ○○○ | ○○○ |
| Palpation of the biceps tendon occurs during the contraction phase | ○○○ | ○○○ |

The psychomotor skill was performed completely and in the appropriate order      0  1  2  3  4  5

The tester had control of the subject and the situation (showed confidence)      0  1  2  3  4  5

Method of performing the skill allowed the tester the ability to determine:
severity, proper progression, and the *fit* in the overall picture (Oral)      0  1  2  3  4  5

In order for a grade of *minimum standard* to be given, the total must be ≥11         **TOTAL =**

I_____I_____I
**Not Acceptable**         **Meets Minimum Standards**      **Exceeds Minimum Standards**

**L:** Laboratory/Classroom Testing
**C:** Clinical/Field Testing
**P:** Practicum Testing
**A:** Assessment/Mock Exam Testing
**S:** Self-Reporting

**Positive Finding:** Pain and/or inability to feel the biceps tendon during contraction
**Involved Structure:** Biceps
**Special Considerations:** N/A
**Reference(s):** Magee; Starkey et al
**Supplies Needed:** N/A

## Special tests
# (ST-U-Test 4)

Peer Review _____ Peer Review _____

Skill Acquisition: _____    Practice Opportunities: _____

*Please demonstrate how you would perform the orthopedic test known as the* **Military Brace Position (Costoclavicular Syndrome Test)** *for the shoulder. You have 2 minutes to complete this task.*

| Tester places athlete and limb in appropriate position | YES | NO |
|---|---|---|
| Seated or standing | ○○○ | ○○○ |
| Arms to the side (relaxed posture) | ○○○ | ○○○ |
| **Tester placed in proper position** | **YES** | **NO** |
| Stands directly behind the athlete | ○○○ | ○○○ |
| Palpates the radial pulse | ○○○ | ○○○ |
| **Tester performs test according to accepted guidelines** | **YES** | **NO** |
| Depresses and retracts the scapula | ○○○ | ○○○ |
| Extends and abducts the shoulder approximately 30 degrees | ○○○ | ○○○ |
| Hyperextends the head | ○○○ | ○○○ |
| Performs assessment bilaterally | ○○○ | ○○○ |

The psychomotor skill was performed completely and in the appropriate order       **0  1  2  3  4  5**

The tester had control of the subject and the situation (showed confidence)       **0  1  2  3  4  5**

Method of performing the skill allowed the tester the ability to determine:
severity, proper progression, and the *fit* in the overall picture (Oral)       **0  1  2  3  4  5**

In order for a grade of *minimum standard* to be given, the total must be ≥11       **TOTAL =**

I_____I_____I
**Not Acceptable**       **Meets Minimum Standards**       **Exceeds Minimum Standards**

**L:** Laboratory/Classroom Testing
**C:** Clinical/Field Testing
**P:** Practicum Testing
**A:** Assessment/Mock Exam Testing
**S:** Self-Reporting

**Positive Finding:** Absence of a radial pulse
**Involved Structure:** Subclavian artery, thoracic outlet syndrome
**Special Considerations:** N/A
**Reference(s):** Starkey et al; Magee
**Supplies Needed:** N/A

## SPECIAL TESTS
# (ST-U-Test 5)

Peer Review _____ Peer Review _____

Skill Acquisition: _____     Practice Opportunities: _____

*Please demonstrate how you would perform the orthopedic test known as the* **Roos Test (Elevated Arm Stress Test)**. *You have 4 minutes to complete this task.*

| Tester places athlete and limb in appropriate position | YES | NO |
|---|---|---|
| Standing | ○○○ | ○○○ |
| Shoulder abducted to 90 degrees | ○○○ | ○○○ |
| Shoulder externally rotated to 90 degrees | ○○○ | ○○○ |
| Elbow flexed to 45 degrees | ○○○ | ○○○ |
| **Tester placed in proper position** | **YES** | **NO** |
| Facing the athlete (observing only) | ○○○ | ○○○ |
| **Tester performs test according to accepted guidelines** | **YES** | **NO** |
| Instructs the athlete to continually open and close hand (make fist, then release) | ○○○ | ○○○ |
| Instructs the athlete to maintain this position for 3 minutes | ○○○ | ○○○ |

The psychomotor skill was performed completely and in the appropriate order    **0  1  2  3  4  5**

The tester had control of the subject and the situation (showed confidence)    **0  1  2  3  4  5**

Method of performing the skill allowed the tester the ability to determine:
severity, proper progression, and the *fit* in the overall picture (Oral)    **0  1  2  3  4  5**

In order for a grade of *minimum standard* to be given, the total must be ≥11    **TOTAL =**

I_____I_____I

**Not Acceptable**     **Meets Minimum Standards**     **Exceeds Minimum Standards**

**L:** Laboratory/Classroom Testing
**C:** Clinical/Field Testing
**P:** Practicum Testing
**A:** Assessment/Mock Exam Testing
**S:** Self-Reporting

**Positive Finding:** Ischemic pain; heaviness and/or weakness
**Involved Structure:** Subclavian artery (indicitive of thoracic outlet syndrome)
**Special Considerations:** N/A
**Reference(s):** Konin et al; Magee
**Supplies Needed:** N/A

## SPECIAL TESTS
# (ST-U-Test 6)

Peer Review _____ Peer Review _____

Skill Acquisition: _____          Practice Opportunities: _____

*This problem allows you the opportunity to demonstrate the special test known as the* **Valsalva's Maneuver**. *You have 2 minutes to complete this task. Please inform the "room captain" when you have completed the task.*

| Tester places athlete and limb in appropriate position | YES | NO |
|---|---|---|
| Seated | OOO | OOO |
| **Tester placed in proper position** | **YES** | **NO** |
| Facing the athlete (observing only) | OOO | OOO |
| **Tester performs test according to accepted guidelines** | **YES** | **NO** |
| Instructs the athlete to take a deep breath and hold throughout | OOO | OOO |
| Instructs the athlete to bear down (as if having a bowel movement) | OOO | OOO |

The psychomotor skill was performed completely and in the appropriate order    **0  1  2  3  4  5**

The tester had control of the subject and the situation (showed confidence)    **0  1  2  3  4  5**

Method of performing the skill allowed the tester the ability to determine:
severity, proper progression, and the *fit* in the overall picture (Oral)    **0  1  2  3  4  5**

In order for a grade of *minimum standard* to be given, the total must be ≥11          **TOTAL =**

I_____I_____I

**Not Acceptable**          **Meets Minimum Standards**     **Exceeds Minimum Standards**

**L:** Laboratory/Classroom Testing
**C:** Clinical/Field Testing
**P:** Practicum Testing
**A:** Assessment/Mock Exam Testing
**S:** Self-Reporting

**Positive Finding:** Increased pain
**Involved Structure:** Possible disc, tumor (space-occupying lesion)
**Special Considerations:** Results are subjective
**Reference(s):** Konin et al; Starkey et al; Magee
**Supplies Needed:** Chair

## SPECIAL TESTS
# (ST-U-Test 7)

Peer Review _____ Peer Review _____

Skill Acquisition: _____    Practice Opportunities: _____

*Please demonstrate how you would perform the orthopedic test known as the* **Speed's Test (Biceps or Straight-Arm Test)** *for the shoulder. You have 2 minutes to complete this task.*

| | YES | NO |
|---|---|---|
| **Tester places athlete and limb in appropriate position** | YES | NO |
| Seated or standing | OOO | OOO |
| Shoulder/elbow placed in anatomical position | OOO | OOO |
| **Tester placed in proper position** | YES | NO |
| Stands to the side, facing the athlete | OOO | OOO |
| Places one finger on the bicipital groove | OOO | OOO |
| Places the other hand on the distal portion of the wrist | OOO | OOO |
| **Tester performs test according to accepted guidelines** | YES | NO |
| Resists flexion of the shoulder to 90 degrees | OOO | OOO |
| Palpates the biceps tendon (bicipital groove) | OOO | OOO |
| Performs break test (90 degrees of shoulder flexion) | OOO | OOO |
| Performs assessment bilaterally | OOO | OOO |

The psychomotor skill was performed completely and in the appropriate order    **0  1  2  3  4  5**

The tester had control of the subject and the situation (showed confidence)    **0  1  2  3  4  5**

Method of performing the skill allowed the tester the ability to determine:
severity, proper progression, and the *fit* in the overall picture (Oral)    **0  1  2  3  4  5**

In order for a grade of *minimum standard* to be given, the total must be ≥11    **TOTAL =**

I_____I_____I

**Not Acceptable**        **Meets Minimum Standards**    **Exceeds Minimum Standards**

**L:** Laboratory/Classroom Testing
**C:** Clinical/Field Testing
**P:** Practicum Testing
**A:** Assessment/Mock Exam Testing
**S:** Self-Reporting

**Positive Finding:** Pain/tenderness (bicipital groove)
**Involved Structure:** Long head of the biceps brachii
**Special Considerations:** N/A
**Reference(s):** Konin et al; Starkey et al; Magee
**Supplies Needed:** N/A

## SPECIAL TESTS
# (ST-U-Test 8)

Peer Review _____ Peer Review _____

Skill Acquisition: _____    Practice Opportunities: _____

*Please demonstrate how you would perform the orthopedic test known as the **Yergason's Test** for the shoulder. You have 2 minutes to complete this task.*

| Tester places athlete and limb in appropriate position | YES | NO |
|---|---|---|
| Seated or standing | ○○○ | ○○○ |
| Elbow flexed to 90 degrees (stabilized against the side of the body) | ○○○ | ○○○ |
| Forearm fully pronated | ○○○ | ○○○ |
| **Tester placed in proper position** | **YES** | **NO** |
| Stands to the side, facing the athlete | ○○○ | ○○○ |
| Places one finger over the bicipital groove | ○○○ | ○○○ |
| Places the other hand around the distal portion of the wrist | ○○○ | ○○○ |
| **Tester performs test according to accepted guidelines** | **YES** | **NO** |
| Resists supination of the forearm through full range of motion | ○○○ | ○○○ |
| Resists external rotation of the shoulder through full range of motion | ○○○ | ○○○ |
| Palpates the biceps tendon bicipital groove (gently) | ○○○ | ○○○ |
| Performs assessment bilaterally | ○○○ | ○○○ |

The psychomotor skill was performed completely and in the appropriate order    0  1  2  3  4  5

The tester had control of the subject and the situation (showed confidence)    0  1  2  3  4  5

Method of performing the skill allowed the tester the ability to determine:
severity, proper progression, and the *fit* in the overall picture (Oral)    0  1  2  3  4  5

In order for a grade of *minimum standard* to be given, the total must be ≥11    **TOTAL =**

I_____I_____I
**Not Acceptable**     **Meets Minimum Standards**     **Exceeds Minimum Standards**

**L:** Laboratory/Classroom Testing
**C:** Clinical/Field Testing
**P:** Practicum Testing
**A:** Assessment/Mock Exam Testing
**S:** Self-Reporting

**Positive Finding:** Pain and/or snapping; biceps tendon popping out of the bicipital groove
**Involved Structure:** Biceps tendon, transverse humeral ligament
**Special Considerations:** N/A
**Reference(s):** Konin et al; Hoppenfeld; Magee; Starkey et al
**Supplies Needed:** Chair

# SPECIAL TESTS
# (ST-U-Test 9)

*This problem allows you the opportunity to demonstrate the* **Hawkins-Kennedy Test for Impingement** *of the shoulder. You have 2 minutes to complete this task.*

| Tester places athlete and limb in appropriate position | YES | NO |
|---|---|---|
| Seated or standing | ooo | ooo |
| Shoulder horizontally flexed to 90 degrees (forward flexion) | ooo | ooo |
| Elbow flexed to 90 degrees | ooo | ooo |
| Forearm fully pronated (palm facing the floor) | ooo | ooo |
| **Tester placed in proper position** | **YES** | **NO** |
| Stands in front, facing the athlete | ooo | ooo |
| Places one hand under the elbow | ooo | ooo |
| Places the other hand over the distal portion of the wrist | ooo | ooo |
| **Tester performs test according to accepted guidelines** | **YES** | **NO** |
| Maintains relaxation of the limb | ooo | ooo |
| Maintains horizontally flexed position (may move into a greater forward flexed position) | ooo | ooo |
| Passively, internally rotates the shoulder | ooo | ooo |
| Performs assessment bilaterally | ooo | ooo |

The psychomotor skill was performed completely and in the appropriate order    0  1  2  3  4  5

The tester had control of the subject and the situation (showed confidence)    0  1  2  3  4  5

Method of performing the skill allowed the tester the ability to determine:
severity, proper progression, and the *fit* in the overall picture (Oral)    0  1  2  3  4  5

In order for a grade of *minimum standard* to be given, the total must be ≥11    TOTAL =

I_____I_____I
**Not Acceptable**    **Meets Minimum Standards**    **Exceeds Minimum Standards**

**L:** Laboratory/Classroom Testing
**C:** Clinical/Field Testing
**P:** Practicum Testing
**A:** Assessment/Mock Exam Testing
**S:** Self-Reporting

**Positive Finding:** Pain
**Involved Structure:** Supraspinatus tendon
**Special Considerations:** N/A
**Reference(s):** Konin et al; Magee; Starkey et al
**Supplies Needed:** N/A

## SPECIAL TESTS
# (ST-U-Test 10)

Peer Review _____ Peer Review _____

Skill Acquisition: _____    Practice Opportunities: _____

*This problem allows you the opportunity to demonstrate the* **Neer Impingement Test (Shoulder Impingement Test)** *of the shoulder. You have 2 minutes to complete this task.*

| Tester places athlete and limb in appropriate position | YES | NO |
|---|---|---|
| Standing or seated | ○○○ | ○○○ |
| Arms placed at athlete's side | ○○○ | ○○○ |
| Shoulder internally rotated, elbow pronated | ○○○ | ○○○ |
| **Tester placed in proper position** | **YES** | **NO** |
| Stands to the side, facing the athlete | ○○○ | ○○○ |
| Places one hand against the scapula | ○○○ | ○○○ |
| Places the other hand under the elbow (supporting the arm) | ○○○ | ○○○ |
| **Tester performs test according to accepted guidelines** | **YES** | **NO** |
| Maintains relaxation of the limb | ○○○ | ○○○ |
| Pushes/jams the greater tuberosity into the border of the acromion | ○○○ | ○○○ |
| Passively flexes the shoulder through a full range of motion | ○○○ | ○○○ |
| Performs assessment bilaterally | ○○○ | ○○○ |

The psychomotor skill was performed completely and in the appropriate order    **0 1 2 3 4 5**

The tester had control of the subject and the situation (showed confidence)    **0 1 2 3 4 5**

Method of performing the skill allowed the tester the ability to determine:
severity, proper progression, and the *fit* in the overall picture (Oral)    **0 1 2 3 4 5**

In order for a grade of *minimum standard* to be given, the total must be ≥11    **TOTAL =**

I_____I_____I

**Not Acceptable**        **Meets Minimum Standards**    **Exceeds Minimum Standards**

**L:** Laboratory/Classroom Testing
**C:** Clinical/Field Testing
**P:** Practicum Testing
**A:** Assessment/Mock Exam Testing
**S:** Self-Reporting

**Positive Finding:** Pain with movement
**Involved Structure:** Supraspinatus; biceps long head tendon
**Special Considerations:** N/A
**Reference(s):** Konin et al; Magee; Starkey et al
**Supplies Needed:** N/A

## SPECIAL TESTS
# (ST-U-Test 11)

Peer Review _____  Peer Review _____

Skill Acquisition: _____    Practice Opportunities: _____

*This problem allows you the opportunity to demonstrate the* **Drop Arm Test (Codman's Test)** *to help rule out rotator cuff pathology. You have 2 minutes to complete this task.*

| Tester places athlete and limb in appropriate position | YES | NO |
|---|---|---|
| Seated or standing | OOO | OOO |
| Arms placed at athlete's side | OOO | OOO |
| Shoulder internally rotated, elbow pronated | OOO | OOO |
| **Tester placed in proper position** | **YES** | **NO** |
| Stands in front, facing the athlete (may stand behind the athlete) | OOO | OOO |
| Places one hand under the wrist | OOO | OOO |
| **Tester performs test according to accepted guidelines** | **YES** | **NO** |
| Passively abducts the shoulder to 90 degrees, then releases arm | OOO | OOO |
| Asks athlete to slowly lower the arm to the side (adduction) | OOO | OOO |
| Performs assessment bilaterally | OOO | OOO |

| | |
|---|---|
| The psychomotor skill was performed completely and in the appropriate order | 0  1  2  3  4  5 |
| The tester had control of the subject and the situation (showed confidence) | 0  1  2  3  4  5 |
| Method of performing the skill allowed the tester the ability to determine: severity, proper progression, and the *fit* in the overall picture (Oral) | 0  1  2  3  4  5 |

In order for a grade of *minimum standard* to be given, the total must be ≥11         **TOTAL =**

I_____I_____I

**Not Acceptable**      **Meets Minimum Standards**      **Exceeds Minimum Standards**

**L:**  Laboratory/Classroom Testing
**C:**  Clinical/Field Testing
**P:**  Practicum Testing
**A:**  Assessment/Mock Exam Testing
**S:**  Self-Reporting

**Positive Finding:** Inability to slowly return the arm to the side
**Involved Structure:** Rotator cuff
**Special Considerations:** N/A
**Reference(s):** Konin et al; Magee; Starkey et al
**Supplies Needed:** N/A

## Special tests
# (ST-U-Test 12)

Peer Review _____ Peer Review _____

Skill Acquisition: _____    Practice Opportunities: _____

*This problem allows you the opportunity to demonstrate the **Pectoralis Major Contracture Test** in order to determine muscle flexibility. You have 2 minutes to complete this task.*

| Tester places athlete and limb in appropriate position | YES | NO |
|---|---|---|
| Supine | ○○○ | ○○○ |
| Athletes clasps both hands behind the head fingers interlocked | ○○○ | ○○○ |
| **Tester placed in proper position** | **YES** | **NO** |
| Stands behind the athlete's head | ○○○ | ○○○ |
| **Tester performs test according to accepted guidelines** | **YES** | **NO** |
| Asks the athlete to relax arms | ○○○ | ○○○ |
| Passively forces the elbows to the table (hyperextension of the shoulder) | ○○○ | ○○○ |

The psychomotor skill was performed completely and in the appropriate order    0 1 2 3 4 5

The tester had control of the subject and the situation (showed confidence)    0 1 2 3 4 5

Method of performing the skill allowed the tester the ability to determine:
severity, proper progression, and the *fit* in the overall picture (Oral)    0 1 2 3 4 5

In order for a grade of *minimum standard* to be given, the total must be ≥11    TOTAL =

I_____I_____I
**Not Acceptable**        **Meets Minimum Standards**        **Exceeds Minimum Standards**

**L:** Laboratory/Classroom Testing
**C:** Clinical/Field Testing
**P:** Practicum Testing
**A:** Assessment/Mock Exam Testing
**S:** Self-Reporting

**Positive Finding:** Elbows unable to touch the table
**Involved Structure:** Pectoralis major
**Special Considerations:** N/A
**Reference(s):** Magee
**Supplies Needed:** Table

# SPECIAL TESTS
# (ST-U-Test 13)

Peer Review _____ Peer Review _____

Skill Acquisition: _____    Practice Opportunities: _____

*This problem allows you the opportunity to demonstrate* **Apley's Scratch Tests** *in order to determine general shoulder flexibility. You have 2 minutes to complete this task.*

| Tester places athlete and limb in appropriate position | YES | NO |
|---|---|---|
| Seated or standing | ○○○ | ○○○ |
| Arms placed at athlete's side | ○○○ | ○○○ |
| **Tester placed in proper position** | **YES** | **NO** |
| Facing the athlete (observing only) | ○○○ | ○○○ |
| **Tester performs test according to accepted guidelines** | **YES** | **NO** |
| Instructs athlete to actively take one hand and touch opposite shoulder (front) | ○○○ | ○○○ |
| Instructs athlete to actively take one hand and touch opposite shoulder (behind head) | ○○○ | ○○○ |
| Instructs athlete to actively take one hand and reach behind and touch opposite scapula | ○○○ | ○○○ |
| Performs assessment bilaterally | ○○○ | ○○○ |

The psychomotor skill was performed completely and in the appropriate order    **0  1  2  3  4  5**

The tester had control of the subject and the situation (showed confidence)    **0  1  2  3  4  5**

Method of performing the skill allowed the tester the ability to determine:
severity, proper progression, and the *fit* in the overall picture (Oral)    **0  1  2  3  4  5**

In order for a grade of *minimum standard* to be given, the total must be ≥11    **TOTAL =**

I_____I_____I
**Not Acceptable        Meets Minimum Standards    Exceeds Minimum Standards**

**L:** Laboratory/Classroom Testing
**C:** Clinical/Field Testing
**P:** Practicum Testing
**A:** Assessment/Mock Exam Testing
**S:** Self-Reporting

**Positive Finding:** Inability to touch opposite shoulder
**Involved Structure:** Structures in and around the glenohumeral joint
**Special Considerations:** N/A
**Reference(s):** Konin; Starkey et al
**Supplies Needed:** N/A

## Special tests
# (ST-U-Test 14)

Peer Review _____  Peer Review _____

Skill Acquisition: _____    Practice Opportunities: _____

*This problem allows you the opportunity to demonstrate **Allen's Test** in order to rule out thoracic outlet syndrome. You have 2 minutes to complete this task.*

| Tester places athlete and limb in appropriate position | YES | NO |
|---|---|---|
| Seated or standing | OOO | OOO |
| Shoulder abducted to 90 degrees | OOO | OOO |
| Shoulder externally rotated to 90 degrees | OOO | OOO |
| Elbow flexed to 90 degrees | OOO | OOO |
| **Tester placed in proper position** | **YES** | **NO** |
| Stands behind the athlete | OOO | OOO |
| Places fingers over the radial pulse (palpate pulse) | OOO | OOO |
| Places the other hand under the elbow (supporting the arm) | OOO | OOO |
| **Tester performs test according to accepted guidelines** | **YES** | **NO** |
| Instructs athlete to look away (laterally rotates toward opposite side) | OOO | OOO |
| Passively horizontally extends the shoulder (horizontal abduction) | OOO | OOO |
| Performs assessment bilaterally | OOO | OOO |

The psychomotor skill was performed completely and in the appropriate order        0  1  2  3  4  5

The tester had control of the subject and the situation (showed confidence)         0  1  2  3  4  5

Method of performing the skill allowed the tester the ability to determine:
severity, proper progression, and the *fit* in the overall picture (Oral)        0  1  2  3  4  5

In order for a grade of *minimum standard* to be given, the total must be ≥11        **TOTAL =**

I_____I_____I

**Not Acceptable**        **Meets Minimum Standards**    **Exceeds Minimum Standards**

**L:** Laboratory/Classroom Testing
**C:** Clinical/Field Testing
**P:** Practicum Testing
**A:** Assessment/Mock Exam Testing
**S:** Self-Reporting

**Positive Finding:** Diminished or absent pulse
**Involved Structure:** Vascular structures, thoracic outlet syndrome
**Special Considerations:** N/A
**Reference(s):** Konin et al; Magee; Starkey et al
**Supplies Needed:** N/A

## SPECIAL TESTS
# (ST-U-Test 15)

Peer Review _____ Peer Review _____

Skill Acquisition: _____    Practice Opportunities: _____

*This problem allows you the opportunity to demonstrate the* **Cozen's Test (Test for Lateral Epicondylitis/Tennis Elbow, Method 1)** *in order to help rule out lateral epicondylitis. You have 2 minutes to complete this task.*

| Tester places athlete and limb in appropriate position | YES | NO |
|---|---|---|
| Seated or standing | ○○○ | ○○○ |
| Elbow flexed to 90 degrees | ○○○ | ○○○ |
| Forearm/elbow placed in full pronation | ○○○ | ○○○ |
| Fingers flexed (make into a fist) | ○○○ | ○○○ |
| **Tester placed in proper position** | **YES** | **NO** |
| Stands in front, facing the athlete | ○○○ | ○○○ |
| Places hand around the wrist | ○○○ | ○○○ |
| Places the other hand under the elbow supporting the arm (palpating lateral epicondyle) | ○○○ | ○○○ |
| **Tester performs test according to accepted guidelines** | **YES** | **NO** |
| Resists wrist extension through a full range of motion | ○○○ | ○○○ |
| Resists radial deviation through a full range of motion | ○○○ | ○○○ |
| Performs assessment bilaterally | ○○○ | ○○○ |

The psychomotor skill was performed completely and in the appropriate order  **0  1  2  3  4  5**

The tester had control of the subject and the situation (showed confidence)  **0  1  2  3  4  5**

Method of performing the skill allowed the tester the ability to determine:
severity, proper progression, and the *fit* in the overall picture (Oral)  **0  1  2  3  4  5**

In order for a grade of *minimum standard* to be given, the total must be ≥11    **TOTAL =**

I_____I_____I
**Not Acceptable**          **Meets Minimum Standards**          **Exceeds Minimum Standards**

**L:** Laboratory/Classroom Testing
**C:** Clinical/Field Testing
**P:** Practicum Testing
**A:** Assessment/Mock Exam Testing
**S:** Self-Reporting

**Positive Finding:** Pain (sudden)
**Involved Structure:** Lateral epicondyle (epicondylitis)
**Special Considerations:** May also resist pronation
**Reference(s):** Starkey; Magee; Konin
**Supplies Needed:** N/A

## SPECIAL TESTS
# (ST-U-Test 16)

Peer Review _____    Peer Review _____

Skill Acquisition: _____    Practice Opportunities: _____

*This problem allows you the opportunity to demonstrate the* **Golfer's Elbow Test (Test for Medial Epicondylitis)** *in order to help rule out medial epicondylitis. You have 2 minutes to complete this task.*

| Tester places athlete and limb in appropriate position | YES | NO |
|---|---|---|
| Seated or standing | ○○○ | ○○○ |
| Elbow flexed to 90 degrees | ○○○ | ○○○ |
| Forearm/elbow placed in full pronation | ○○○ | ○○○ |
| Fingers flexed (make into a fist) | ○○○ | ○○○ |
| **Tester placed in proper position** | **YES** | **NO** |
| Stands in front, facing the athlete | ○○○ | ○○○ |
| Places hand around the wrist | ○○○ | ○○○ |
| Places the other hand under the elbow supporting the arm (palpating medial epicondyle) | ○○○ | ○○○ |
| **Tester performs test according to accepted guidelines** | **YES** | **NO** |
| Passively supinates the forearm through a full range of motion | ○○○ | ○○○ |
| Passively extend the elbow through a full range of motion | ○○○ | ○○○ |
| Passively extend the wrist through a full range of motion | ○○○ | ○○○ |
| Performs assessment bilaterally | ○○○ | ○○○ |

The psychomotor skill was performed completely and in the appropriate order    **0  1  2  3  4  5**

The tester had control of the subject and the situation (showed confidence)    **0  1  2  3  4  5**

Method of performing the skill allowed the tester the ability to determine:
severity, proper progression, and the *fit* in the overall picture (Oral)    **0  1  2  3  4  5**

In order for a grade of *minimum standard* to be given, the total must be ≥11    **TOTAL =**

I_____I_____I
**Not Acceptable**        **Meets Minimum Standards**        **Exceeds Minimum Standards**

**L:** Laboratory/Classroom Testing
**C:** Clinical/Field Testing
**P:** Practicum Testing
**A:** Assessment/Mock Exam Testing
**S:** Self-Reporting

**Positive Finding:** Pain
**Involved Structure:** Medial epicondyle (epicondylitis)
**Special Considerations:** N/A
**Reference(s):** Magee
**Supplies Needed:** N/A

## SPECIAL TESTS
# (ST-U-Test 17)

Peer Review _____ Peer Review _____

Skill Acquisition: _____     Practice Opportunities: _____

*Please demonstrate the* **Tinel's Sign** *in order to rule out a possible injury to the ulnar nerve (**elbow**). You have 2 minutes to complete this task.*

| Tester places athlete and limb in appropriate position | YES | NO |
|---|---|---|
| Standing or seated | OOO | OOO |
| Elbow placed in slight flexion | OOO | OOO |
| **Tester placed in proper position** | **YES** | **NO** |
| Stands in front, facing the athlete | OOO | OOO |
| Places hand around the wrist supporting the arm | OOO | OOO |
| Places the other hand against the medial aspect of the elbow | OOO | OOO |
| **Tester performs test according to accepted guidelines** | **YES** | **NO** |
| Applies pressure (tapping motion) over the ulnar nerve (between the olecranon process and medial epicondyle) | OOO | OOO |
| Performs assessment bilaterally | OOO | OOO |

The psychomotor skill was performed completely and in the appropriate order    0  1  2  3  4  5

The tester had control of the subject and the situation (showed confidence)    0  1  2  3  4  5

Method of performing the skill allowed the tester the ability to determine:
severity, proper progression, and the *fit* in the overall picture (Oral)    0  1  2  3  4  5

In order for a grade of *minimum standard* to be given, the total must be ≥11    **TOTAL =**

I_____I_____I

**Not Acceptable**    **Meets Minimum Standards**    **Exceeds Minimum Standards**

**L:** Laboratory/Classroom Testing
**C:** Clinical/Field Testing
**P:** Practicum Testing
**A:** Assessment/Mock Exam Testing
**S:** Self-Reporting

**Positive Finding:** Tingling/pain
**Involved Structure:** Ulnar nerve
**Special Considerations:** N/A
**Reference(s):** Konin et al; Magee
**Supplies Needed:** N/A

## Special tests
# (ST-U-Test 18)

Peer Review _____ Peer Review _____

Skill Acquisition: _____    Practice Opportunities: _____

*This problem allows you the opportunity to demonstrate the* **Pinch Grip Test** *in order to help rule out injury to the anterior interosseous nerve. You have 2 minutes to complete this task.*

| | YES | NO |
|---|---|---|
| **Tester places athlete and limb in appropriate position** | YES | NO |
| Seated or standing | ○○○ | ○○○ |
| **Tester placed in proper position** | YES | NO |
| Facing the athlete (observing only) | ○○○ | ○○○ |
| **Tester performs test according to accepted guidelines** | YES | NO |
| Instructs the athlete to pinch the tips of the thumb and index finger together (tip-to-tip pinch) | ○○○ | ○○○ |
| Performs assessment bilaterally | ○○○ | ○○○ |

The psychomotor skill was performed completely and in the appropriate order    **0 1 2 3 4 5**

The tester had control of the subject and the situation (showed confidence)    **0 1 2 3 4 5**

Method of performing the skill allowed the tester the ability to determine:
severity, proper progression, and the *fit* in the overall picture (Oral)    **0 1 2 3 4 5**

In order for a grade of *minimum standard* to be given, the total must be ≥11    **TOTAL =**

I_____I_____I

**Not Acceptable**        **Meets Minimum Standards**    **Exceeds Minimum Standards**

**L:** Laboratory/Classroom Testing
**C:** Clinical/Field Testing
**P:** Practicum Testing
**A:** Assessment/Mock Exam Testing
**S:** Self-Reporting

**Positive Finding:** Inability to touch tips together
**Involved Structure:** Anterior interosseous nerve
(branch of the median nerve)
**Special Considerations:** N/A
**Reference(s):** Konin et al; Magee
**Supplies Needed:** N/A

## SPECIAL TESTS
# (ST-U-Test 19)

Peer Review _____ Peer Review _____

Skill Acquisition: _____    Practice Opportunities: _____

*This problem allows you the opportunity to demonstrate **Finkelstein's Test** in order to help rule out de Quervain's disease or Hoffmann's disease. You have 2 minutes to complete this task.*

| Tester places athlete and limb in appropriate position | YES | NO |
|---|---|---|
| Standing or seated | ○○○ | ○○○ |
| Athlete is asked to form a fist around the thumb (fist with thumb inside) | ○○○ | ○○○ |
| **Tester placed in proper position** | **YES** | **NO** |
| Stands in front, facing the athlete | ○○○ | ○○○ |
| Places hand under the forearm supporting the arm | ○○○ | ○○○ |
| Places the other hand around the fist | ○○○ | ○○○ |
| **Tester performs test according to accepted guidelines** | **YES** | **NO** |
| Maintains relaxation of the involved limb | ○○○ | ○○○ |
| Passively deviates the wrist toward the ulna (ulnar deviation) | ○○○ | ○○○ |
| Performs assessment bilaterally | ○○○ | ○○○ |

The psychomotor skill was performed completely and in the appropriate order    0 1 2 3 4 5

The tester had control of the subject and the situation (showed confidence)    0 1 2 3 4 5

Method of performing the skill allowed the tester the ability to determine: severity, proper progression, and the *fit* in the overall picture (Oral)    0 1 2 3 4 5

In order for a grade of *minimum standard* to be given, the total must be ≥11    **TOTAL =**

I_____I_____I

**Not Acceptable**        **Meets Minimum Standards**    **Exceeds Minimum Standards**

**L:** Laboratory/Classroom Testing
**C:** Clinical/Field Testing
**P:** Practicum Testing
**A:** Assessment/Mock Exam Testing
**S:** Self-Reporting

**Positive Finding:** Pain
**Involved Structure:** Abductor pollicis longus, extensor pollicis brevis
**Special Considerations:** N/A
**Reference(s):** Konin et al; Starkey et al; Magee
**Supplies Needed:** N/A

## SPECIAL TESTS
# (ST-U-Test 20)

Peer Review _____ Peer Review _____

Skill Acquisition: _____    Practice Opportunities: _____

*Please demonstrate the **Tinel's Sign** in order to rule out a possible injury to the median nerve (**wrist**) such as carpal tunnel syndrome). You have 2 minutes to complete this task.*

| Tester places athlete and limb in appropriate position | YES | NO |
|---|---|---|
| Seated | ○○○ | ○○○ |
| Elbow flexed to approximately 90 degrees | ○○○ | ○○○ |
| Forearm placed in full supination (palm up) | ○○○ | ○○○ |
| Forearm resting on the table (supporting surface) | ○○○ | ○○○ |
| **Tester placed in proper position** | YES | NO |
| Sits to the involved side, facing the athlete | ○○○ | ○○○ |
| Places one hand over the middle portion of the forearm | ○○○ | ○○○ |
| Places the other hand over the carpal tunnel area | ○○○ | ○○○ |
| **Tester performs test according to accepted guidelines** | YES | NO |
| Applies pressure (tapping motion) over the carpal tunnel area (distal forearm) | ○○○ | ○○○ |
| Performs assessment bilaterally | ○○ | ○○ |

The psychomotor skill was performed completely and in the appropriate order     0  1  2  3  4  5

The tester had control of the subject and the situation (showed confidence)     0  1  2  3  4  5

Method of performing the skill allowed the tester the ability to determine:
severity, proper progression, and the *fit* in the overall picture (Oral)     0  1  2  3  4  5

In order for a grade of *minimum standard* to be given, the total must be ≥11     **TOTAL =**

I_____I_____I
**Not Acceptable**     **Meets Minimum Standards**     **Exceeds Minimum Standards**

**L:** Laboratory/Classroom Testing
**C:** Clinical/Field Testing
**P:** Practicum Testing
**A:** Assessment/Mock Exam Testing
**S:** Self-Reporting

**Positive Finding:** Tingling and pain
**Involved Structure:** Median nerve
**Special Considerations:** N/A
**Reference(s):** Konin et al; Magee
**Supplies Needed:** Chair/table

# SPECIAL TESTS
# (ST-U-Test 21)

Peer Review _____ Peer Review _____

Skill Acquisition: _____    Practice Opportunities: _____

*This problem allows you the opportunity to demonstrate **Phalen's Test (Wrist Flexion Test)** for the wrist. You have 3 minutes to perform this task.*

| Tester places athlete and limb in appropriate position | YES | NO |
|---|---|---|
| Standing or seated | OOO | OOO |
| Shoulders flexed to 90 degrees, elbows flexed to 90 degrees, wrists flexed to 90 degrees | OOO | OOO |
| Dorsal aspect of both hands are in complete contact | OOO | OOO |
| **Tester placed in proper position** | **YES** | **NO** |
| Stands in front, facing the athlete | OOO | OOO |
| Places hand around one wrist | OOO | OOO |
| Places the other hand around the other wrist | OOO | OOO |
| **Tester performs test according to accepted guidelines** | **YES** | **NO** |
| Applies steady compressive force inward (pushes wrist together) | OOO | OOO |
| Holds compression for 1 minute | OOO | OOO |

The psychomotor skill was performed completely and in the appropriate order    0 1 2 3 4 5

The tester had control of the subject and the situation (showed confidence)    0 1 2 3 4 5

Method of performing the skill allowed the tester the ability to determine:
severity, proper progression, and the *fit* in the overall picture (Oral)    0 1 2 3 4 5

In order for a grade of *minimum standard* to be given, the total must be ≥11    **TOTAL =**

I_____I_____I

**Not Acceptable**    **Meets Minimum Standards**    **Exceeds Minimum Standards**

**L:** Laboratory/Classroom Testing
**C:** Clinical/Field Testing
**P:** Practicum Testing
**A:** Assessment/Mock Exam Testing
**S:** Self-Reporting

**Positive Finding:** Tingling and/or numbness
**Involved Structure:** Median nerve, carpal tunnel syndrome
**Special Considerations:** N/A
**Reference(s):** Konin et al; Magee; Starkey et al
**Supplies Needed:** N/A

## SPECIAL TESTS
# (ST-U-Test 22)

Peer Review _____ Peer Review _____

Skill Acquisition: _____    Practice Opportunities: _____

*This problem allows you the opportunity to demonstrate the* **Foraminal Compression Test (Spurling's Test/Cervical Compression Test)** *in order to confirm pressure on a nerve root. You have 3 minutes to perform this task. Please inform the examiner when you have completed the task.*

| Tester places athlete and limb in appropriate position | YES | NO |
|---|---|---|
| Seated | OOO | OOO |
|   Stage 1: Head is placed in a neutral position (cervical compression test) | OOO | OOO |
|   Stage 2: Head is placed in a slightly extended position | OOO | OOO |
|   Stage 3: Head is place in a slightly extended position and laterally flexes to the involved side (Spurling's test) | OOO | OOO |
| **Tester placed in proper position** | **YES** | **NO** |
| Stands behind the athlete | OOO | OOO |
| Places both hands on top of the head (fingers interlocked) | OOO | OOO |
| **Tester performs test according to accepted guidelines** | **YES** | **NO** |
| Maintains relaxation of the head | OOO | OOO |
| Applies a compressive force downward: Stage 1, Stage 2, Stage 3 | OOO | OOO |

The psychomotor skill was performed completely and in the appropriate order    **0 1 2 3 4 5**

The tester had control of the subject and the situation (showed confidence)    **0 1 2 3 4 5**

Method of performing the skill allowed the tester the ability to determine:
severity, proper progression, and the *fit* in the overall picture (Oral)    **0 1 2 3 4 5**

In order for a grade of *minimum standard* to be given, the total must be ≥11    **TOTAL =**

I_____I_____I
**Not Acceptable**     **Meets Minimum Standards**     **Exceeds Minimum Standards**

**L:** Laboratory/Classroom Testing
**C:** Clinical/Field Testing
**P:** Practicum Testing
**A:** Assessment/Mock Exam Testing
**S:** Self-Reporting

**Positive Finding:** Radiating pain
**Involved Structure:** Nerve root(s)
**Special Considerations:** Several medical conditions warrant precautions when applying pressure
**Reference(s):** Konin et al; Magee; Starkey et al
**Supplies Needed:** Chair

## SPECIAL TESTS
# (ST-U-Test 23)

Peer Review _____ Peer Review _____

Skill Acquisition: _____    Practice Opportunities: _____

*This problem allows you the opportunity to demonstrate the* **Foraminal Distraction Test (Cervical Distraction Test)** *in order to confirm pressure on a nerve root. You have 2 minutes to perform this task. Please inform the examiner when you have completed the task.*

| Tester places athlete and limb in appropriate position | YES | NO |
|---|---|---|
| Seated or supine | OOO | OOO |
| **Tester placed in proper position** | **YES** | **NO** |
| Stands behind the athlete | OOO | OOO |
| Places one hand under the athlete's chin | OOO | OOO |
| Places the other hand against the base of the occiput | OOO | OOO |
| **Tester performs test according to accepted guidelines** | **YES** | **NO** |
| Maintains relaxation of the head | OOO | OOO |
| Applies a distractive force upward (slowly lifts or pulls the head) | OOO | OOO |

| | |
|---|---|
| The psychomotor skill was performed completely and in the appropriate order | 0  1  2  3  4  5 |
| The tester had control of the subject and the situation (showed confidence) | 0  1  2  3  4  5 |
| Method of performing the skill allowed the tester the ability to determine: severity, proper progression, and the *fit* in the overall picture (Oral) | 0  1  2  3  4  5 |

In order for a grade of *minimum standard* to be given, the total must be ≥11          **TOTAL =**

I_____I_____I

**Not Acceptable**          **Meets Minimum Standards**          **Exceeds Minimum Standards**

**L:** Laboratory/Classroom Testing
**C:** Clinical/Field Testing
**P:** Practicum Testing
**A:** Assessment/Mock Exam Testing
**S:** Self-Reporting

**Positive Finding:** Pain decreases
**Involved Structure:** Nerve root
**Special Considerations:** Distraction should not be performed if there are any signs of instability
**Reference(s):** Konin et al; Magee; Starkey et al
**Supplies Needed:** Chair and/or table

## SPECIAL TESTS
# (ST-U-Test 24)

Peer Review _____ Peer Review _____

Skill Acquisition: _____    Practice Opportunities: _____

*This problem allows you the opportunity to demonstrate the* **Shoulder Abduction Test** *in order to help rule out a herniated disc or nerve root compression. You have 2 minutes to complete this task. Please inform the examiner when you have completed the task.*

| | YES | NO |
|---|---|---|
| **Tester places athlete and limb in appropriate position** | **YES** | **NO** |
| Seated or standing | ○○○ | ○○○ |
| **Tester placed in proper position** | **YES** | **NO** |
| Facing the athlete (observing only) | ○○○ | ○○○ |
| **Tester performs test according to accepted guidelines** | **YES** | **NO** |
| Instructs the athlete to actively abduct the shoulder | ○○○ | ○○○ |
| Instructs the athlete to flex elbow by placing the palm of the hand on top of the head | ○○○ | ○○○ |
| Performs assessment bilaterally | ○○○ | ○○○ |

The psychomotor skill was performed completely and in the appropriate order    **0  1  2  3  4  5**

The tester had control of the subject and the situation (showed confidence)    **0  1  2  3  4  5**

Method of performing the skill allowed the tester the ability to determine:
severity, proper progression, and the *fit* in the overall picture (Oral)    **0  1  2  3  4  5**

In order for a grade of *minimum standard* to be given, the total must be ≥11    **TOTAL =**

I_____I_____I
**Not Acceptable**        **Meets Minimum Standards**    **Exceeds Minimum Standards**

**L:** Laboratory/Classroom Testing
**C:** Clinical/Field Testing
**P:** Practicum Testing
**A:** Assessment/Mock Exam Testing
**S:** Self-Reporting

**Positive Finding:** Decreased symptoms (pain)
**Involved Structure:** Nerve root/herniated disc
**Special Considerations:** N/A
**Reference(s):** Starkey et al
**Supplies Needed:** N/A

# SPECIAL TESTS
# (ST-U-Test 25)

Peer Review _____ Peer Review _____

Skill Acquisition: _____    Practice Opportunities: _____

*This problem allows you the opportunity to demonstrate the* **Brachial Plexus Tension Test (Brachial Plexus Traction Test/Shoulder Depression Test)**. *You have 2 minutes to complete this task. Please inform the examiner when you have completed the task.*

| Tester places athlete and limb in appropriate position | YES | NO |
|---|---|---|
| Standing or seated | OOO | OOO |
| **Tester placed in proper position** | **YES** | **NO** |
| Stands behind the athlete | OOO | OOO |
| Places one hand on the side of the athlete's head (involved side) | OOO | OOO |
| Places the other hand on top of the acromioclavicular joint (involved side) | OOO | OOO |
| **Tester performs test according to accepted guidelines** | **YES** | **NO** |
| Maintains relaxation of the head, neck, and shoulder area | OOO | OOO |
| Passively laterally flexes the head (away from the shoulder) | OOO | OOO |
| Depresses the shoulder (away from the head) | OOO | OOO |

| | |
|---|---|
| The psychomotor skill was performed completely and in the appropriate order | 0  1  2  3  **4**  5 |
| The tester had control of the subject and the situation (showed confidence) | 0  1  2  3  4  5 |
| Method of performing the skill allowed the tester the ability to determine: severity, proper progression, and the *fit* in the overall picture (Oral) | 0  1  2  3  4  5 |

In order for a grade of *minimum standard* to be given, the total must be ≥11    TOTAL =

I_____I_____I
**Not Acceptable**    **Meets Minimum Standards**    **Exceeds Minimum Standards**

**L:** Laboratory/Classroom Testing
**C:** Clinical/Field Testing
**P:** Practicum Testing
**A:** Assessment/Mock Exam Testing
**S:** Self-Reporting

**Positive Finding:** Pain (radiating)
**Involved Structure:** Brachial plexus/nerve root
**Special Considerations:** N/A
**Reference(s):** Starkey et al; Shultz et al
**Supplies Needed:** N/A

## SPECIAL TESTS
# (ST-U-Test 26)

Peer Review _____ Peer Review _____

Skill Acquisition: _____    Practice Opportunities: _____

*This problem allows you the opportunity to demonstrate* **Tinel's Sign for the Cervical Spine** *to help rule out problems to the brachial plexus. You have 2 minutes to complete this task. Please inform the examiner when you have completed the task.*

| Tester places athlete and limb in appropriate position | YES | NO |
|---|---|---|
| Seated | OOO | OOO |
| Head slightly flexed | OOO | OOO |
| **Tester placed in proper position** | **YES** | **NO** |
| Stands behind the athlete | OOO | OOO |
| Places one hand over the transverse processes (each of the cervical vertebra) | OOO | OOO |
| **Tester performs test according to accepted guidelines** | **YES** | **NO** |
| Applies pressure (tapping motion) over each transverse process | OOO | OOO |
| Taps multiple vertebrae | OOO | OOO |
| Performs assessment on both sides of the vertebrae | OOO | OOO |

The psychomotor skill was performed completely and in the appropriate order    **0  1  2  3  4  5**

The tester had control of the subject and the situation (showed confidence)    **0  1  2  3  4  5**

Method of performing the skill allowed the tester the ability to determine:
severity, proper progression, and the *fit* in the overall picture (Oral)    **0  1  2  3  4  5**

In order for a grade of *minimum standard* to be given, the total must be ≥11    **TOTAL =**

I_____I_____I
**Not Acceptable**        **Meets Minimum Standards**    **Exceeds Minimum Standards**

**L:** Laboratory/Classroom Testing
**C:** Clinical/Field Testing
**P:** Practicum Testing
**A:** Assessment/Mock Exam Testing
**S:** Self-Reporting

**Positive Finding:** Pain (radiating)
**Involved Structure:** Brachial plexus
**Special Considerations:** N/A
**Reference(s):** Shultz et al
**Supplies Needed:** Chair

## SPECIAL TESTS
# (ST-U-Test 27)

Peer Review _____    Peer Review _____

Skill Acquisition: _____    Practice Opportunities: _____

*This problem allows you the opportunity to demonstrate the* **Vertebral Artery Test.** *You have 2 minutes to complete this task. Please inform the examiner when you have completed the task.*

| Tester places athlete and limb in appropriate position | YES | NO |
|---|---|---|
| Supine | OOO | OOO |
| Head positioned off the table | OOO | OOO |
| **Tester placed in proper position** | **YES** | **NO** |
| Standing or seated behind the athlete (at the head) | OOO | OOO |
| Places both hands under the occiput (holding the head) | OOO | OOO |
| **Tester performs test according to accepted guidelines** | **YES** | **NO** |
| Maintains relaxation of the head, neck, and shoulder area | OOO | OOO |
| Passively extends and laterally flexes the head | OOO | OOO |
| Passively laterally rotates the head | OOO | OOO |
| Maintains the position for 30 seconds | OOO | OOO |
| Performs assessment to the opposite side | OOO | OOO |

The psychomotor skill was performed completely and in the appropriate order    **0  1  2  3  4  5**

The tester had control of the subject and the situation (showed confidence)    **0  1  2  3  4  5**

Method of performing the skill allowed the tester the ability to determine:
severity, proper progression, and the *fit* in the overall picture (Oral)    **0  1  2  3  4  5**

In order for a grade of *minimum standard* to be given, the total must be ≥11    **TOTAL =**

I_____I_____I
**Not Acceptable**          **Meets Minimum Standards**          **Exceeds Minimum Standards**

**L:** Laboratory/Classroom Testing
**C:** Clinical/Field Testing
**P:** Practicum Testing
**A:** Assessment/Mock Exam Testing
**S:** Self-Reporting

**Positive Finding:** Dizziness, confusion, pupil changes
**Involved Structure:** Vertebral artery
**Special Considerations:** Positive test-refer to a physician
**Reference(s):** Starkey et al
**Supplies Needed:** Table

## SPECIAL TESTS
# (ST-L-Test 1)

Peer Review _____ Peer Review _____

Skill Acquisition: _____    Practice Opportunities: _____

*This problem allows you the opportunity to demonstrate* **Thompson's Test (Simmonds' Test)**. *You have 2 minutes to complete this task.*

| Tester places athlete and limb in appropriate position | YES | NO |
|---|---|---|
| Prone with feet over the edge of the table | ○○○ | ○○○ |
| **Tester placed in proper position** | **YES** | **NO** |
| Stands to the side of the athlete | ○○○ | ○○○ |
| **Tester performs test according to accepted guidelines** | **YES** | **NO** |
| Squeezes belly of the calf muscle (gastrocnemius/soleus) | ○○○ | ○○○ |
| Maintains relaxation of the limb | ○○○ | ○○○ |
| Performs assessment bilaterally | ○○○ | ○○○ |

The psychomotor skill was performed completely and in the appropriate order    **0  1  2  3  4  5**

The tester had control of the subject and the situation (showed confidence)    **0  1  2  3  4  5**

Method of performing the skill allowed the tester the ability to determine:
severity, proper progression, and the *fit* in the overall picture (Oral)    **0  1  2  3  4  5**

In order for a grade of *minimum standard* to be given, the total must be ≥11    **TOTAL =**

I_____I_____I

**Not Acceptable**        **Meets Minimum Standards**        **Exceeds Minimum Standards**

**L:** Laboratory/Classroom Testing
**C:** Clinical/Field Testing
**P:** Practicum Testing
**A:** Assessment/Mock Exam Testing
**S:** Self-Reporting

**Positive Finding:** Foot does not plantar flex
**Involved Structure:** Achilles' tendon (rupture)
**Special Considerations:** N/A
**Reference(s):** Konin et al; Magee; Starkey et al
**Supplies Needed:** Table

# SPECIAL TESTS
## (ST-L-Test 2)

Peer Review _____ Peer Review _____

Skill Acquisition: _____     Practice Opportunities: _____

*This problem allows you the opportunity to demonstrate the* **Percussion (Tap) Test** *to rule out a fracture to the* **ankle**. *You have 2 minutes to complete this task.*

| Tester places athlete and limb in appropriate position | YES | NO |
|---|---|---|
| Supine with foot off the table | ооо | ооо |
| Knee placed in full extension | ооо | ооо |
| **Tester placed in proper position** | **YES** | **NO** |
| Stands to the side of the athlete | ооо | ооо |
| Places one hand on the foot | ооо | ооо |
| Places the other hand in position to tap the heel | ооо | ооо |
| **Tester performs test according to accepted guidelines** | **YES** | **NO** |
| Passively dorsiflexes the foot | ооо | ооо |
| Taps firmly on the bottom of the heel (calcaneus) | ооо | ооо |

The psychomotor skill was performed completely and in the appropriate order       0  1  2  3  4  5

The tester had control of the subject and the situation (showed confidence)       0  1  2  3  4  5

Method of performing the skill allowed the tester the ability to determine:
severity, proper progression, and the *fit* in the overall picture (Oral)       0  1  2  3  4  5

In order for a grade of *minimum standard* to be given, the total must be ≥11       **TOTAL =**

I_____I_____I

**Not Acceptable**          **Meets Minimum Standards**          **Exceeds Minimum Standards**

L: Laboratory/Classroom Testing
C: Clinical/Field Testing
P: Practicum Testing
A: Assessment/Mock Exam Testing
S: Self-Reporting

**Positive Finding:** Pain at the site of the injury
**Involved Structure:** Bone (fracture)
**Special Considerations:** Do not attempt if obvious deformity exists
**Reference(s):** Konin
**Supplies Needed:** Table

## Special Tests
# (ST-L-Test 3)

Peer Review _____ Peer Review _____

Skill Acquisition: _____    Practice Opportunities: _____

*This problem allows you the opportunity to demonstrate the **Compression Test** to rule out a fracture to the **tibia**. You have 2 minutes to complete this task.*

| Tester places athlete and limb in appropriate position | YES | NO |
|---|---|---|
| Supine with foot off the table | OOO | OOO |
| Knee placed in full extension | OOO | OOO |
| **Tester placed in proper position** | **YES** | **NO** |
| Stands to the side of the athlete | OOO | OOO |
| Places both hands around the lower leg (tibia/fibula) | OOO | OOO |
| **Tester performs test according to accepted guidelines** | **YES** | **NO** |
| Squeezes the tibia and fibula together (proximal to the injury site) | OOO | OOO |
| Squeezes the tibia and fibula together (distal to the injury site) | OOO | OOO |

The psychomotor skill was performed completely and in the appropriate order    **0  1  2  3  4  5**

The tester had control of the subject and the situation (showed confidence)    **0  1  2  3  4  5**

Method of performing the skill allowed the tester the ability to determine:
severity, proper progression, and the *fit* in the overall picture (Oral)    **0  1  2  3  4  5**

In order for a grade of *minimum standard* to be given, the total must be ≥11    **TOTAL =**

I_____I_____I

**Not Acceptable**          **Meets Minimum Standards**          **Exceeds Minimum Standards**

**L:** Laboratory/Classroom Testing
**C:** Clinical/Field Testing
**P:** Practicum Testing
**A:** Assessment/Mock Exam Testing
**S:** Self-Reporting

**Positive Finding:** Pain at the site of the injury
**Involved Structure:** Bone (fracture)
**Special Considerations:** Do not attempt if obvious deformity exists
**Reference(s):** Konin
**Supplies Needed:** Table

# SPECIAL TESTS
## (ST-L-Test 4)

Peer Review _____   Peer Review _____

Skill Acquisition: _____   Practice Opportunities: _____

*This problem allows you the opportunity to demonstrate* **Homan's Sign**. *You have 2 minutes to complete this task.*

| Tester places athlete and limb in appropriate position | YES | NO |
|---|---|---|
| Supine | ○○○ | ○○○ |
| Knee placed in full extension | ○○○ | ○○○ |
| **Tester placed in proper position** | **YES** | **NO** |
| Stands to the side of the athlete | ○○○ | ○○○ |
| Places one hand over the lower leg (supporting the limb) | ○○○ | ○○○ |
| Places the other hand on the plantar surface of the foot | ○○○ | ○○○ |
| **Tester performs test according to accepted guidelines** | **YES** | **NO** |
| Passively dorsiflexes the foot | ○○○ | ○○○ |
| Maintains relaxation of the limb | ○○○ | ○○○ |
| Performs assessment bilaterally | ○○○ | ○○○ |

The psychomotor skill was performed completely and in the appropriate order    0 1 2 3 4 5

The tester had control of the subject and the situation (showed confidence)    0 1 2 3 4 5

Method of performing the skill allowed the tester the ability to determine:
severity, proper progression, and the *fit* in the overall picture (Oral)    0 1 2 3 4 5

In order for a grade of *minimum standard* to be given, the total must be ≥11    **TOTAL =**

I_____I_____I

**Not Acceptable**     **Meets Minimum Standards**    **Exceeds Minimum Standards**

**L:** Laboratory/Classroom Testing
**C:** Clinical/Field Testing
**P:** Practicum Testing
**A:** Assessment/Mock Exam Testing
**S:** Self-Reporting

**Positive Finding:** Pain in the calf area (gastrocnemius/soleus complex)
**Involved Structure:** Thrombophlebitis (possible)
**Special Considerations:** Rule out muscle injury; check dorsalis pedis pulse
**Reference(s):** Konin; Magee; Starkey
**Supplies Needed:** Supine

## SPECIAL TESTS
# (ST-L-Test 5)

Peer Review _____ Peer Review _____

Skill Acquisition: _____        Practice Opportunities: _____

*This problem allows you the opportunity to demonstrate the* **Tinel's Sign at the Ankle (Percussion Sign)**. *You have 2 minutes to complete this task.*

| | YES | NO |
|---|---|---|
| **Tester places athlete and limb in appropriate position** | YES | NO |
| Foot placed in a stable position (seated, prone, etc) | OOO | OOO |
| **Tester placed in proper position** | YES | NO |
| Stands to the side of the limb | OOO | OOO |
| Places one hand on the lower leg | OOO | OOO |
| Places the other hand in position to tap the area around the medial malleolus | OOO | OOO |
| **Tester performs test according to accepted guidelines** | YES | NO |
| Taps firmly on the dorsum of the ankle (anterior tibial branch of the deep peroneal nerve) | OOO | OOO |
| Taps firmly behind the medial malleolus (posterior tibial nerve) | OOO | OOO |
| Performs assessment bilaterally | OOO | OOO |

The psychomotor skill was performed completely and in the appropriate order      0  1  2  3  4  5

The tester had control of the subject and the situation (showed confidence)      0  1  2  3  4  5

Method of performing the skill allowed the tester the ability to determine:
severity, proper progression, and the *fit* in the overall picture (Oral)      0  1  2  3  4  5

In order for a grade of *minimum standard* to be given, the total must be ≥11      **TOTAL =**

I_____I_____I
**Not Acceptable**      **Meets Minimum Standards**      **Exceeds Minimum Standards**

**L:** Laboratory/Classroom Testing
**C:** Clinical/Field Testing
**P:** Practicum Testing
**A:** Assessment/Mock Exam Testing
**S:** Self-Reporting

**Positive Finding:** Tingling and/or paresthesia
**Involved Structure:** Anterior tibial branch of the deep peroneal nerve, posterior tibial nerve
**Special Considerations:** N/A
**Reference(s):** Magee
**Supplies Needed:** Supporting surface (table, floor)

# SPECIAL TESTS
# (ST-L-Test 6)

Skill Acquisition: _____    Practice Opportunities: _____

*This problem allows you the opportunity to demonstrate* **McMurray's Test for the Knee**. *You have 2 minutes to complete this task.*

| Tester places athlete and limb in appropriate position | YES | NO |
|---|---|---|
| Supine | OOO | OOO |
| Knee flexed to 90 degrees or knee extended to 0 degrees (starting with either knee) | OOO | OOO |
| **Tester placed in proper position** | **YES** | **NO** |
| Stands to the side of the athlete | OOO | OOO |
| Grasps the involved foot (heel) with one hand | OOO | OOO |
| Places the other hand in the position to palpate and support the knee | OOO | OOO |
| **Tester performs test according to accepted guidelines** | **YES** | **NO** |
| Passively medially rotates the knee while palpating the lateral joint line | OOO | OOO |
| Applies valgus stress to the knee | OOO | OOO |
| Passively moves the knee through a figure-8 motion (extension and flexion) | OOO | OOO |
| Passively laterally rotates the knee while palpating the medial joint line | OOO | OOO |
| Applies a varus stress to the knee | OOO | OOO |
| Passively moves the knee through a figure-8 motion (extension and flexion) | OOO | OOO |
| Maintains relaxation of the limb | OOO | OOO |
| Performs assessment bilaterally | OOO | OOO |

The psychomotor skill was performed completely and in the appropriate order      0  1  2  3  4  5

The tester had control of the subject and the situation (showed confidence)      0  1  2  3  4  5

Method of performing the skill allowed the tester the ability to determine:
severity, proper progression, and the *fit* in the overall picture (Oral)      0  1  2  3  4  5

In order for a grade of *minimum standard* to be given, the total must be ≥11      **TOTAL =**

|_____|_____|

**Not Acceptable**      **Meets Minimum Standards**      **Exceeds Minimum Standards**

**L:** Laboratory/Classroom Testing
**C:** Clinical/Field Testing
**P:** Practicum Testing
**A:** Assessment/Mock Exam Testing
**S:** Self-Reporting

**Positive Finding:** Clicking or locking within knee joint
**Involved Structure:** Meniscus (medial/lateral)
**Special Considerations:** Rule out patella femoral problems
**Reference(s):** Konin et al; Magee; Starkey et al
**Supplies Needed:** Table

## SPECIAL TESTS
# (ST-L-Test 7)

Skill Acquisition: _____    Practice Opportunities: _____

*This problem allows you the opportunity to demonstrate* **Steinman's Tenderness Displacement Test (First Steinman's Sign)**. *You have 2 minutes to complete this task.*

| Tester places athlete and limb in appropriate position | YES | NO |
|---|---|---|
| Supine | OOO | OOO |
| Knee placed in full extension (0 degrees) | OOO | OOO |
| **Tester placed in proper position** | **YES** | **NO** |
| Stands to the side of the athlete | OOO | OOO |
| Grasps the involved foot (heel) with one hand | OOO | OOO |
| Places the other hand in the position to support the knee | OOO | OOO |
| **Tester performs test according to accepted guidelines** | **YES** | **NO** |
| Passively moves the knee into full flexion | OOO | OOO |
| Passively rotates the knee medially | OOO | OOO |
| Passively rotates the knee laterally | OOO | OOO |
| Repeats medial and lateral rotation | OOO | OOO |
| Maintains relaxation of the limb | OOO | OOO |
| Performs assessment bilaterally | OOO | OOO |

The psychomotor skill was performed completely and in the appropriate order    **0  1  2  3  4  5**

The tester had control of the subject and the situation (showed confidence)    **0  1  2  3  4  5**

Method of performing the skill allowed the tester the ability to determine:
severity, proper progression, and the *fit* in the overall picture (Oral)    **0  1  2  3  4  5**

In order for a grade of *minimum standard* to be given, the total must be ≥11    **TOTAL =**

I_____I_____I

**Not Acceptable**          **Meets Minimum Standards**          **Exceeds Minimum Standards**

**L:** Laboratory/Classroom Testing
**C:** Clinical/Field Testing
**P:** Practicum Testing
**A:** Assessment/Mock Exam Testing
**S:** Self-Reporting

**Positive Finding:** Pain during rotation, lacks full flexion
**Involved Structure:** Meniscus (medial/lateral)
**Special Considerations:** N/A
**Reference(s):** Magee
**Supplies Needed:** Table

# SPECIAL TESTS
# (ST-L-Test 8)

Peer Review _____ Peer Review _____

Skill Acquisition: _____    Practice Opportunities: _____

*This problem allows you the opportunity to demonstrate the* **Patellofemoral Grind Test (Clarke's Test/Patella Hold/Zohler's Sign)** *for the knee. You have 2 minutes to complete this task.*

| Tester places athlete and limb in appropriate position | YES | NO |
|---|---|---|
| Supine | OOO | OOO |
| Knee placed in full extension (heels on the table) | OOO | OOO |
| **Tester placed in proper position** | **YES** | **NO** |
| Stands to the side of the athlete | OOO | OOO |
| Places hand over the superior pole of the patella (web of the hand) | OOO | OOO |
| **Tester performs test according to accepted guidelines** | **YES** | **NO** |
| Applies downward-inferior pressure on the patella | OOO | OOO |
| Instructs the athlete to actively contract the quadriceps | OOO | OOO |
| Performs the assessment bilaterally | OOO | OOO |

| | |
|---|---|
| The psychomotor skill was performed completely and in the appropriate order | 0  1  2  3  4  5 |
| The tester had control of the subject and the situation (showed confidence) | 0  1  2  3  4  5 |
| Method of performing the skill allowed the tester the ability to determine: severity, proper progression, and the *fit* in the overall picture (Oral) | 0  1  2  3  4  5 |

In order for a grade of *minimum standard* to be given, the total must be ≥11          **TOTAL =**

I_____I_____I

**Not Acceptable**          **Meets Minimum Standards**          **Exceeds Minimum Standards**

**L:** Laboratory/Classroom Testing
**C:** Clinical/Field Testing
**P:** Practicum Testing
**A:** Assessment/Mock Exam Testing
**S:** Self-Reporting

**Positive Finding:** Pain/crepitation
**Involved Structure:** Patella
**Special Considerations:** N/A
**Reference(s):** Konin et al; Magee
**Supplies Needed:** N/A

## SPECIAL TESTS
# (ST-L-Test 9)

Peer Review _____ Peer Review _____

Skill Acquisition: _____    Practice Opportunities: _____

*This problem allows you the opportunity to demonstrate the* **Patellar Apprehension Test (Fairbank's Apprehension Test)**. *You have 2 minutes to complete this task.*

| Tester places athlete and limb in appropriate position | YES | NO |
|---|---|---|
| Supine | ○○○ | ○○○ |
| Knee placed in full extension (heels on the table) | ○○○ | ○○○ |
| **Tester placed in proper position** | **YES** | **NO** |
| Stands to the side of the athlete | ○○○ | ○○○ |
| Places thumbs over the medial border of the patella | ○○○ | ○○○ |
| **Tester performs test according to accepted guidelines** | **YES** | **NO** |
| Passively moves the patella in a lateral direction | ○○○ | ○○○ |
| Performs assessment bilaterally | ○○○ | ○○○ |

The psychomotor skill was performed completely and in the appropriate order      **0  1  2  3  4  5**

The tester had control of the subject and the situation (showed confidence)      **0  1  2  3  4  5**

Method of performing the skill allowed the tester the ability to determine:
severity, proper progression, and the *fit* in the overall picture (Oral)      **0  1  2  3  4  5**

In order for a grade of *minimum standard* to be given, the total must be ≥11      **TOTAL =**

I_____I_____I
**Not Acceptable        Meets Minimum Standards        Exceeds Minimum Standards**

**L:** Laboratory/Classroom Testing
**C:** Clinical/Field Testing
**P:** Practicum Testing
**A:** Assessment/Mock Exam Testing
**S:** Self-Reporting

**Positive Finding:** Pain, apprehension, tightening of the quads
**Involved Structure:** Patella
**Special Considerations:** N/A
**Reference(s):** Konin et al; Magee
**Supplies Needed:** Table

# SPECIAL TESTS
# (ST-L-Test 10)

Peer Review _____ Peer Review _____

Skill Acquisition: _____    Practice Opportunities: _____

*This problem allows you the opportunity to demonstrate the* **Ballottable Patella (Patella Tap Test)**. *You have 2 minutes to complete this task.*

| Tester places athlete and limb in appropriate position | YES | NO |
|---|---|---|
| Supine | OOO | OOO |
| Knee placed in full extension (heels on the table) | OOO | OOO |
| **Tester placed in proper position** | **YES** | **NO** |
| Stands to the side of the athlete | OOO | OOO |
| Places one hand over the suprapatellar pouch (just above the superior pole of the patella) | OOO | OOO |
| Places the other hand over the central portion of the patella | OOO | OOO |
| **Tester performs test according to accepted guidelines** | **YES** | **NO** |
| Applies downward pressure on the patella | OOO | OOO |
| Maintains relaxation of the limb | OOO | OOO |
| Performs assessment bilaterally | OOO | OOO |

The psychomotor skill was performed completely and in the appropriate order   0 1 2 3 4 5

The tester had control of the subject and the situation (showed confidence)   0 1 2 3 4 5

Method of performing the skill allowed the tester the ability to determine: severity, proper progression, and the *fit* in the overall picture (Oral)   0 1 2 3 4 5

In order for a grade of *minimum standard* to be given, the total must be ≥11    TOTAL = 

I_____I_____I

**Not Acceptable**     **Meets Minimum Standards**     **Exceeds Minimum Standards**

**L:** Laboratory/Classroom Testing
**C:** Clinical/Field Testing
**P:** Practicum Testing
**A:** Assessment/Mock Exam Testing
**S:** Self-Reporting

**Positive Finding:** Rebound of the patella
**Involved Structure:** Joint (effusion)
**Special Considerations:** Measure thigh girth
**Reference(s):** Konin et al; Starkey et al
**Supplies Needed:** Table

## SPECIAL TESTS
# (ST-L-Test 11)

Peer Review _____ Peer Review _____

Skill Acquisition: _____     Practice Opportunities: _____

*This problem allows you the opportunity to demonstrate the **Sweep Test**. You have 2 minutes to complete this task.*

| Tester places athlete and limb in appropriate position | YES | NO |
|---|---|---|
| Supine | ○○○ | ○○○ |
| Knee placed in full extension (heels on the table) | ○○○ | ○○○ |
| **Tester placed in proper position** | **YES** | **NO** |
| Stands to the side of the athlete | ○○○ | ○○○ |
| Places hands on the medial side of the patella | ○○○ | ○○○ |
| **Tester performs test according to accepted guidelines** | **YES** | **NO** |
| Pushes edema/swelling proximally and/or laterally ("milking") | ○○○ | ○○○ |
| Applies pressure to the lateral aspect of the knee | ○○○ | ○○○ |
| Maintains relaxation of the limb | ○○○ | ○○○ |
| Performs assessment bilaterally | ○○○ | ○○○ |

The psychomotor skill was performed completely and in the appropriate order    0 1 2 3 4 5

The tester had control of the subject and the situation (showed confidence)    0 1 2 3 4 5

Method of performing the skill allowed the tester the ability to determine:
severity, proper progression, and the *fit* in the overall picture (Oral)    0 1 2 3 4 5

In order for a grade of *minimum standard* to be given, the total must be ≥11    **TOTAL =**

I_____I_____I
**Not Acceptable**      **Meets Minimum Standards**      **Exceeds Minimum Standards**

**L:** Laboratory/Classroom Testing
**C:** Clinical/Field Testing
**P:** Practicum Testing
**A:** Assessment/Mock Exam Testing
**S:** Self-Reporting

**Positive Finding:** Fluid reforms on the medial side
**Involved Structure:** Intracapsular swelling
**Special Considerations:** N/A
**Reference(s):** Starkey et al
**Supplies Needed:** Table

## SPECIAL TESTS
# (ST-L-Test 12)

Peer Review _____ Peer Review _____

Skill Acquisition: _____    Practice Opportunities: _____

*This problem allows you the opportunity to demonstrate the* **Bounce Home Test** *for the knee. You have 2 minutes to complete this task.*

| Tester places athlete and limb in appropriate position | YES | NO |
|---|---|---|
| Supine | ○○○ | ○○○ |
| Knee placed into slight flexion | ○○○ | ○○○ |
| **Tester placed in proper position** | **YES** | **NO** |
| Stands to the side of the athlete | ○○○ | ○○○ |
| Places one hand under the heel of the involved limb | ○○○ | ○○○ |
| Places other hand under the knee joint | ○○○ | ○○○ |
| **Tester performs test according to accepted guidelines** | **YES** | **NO** |
| Passively flexes the knee (approximately 30 degrees) | ○○○ | ○○○ |
| Allows the knee to fall to neutral (gravity) | ○○○ | ○○○ |
| Maintains relaxation of the limb | ○○○ | ○○○ |
| Performs assessment bilaterally | ○○○ | ○○○ |

The psychomotor skill was performed completely and in the appropriate order     0  1  2  3  4  5

The tester had control of the subject and the situation (showed confidence)     0  1  2  3  4  5

Method of performing the skill allowed the tester the ability to determine:
severity, proper progression, and the *fit* in the overall picture (Oral)     0  1  2  3  4  5

In order for a grade of *minimum standard* to be given, the total must be ≥11     **TOTAL =**

|_____|_____|
**Not Acceptable**          **Meets Minimum Standards**          **Exceeds Minimum Standards**

**L:** Laboratory/Classroom Testing
**C:** Clinical/Field Testing
**P:** Practicum Testing
**A:** Assessment/Mock Exam Testing
**S:** Self-Reporting

**Positive Finding:** Rubbery end-feel, springy block, lacks full extension
**Involved Structure:** Structural block; meniscus
**Special Considerations:** N/A
**Reference(s):** Konin et al; Magee
**Supplies Needed:** Table

## SPECIAL TESTS
# (ST-L-Test 13)

Peer Review _____ Peer Review _____

Skill Acquisition: _____    Practice Opportunities: _____

*This problem allows you the opportunity to demonstrate* **Apley's Compression Test** *for the knee. You have 2 minutes to complete this task.*

| Tester places athlete and limb in appropriate position | YES | NO |
|---|---|---|
| Prone | ○○○ | ○○○ |
| Knee flexed to 90 degrees | ○○○ | ○○○ |
| **Tester placed in proper position** | **YES** | **NO** |
| Stands to the side of the athlete | ○○○ | ○○○ |
| Places one hand over the posterior femur (may stabilize with knee) | ○○○ | ○○○ |
| Grasps other hand around the distal portion of the tibia/fibula | ○○○ | ○○○ |
| **Tester performs test according to accepted guidelines** | **YES** | **NO** |
| Applies downward pressure of the tibia/fibula (compressing the knee joint) | ○○○ | ○○○ |
| Simultaneously medially/laterally rotates the tibia | ○○○ | ○○○ |
| Maintains relaxation of the limb | ○○○ | ○○○ |
| Performs assessment bilaterally | ○○○ | ○○○ |

The psychomotor skill was performed completely and in the appropriate order     **0  1  2  3  4  5**

The tester had control of the subject and the situation (showed confidence)     **0  1  2  3  4  5**

Method of performing the skill allowed the tester the ability to determine:
severity, proper progression, and the *fit* in the overall picture (Oral)     **0  1  2  3  4  5**

In order for a grade of *minimum standard* to be given, the total must be ≥11     **TOTAL =**

|_____|_____|
**Not Acceptable**        **Meets Minimum Standards**    **Exceeds Minimum Standards**

**L:** Laboratory/Classroom Testing
**C:** Clinical/Field Testing
**P:** Practicum Testing
**A:** Assessment/Mock Exam Testing
**S:** Self-Reporting

**Positive Finding:** Pain, clicking, restriction
**Involved Structure:** Meniscus
**Special Considerations:** Combine with Apley's distraction test
**Reference(s):** Konin et al; Magee; Starkey et al
**Supplies Needed:** Table

# SPECIAL TESTS
# (ST-L-Test 14)

Peer Review _____ Peer Review _____

Skill Acquisition: _____    Practice Opportunities: _____

*This problem allows you the opportunity to demonstrate* **Apley's Distraction Test** *for the knee. You have 2 minutes to complete this task.*

| Tester places athlete and limb in appropriate position | YES | NO |
|---|---|---|
| Prone | OOO | OOO |
| Knee flexed to 90 degrees | OOO | OOO |
| **Tester placed in proper position** | **YES** | **NO** |
| Stands to the side of the athlete | OOO | OOO |
| Places one hand over posterior femur (may stabilize with knee) | OOO | OOO |
| Grasp other hand around the distal portion of the tibia/fibula | OOO | OOO |
| **Tester performs test according to accepted guidelines** | **YES** | **NO** |
| Applies upward pressure of the tibia/fibula (distracting the knee) | OOO | OOO |
| Simultaneously medially/laterally rotates the tibia | OOO | OOO |
| Maintains relaxation of the limb | OOO | OOO |
| Performs assessment bilaterally | OOO | OOO |

The psychomotor skill was performed completely and in the appropriate order    **0  1  2  3  4  5**

The tester had control of the subject and the situation (showed confidence)    **0  1  2  3  4  5**

Method of performing the skill allowed the tester the ability to determine:
severity, proper progression, and the *fit* in the overall picture (Oral)    **0  1  2  3  4  5**

In order for a grade of *minimum standard* to be given, the total must be ≥11    **TOTAL =**

I_____I_____I
   **Not Acceptable**      **Meets Minimum Standards**      **Exceeds Minimum Standards**

**L:** Laboratory/Classroom Testing
**C:** Clinical/Field Testing
**P:** Practicum Testing
**A:** Assessment/Mock Exam Testing
**S:** Self-Reporting

**Positive Finding:** Pain
**Involved Structure:** General ligamentous meniscus (pain goes away)
**Special Considerations:** Combine with Apley's compression test
**Reference(s):** Konin et al; Magee; Starkey et al
**Supplies Needed:** Table

## SPECIAL TESTS
# (ST-L-Test 15)

Peer Review _____ Peer Review _____

Skill Acquisition: _____    Practice Opportunities: _____

*This problem allows you the opportunity to demonstrate the **FABER Test (Figure-Four Test/Patrick's Test/Jansen's Test)**. You have 2 minutes to complete this task.*

| Tester places athlete and limb in appropriate position | YES | NO |
|---|---|---|
| Supine | OOO | OOO |
| Hip **f**lexed, **ab**ducted, and **e**xternally **r**otated (FABER)-figure-four position | OOO | OOO |
| Foot placed on opposite knee (above the superior pole of the patella) | OOO | OOO |
| **Tester placed in proper position** | **YES** | **NO** |
| Stands to the side of the athlete | OOO | OOO |
| Places one hand on the ASIS (opposite the involved side) | OOO | OOO |
| Places the other hand on the involved knee | OOO | OOO |
| **Tester performs test according to accepted guidelines** | **YES** | **NO** |
| Slowly press the knee toward the table | OOO | OOO |
| Maintains relaxation of the limb | OOO | OOO |
| Performs assessment bilaterally | OOO | OOO |

The psychomotor skill was performed completely and in the appropriate order    **0  1  2  3  4  5**

The tester had control of the subject and the situation (showed confidence)    **0  1  2  3  4  5**

Method of performing the skill allowed the tester the ability to determine:
severity, proper progression, and the *fit* in the overall picture (Oral)    **0  1  2  3  4  5**

In order for a grade of *minimum standard* to be given, the total must be ≥11    **TOTAL =**

I_____I_____I
**Not Acceptable**         **Meets Minimum Standards**    **Exceeds Minimum Standards**

**L:** Laboratory/Classroom Testing
**C:** Clinical/Field Testing
**P:** Practicum Testing
**A:** Assessment/Mock Exam Testing
**S:** Self-Reporting

**Positive Finding:** Knee does not move to the table (ideal parallel to the table)
**Involved Structure:** Iliopsoas, sacroiliac joint
**Special Considerations:** N/A
**Reference(s):** Konin et al; Magee; Starkey et al
**Supplies Needed:** Table

# SPECIAL TESTS
# (ST-L-Test 16)

Peer Review _____ Peer Review _____

Skill Acquisition: _____    Practice Opportunities: _____

*This problem allows you the opportunity to demonstrate the* **Gaenslen's Test***. You have 2 minutes to complete this task.*

| Tester places athlete and limb in appropriate position | YES | NO |
|---|---|---|
| Side lying | ○○○ | ○○○ |
| Hip hyperextended (upper limb) | ○○○ | ○○○ |
| Hip/knee flexed (lower limb) with leg held against chest | ○○○ | ○○○ |
| **Tester placed in proper position** | **YES** | **NO** |
| Stands behind the athlete | ○○○ | ○○○ |
| Places one hand on the pelvis (stabilize) | ○○○ | ○○○ |
| Places other hand against the anterior knee | ○○○ | ○○○ |
| **Tester performs test according to accepted guidelines** | **YES** | **NO** |
| Passively extends the hip (over pressure) | ○○○ | ○○○ |
| Maintains relaxation of the limb | ○○○ | ○○○ |
| Performs assessment bilaterally | ○○○ | ○○○ |

| | |
|---|---|
| The psychomotor skill was performed completely and in the appropriate order | 0  1  2  3  4  5 |
| The tester had control of the subject and the situation (showed confidence) | 0  1  2  3  4  5 |
| Method of performing the skill allowed the tester the ability to determine: severity, proper progression, and the *fit* in the overall picture (Oral) | 0  1  2  3  4  5 |

In order for a grade of *minimum standard* to be given, the total must be ≥11        **TOTAL =**

I_____I_____I

**Not Acceptable**          **Meets Minimum Standards**          **Exceeds Minimum Standards**

**L:** Laboratory/Classroom Testing
**C:** Clinical/Field Testing
**P:** Practicum Testing
**A:** Assessment/Mock Exam Testing
**S:** Self-Reporting

**Positive Finding:** Pain
**Involved Structure:** Sacroiliac joint, hip
**Special Considerations:** May be done supine (leg hanging off the table)
**Reference(s):** Magee
**Supplies Needed:** Table

## SPECIAL TESTS
# (ST-L-Test 17)

Peer Review _____ Peer Review _____

Skill Acquisition: _____    Practice Opportunities: _____

*This problem allows you the opportunity to demonstrate the* **Sacroiliac Compression Test (Gapping Test/ Transverse Anterior Stress Test)**. *You have 2 minutes to complete this task.*

| Tester places athlete and limb in appropriate position | YES | NO |
|---|---|---|
| Supine | ooo | ooo |
| **Tester placed in proper position** | **YES** | **NO** |
| Stands behind the athlete | ooo | ooo |
| Places hands over the ASIS (X pattern/cross-arm pattern) | ooo | ooo |
| **Tester performs test according to accepted guidelines** | **YES** | **NO** |
| Applies downward and outward pressure (attempting to spread the ASIS) | ooo | ooo |
| Asks the athlete to relax | ooo | ooo |
| Performs assessment bilaterally | ooo | ooo |

The psychomotor skill was performed completely and in the appropriate order    0  1  2  3  4  5

The tester had control of the subject and the situation (showed confidence)    0  1  2  3  4  5

Method of performing the skill allowed the tester the ability to determine:
severity, proper progression, and the *fit* in the overall picture (Oral)    0  1  2  3  4  5

In order for a grade of *minimum standard* to be given, the total must be ≥11    **TOTAL =**

I_____I_____I
**Not Acceptable**          **Meets Minimum Standards**      **Exceeds Minimum Standards**

**L:** Laboratory/Classroom Testing
**C:** Clinical/Field Testing
**P:** Practicum Testing
**A:** Assessment/Mock Exam Testing
**S:** Self-Reporting

**Positive Finding:** Pain (sacroiliac area)
**Involved Structure:** Sacroiliac joint
**Special Considerations:** N/A
**Reference(s):** Starkey et al; Magee
**Supplies Needed:** Table

# SPECIAL TESTS
# (ST-L-Test 18)

Peer Review _____ Peer Review _____

Skill Acquisition: _____        Practice Opportunities: _____

*This problem allows you the opportunity to demonstrate the* **Sacroiliac Distraction Test (Approximation Test/ Transverse Posterior Stress Test)**. *You have 2 minutes to complete this task.*

| | YES | NO |
|---|---|---|
| **Tester places athlete and limb in appropriate position** | YES | NO |
| Side lying | OOO | OOO |
| **Tester placed in proper position** | YES | NO |
| Stands behind the athlete | OOO | OOO |
| Places both hands over the lateral aspect of the pelvis (iliac crest) | OOO | OOO |
| **Tester performs test according to accepted guidelines** | YES | NO |
| Applies downward pressure (pushing toward the table) | OOO | OOO |
| Asks the athlete to relax | OOO | OOO |
| Performs assessment bilaterally | OOO | OOO |

The psychomotor skill was performed completely and in the appropriate order     0 1 2 3 4 5

The tester had control of the subject and the situation (showed confidence)     0 1 2 3 4 5

Method of performing the skill allowed the tester the ability to determine:
severity, proper progression, and the *fit* in the overall picture (Oral)     0 1 2 3 4 5

In order for a grade of *minimum standard* to be given, the total must be ≥11     **TOTAL =**

I_____I_____I

**Not Acceptable          Meets Minimum Standards          Exceeds Minimum Standards**

**L:** Laboratory/Classroom Testing
**C:** Clinical/Field Testing
**P:** Practicum Testing
**A:** Assessment/Mock Exam Testing
**S:** Self-Reporting

**Positive Finding:** Pain (sacroiliac area)
**Involved Structure:** Sacroiliac joint
**Special Considerations:** N/A
**Reference(s):** Starkey et al; Magee
**Supplies Needed:** Table

## SPECIAL TESTS
# (ST-L-Test 19)

Peer Review _____ Peer Review _____

Skill Acquisition: _____    Practice Opportunities: _____

*This problem allows you the opportunity to demonstrate the* **Tripod Sign (Hamstrings Contracture, Method 2)** *for hamstring flexibility. You have 2 minutes to complete this task.*

| Tester places athlete and limb in appropriate position | YES | NO |
|---|---|---|
| Seated | ○○○ | ○○○ |
| Knees flexed to 90 degrees (hanging over the edge of the table) | ○○○ | ○○○ |
| **Tester placed in proper position** | **YES** | **NO** |
| Stands to the side of the athlete | ○○○ | ○○○ |
| Places hand around the distal aspect of the lower leg | ○○○ | ○○○ |
| Places the other hand over the distal aspect of the femur (above the knee) | ○○○ | ○○○ |
| **Tester performs test according to accepted guidelines** | **YES** | **NO** |
| Passively extends the knee | ○○○ | ○○○ |
| Maintains relaxation of the limb | ○○○ | ○○○ |
| Performs assessment bilaterally | ○○○ | ○○○ |

The psychomotor skill was performed completely and in the appropriate order    0 1 2 3 4 5

The tester had control of the subject and the situation (showed confidence)    0 1 2 3 4 5

Method of performing the skill allowed the tester the ability to determine:
severity, proper progression, and the *fit* in the overall picture (Oral)    0 1 2 3 4 5

In order for a grade of *minimum standard* to be given, the total must be ≥11    **TOTAL =**

I_____I_____I
**Not Acceptable**      **Meets Minimum Standards**      **Exceeds Minimum Standards**

**L:** Laboratory/Classroom Testing
**C:** Clinical/Field Testing
**P:** Practicum Testing
**A:** Assessment/Mock Exam Testing
**S:** Self-Reporting

**Positive Finding:** Hyperextends the trunk
**Involved Structure:** Hamstrings
**Special Considerations:** N/A
**Reference(s):** Magee
**Supplies Needed:** Table

# SPECIAL TESTS
# (ST-L-Test 20)

Peer Review _____ Peer Review _____

Skill Acquisition: _____    Practice Opportunities: _____

*This problem allows you the opportunity to demonstrate the* **Ely's Test (Tight Rectus Femoris, Method 2)**. *You have 2 minutes to complete this task.*

| Tester places athlete and limb in appropriate position | YES | NO |
|---|---|---|
| Prone | ○○○ | ○○○ |
| Knees extended | ○○○ | ○○○ |
| **Tester placed in proper position** | **YES** | **NO** |
| Stands to the side of the athlete | ○○○ | ○○○ |
| Places hand around distal aspect of the lower leg | ○○○ | ○○○ |
| Places the other over the distal aspect of the femur (above the knee) | ○○○ | ○○○ |
| **Tester performs test according to accepted guidelines** | **YES** | **NO** |
| Passively flexes the knee (overpressure) | ○○○ | ○○○ |
| Maintains relaxation of the limb | ○○○ | ○○○ |
| Performs assessment bilaterally | ○○○ | ○○○ |

The psychomotor skill was performed completely and in the appropriate order    0 1 2 3 4 5

The tester had control of the subject and the situation (showed confidence)    0 1 2 3 4 5

Method of performing the skill allowed the tester the ability to determine:
severity, proper progression, and the *fit* in the overall picture (Oral)    0 1 2 3 4 5

In order for a grade of *minimum standard* to be given, the total must be ≥11    **TOTAL =**

I_____I_____I
**Not Acceptable**          **Meets Minimum Standards**      **Exceeds Minimum Standards**

**L:** Laboratory/Classroom Testing
**C:** Clinical/Field Testing
**P:** Practicum Testing
**A:** Assessment/Mock Exam Testing
**S:** Self-Reporting

**Positive Finding:** Hip moves off the table on the involved side
**Involved Structure:** Rectus femoris
**Special Considerations:** N/A
**Reference(s):** Konin et al; Magee
**Supplies Needed:** Table

## SPECIAL TESTS
# (ST-L-Test 21)

Peer Review _____ Peer Review _____

Skill Acquisition: _____     Practice Opportunities: _____

*This problem allows you the opportunity to demonstrate the* **Femoral Nerve Traction Test***. You have 2 minutes to complete this task.*

| Tester places athlete and limb in appropriate position | YES | NO |
|---|---|---|
| Side lying | ooo | ooo |
| Torso, hip, and leg in straight alignment | ooo | ooo |
| Hip/knee slightly flexed (bottom leg uninvolved limb) | ooo | ooo |
| Head slightly flexed | ooo | ooo |
| **Tester placed in proper position** | **YES** | **NO** |
| Stands behind the athlete | ooo | ooo |
| Places hand under the knee (supporting the lower leg) | ooo | ooo |
| Places the other hand over the lateral aspect of the pelvis (iliac crest) | ooo | ooo |
| **Tester performs test according to accepted guidelines** | **YES** | **NO** |
| Passively extends the hip | ooo | ooo |
| Passively flexes the knee | ooo | ooo |
| Maintains relaxation of the limb | ooo | ooo |
| Performs assessment bilaterally | ooo | ooo |

The psychomotor skill was performed completely and in the appropriate order     0 1 2 3 4 5

The tester had control of the subject and the situation (showed confidence)     0 1 2 3 4 5

Method of performing the skill allowed the tester the ability to determine:
severity, proper progression, and the *fit* in the overall picture (Oral)     0 1 2 3 4 5

In order for a grade of *minimum standard* to be given, the total must be ≥11     **TOTAL =**

I_____I_____I

**Not Acceptable**     **Meets Minimum Standards**     **Exceeds Minimum Standards**

**L:** Laboratory/Classroom Testing
**C:** Clinical/Field Testing
**P:** Practicum Testing
**A:** Assessment/Mock Exam Testing
**S:** Self-Reporting

**Positive Finding:** Pain shooting down the anterior thigh
**Involved Structure:** Femoral nerve
**Special Considerations:** May also serve as a traction test for L2-L4
**Reference(s):** Magee
**Supplies Needed:** N/A

## SPECIAL TESTS
# (ST-L-Test 22)

Peer Review _____ , ___ Peer Review _____

Skill Acquisition: _____    Practice Opportunities: _____

*This problem allows you the opportunity to demonstrate the* **Trendelenburg Test (Trendelenburg Sign)**. *You have 2 minutes to complete this task.*

| | YES | NO |
|---|---|---|
| **Tester places athlete and limb in appropriate position** | YES | NO |
| Standing | ○○○ | ○○○ |
| **Tester placed in proper position** | YES | NO |
| Stands behind the athlete (observing only movement of the pelvis) | ○○○ | ○○○ |
| **Tester performs test according to accepted guidelines** | YES | NO |
| Instructs the athlete to balance on one leg (10 seconds) | ○○○ | ○○○ |
| Performs assessment bilaterally | ○○○ | ○○○ |

The psychomotor skill was performed completely and in the appropriate order    0  1  2  3  4  5

The tester had control of the subject and the situation (showed confidence)    0  1  2  3  4  5

Method of performing the skill allowed the tester the ability to determine:
severity, proper progression, and the *fit* in the overall picture (Oral)    0  1  2  3  4  5

In order for a grade of *minimum standard* to be given, the total must be ≥11    **TOTAL =**

I_____I_____I
**Not Acceptable**          **Meets Minimum Standards**    **Exceeds Minimum Standards**

**L:** Laboratory/Classroom Testing
**C:** Clinical/Field Testing
**P:** Practicum Testing
**A:** Assessment/Mock Exam Testing
**S:** Self-Reporting

**Positive Finding:** Pelvis on the unsupported side/ nonstance leg drops
**Involved Structure:** Gluteus medius (weakness)
**Special Considerations:** May view from the front
**Reference(s):** Konin et al; Magee; Starkey et al
**Supplies Needed:** N/A

## SPECIAL TESTS
# (ST-L-Test 23)

Peer Review _____ Peer Review _____

Skill Acquisition: _____    Practice Opportunities: _____

*This problem allows you the opportunity to demonstrate the* **Thomas Test**. *You have 2 minutes to complete this task.*

| Tester places athlete and limb in appropriate position | YES | NO |
|---|---|---|
| Supine | ○○○ | ○○○ |
| Hips/knees in full extension | ○○○ | ○○○ |
| **Tester placed in proper position** | **YES** | **NO** |
| Stands to the side of the athlete | ○○○ | ○○○ |
| Places one hand over the pelvis (monitors lumbar lordosis and/or pelvic tilt) | ○○○ | ○○○ |
| Places the other hand around the knee | ○○○ | ○○○ |
| **Tester performs test according to accepted guidelines** | **YES** | **NO** |
| Passively flexes the hip and knee—overpressure (opposite limb is the involved hip) | ○○○ | ○○○ |
| Maintains relaxation of the limb | ○○○ | ○○○ |
| Performs assessment bilaterally | ○○○ | ○○○ |

The psychomotor skill was performed completely and in the appropriate order    **0  1  2  3  4  5**

The tester had control of the subject and the situation (showed confidence)    **0  1  2  3  4  5**

Method of performing the skill allowed the tester the ability to determine:
severity, proper progression, and the *fit* in the overall picture (Oral)    **0  1  2  3  4  5**

In order for a grade of *minimum standard* to be given, the total must be ≥11    **TOTAL =**

I_____I_____I
**Not Acceptable**    **Meets Minimum Standards**    **Exceeds Minimum Standards**

**L:** Laboratory/Classroom Testing
**C:** Clinical/Field Testing
**P:** Practicum Testing
**A:** Assessment/Mock Exam Testing
**S:** Self-Reporting

**Positive Finding:** Opposite leg comes off the table
**Involved Structure:** Iliopsoas, rectus femoris
**Special Considerations:** Starting position may be full flexion, move to extension
**Reference(s):** Konin et al; Magee; Starkey et al
**Supplies Needed:** Table

# SPECIAL TESTS
# (ST-L-Test 24)

Skill Acquisition: _____    Practice Opportunities: _____

*This problem allows you the opportunity to demonstrate the **Rectus Femoris Contracture Test, Method 1**. You have 2 minutes to complete this task.*

| Tester places athlete and limb in appropriate position | YES | NO |
|---|---|---|
| Supine | ○○○ | ○○○ |
| Knees flexed to 90 degrees (legs off the edge of the table) | ○○○ | ○○○ |
| **Tester placed in proper position** | **YES** | **NO** |
| Stands to the side of the athlete (observing only) | ○○○ | ○○○ |
| **Tester performs test according to accepted guidelines** | **YES** | **NO** |
| Instructs the athlete to actively flex the hip and knee of the opposite side (may be done passively by the tester) | ○○○ | ○○○ |
| Performs assessment bilaterally | ○○○ | ○○○ |

| | |
|---|---|
| The psychomotor skill was performed completely and in the appropriate order | 0  1  2  3  4  5 |
| The tester had control of the subject and the situation (showed confidence) | 0  1  2  3  4  5 |
| Method of performing the skill allowed the tester the ability to determine: severity, proper progression, and the *fit* in the overall picture (Oral) | 0  1  2  3  4  5 |

In order for a grade of *minimum standard* to be given, the total must be ≥11          TOTAL =

I_____I_____I

Not Acceptable          Meets Minimum Standards          Exceeds Minimum Standards

**L:** Laboratory/Classroom Testing
**C:** Clinical/Field Testing
**P:** Practicum Testing
**A:** Assessment/Mock Exam Testing
**S:** Self-Reporting

**Positive Finding:** Opposite leg moves into an extended position (flexion and extension)
**Involved Structure:** Iliopsoas, rectus femoris
**Special Considerations:** N/A
**Reference(s):** Konin et al; Magee
**Supplies Needed:** Table

## SPECIAL TESTS
# (ST-L-Test 25)

Peer Review _____ Peer Review _____

Skill Acquisition: _____    Practice Opportunities: _____

*This problem allows you the opportunity to demonstrate **Ober's Test**. You have 2 minutes to complete this task.*

| Tester places athlete and limb in appropriate position | YES | NO |
|---|---|---|
| Side lying (involved limb on top) | ○○○ | ○○○ |
| Hip/knee of the opposite limb is flexed | ○○○ | ○○○ |
| **Tester placed in proper position** | **YES** | **NO** |
| Stands behind the athlete | ○○○ | ○○○ |
| Places hand over the lateral aspect of the pelvis (prevent rolling/stabilize) | ○○○ | ○○○ |
| Places the other hand under the lower leg (support) | ○○○ | ○○○ |
| **Tester performs test according to accepted guidelines** | **YES** | **NO** |
| Passively abducts and extends the hip | ○○○ | ○○○ |
| Instructs the athlete to slowly lower the hip (adduction) | ○○○ | ○○○ |
| Performs assessment bilaterally | ○○○ | ○○○ |

The psychomotor skill was performed completely and in the appropriate order    **0 1 2 3 4 5**

The tester had control of the subject and the situation (showed confidence)    **0 1 2 3 4 5**

Method of performing the skill allowed the tester the ability to determine:
severity, proper progression, and the *fit* in the overall picture (Oral)    **0 1 2 3 4 5**

In order for a grade of *minimum standard* to be given, the total must be ≥11    **TOTAL =**

I_____I_____I

**Not Acceptable**          **Meets Minimum Standards**          **Exceeds Minimum Standards**

**L:** Laboratory/Classroom Testing
**C:** Clinical/Field Testing
**P:** Practicum Testing
**A:** Assessment/Mock Exam Testing
**S:** Self-Reporting

**Positive Finding:** Unable to adduct the hip
**Involved Structure:** Iliotibial band, tensor fasciae latae
**Special Considerations:** N/A
**Reference(s):** Konin et al; Magee; Starkey et al
**Supplies Needed:** Table

# SPECIAL TESTS
# (ST-L-Test 26)

Peer Review _____ Peer Review _____

Skill Acquisition: _____    Practice Opportunities: _____

*This problem allows you the opportunity to demonstrate **Noble's Compression Test (Noble's Test)** in order to help rule out iliotibial band friction syndrome. You have 2 minutes to complete this task.*

| Tester places athlete and limb in appropriate position | YES | NO |
|---|---|---|
| Supine | ○○○ | ○○○ |
| Knee flexed to 90 degrees | ○○○ | ○○○ |
| **Tester placed in proper position** | **YES** | **NO** |
| Stands to the side of the athlete | ○○○ | ○○○ |
| Places thumb and/or fingers over the lateral femoral epicondyle | ○○○ | ○○○ |
| Places other hand under the knee for support | ○○○ | ○○○ |
| **Tester performs test according to accepted guidelines** | **YES** | **NO** |
| Applies pressure over the lateral femoral epicondyle | ○○○ | ○○○ |
| Instructs the athlete to actively extend the knee at slow pace (may be performed passively) | ○○○ | ○○○ |
| Performs assessment bilaterally | ○○○ | ○○○ |

The psychomotor skill was performed completely and in the appropriate order    0 1 2 3 4 5

The tester had control of the subject and the situation (showed confidence)    0 1 2 3 4 5

Method of performing the skill allowed the tester the ability to determine:
severity, proper progression, and the *fit* in the overall picture (Oral)    0 1 2 3 4 5

In order for a grade of *minimum standard* to be given, the total must be ≥11    TOTAL =

I_____I_____I
**Not Acceptable**      **Meets Minimum Standards**      **Exceeds Minimum Standards**

**L:** Laboratory/Classroom Testing
**C:** Clinical/Field Testing
**P:** Practicum Testing
**A:** Assessment/Mock Exam Testing
**S:** Self-Reporting

**Positive Finding:** Increased pain around 30 degrees of extension
**Involved Structure:** Iliotibial band
**Special Considerations:** N/A
**Reference(s):** Magee; Starkey et al
**Supplies Needed:** Table

## SPECIAL TESTS
# (ST-L-Test 27)

Peer Review _____ Peer Review _____

Skill Acquisition: _____    Practice Opportunities: _____

*This problem allows you the opportunity to demonstrate the **Piriformis Test**. You have 2 minutes to complete this task.*

| Tester places athlete and limb in appropriate position | YES | NO |
|---|---|---|
| Side lying near the edge to the table (involved side on top) | OOO | OOO |
| Hip flexed to 60 degrees | OOO | OOO |
| Knee in slight flexion | OOO | OOO |
| **Tester placed in proper position** | **YES** | **NO** |
| Stands behind the athlete | OOO | OOO |
| Places hand over the lateral aspect of the pelvis (prevent rolling/stabilize) | OOO | OOO |
| Places the other hand over the knee | OOO | OOO |
| **Tester performs test according to accepted guidelines** | **YES** | **NO** |
| Applies a downward pressure on the knee | OOO | OOO |
| Maintains relaxation of the limb | OOO | OOO |
| Performs assessment bilaterally | OOO | OOO |

The psychomotor skill was performed completely and in the appropriate order    0 1 2 3 4 5

The tester had control of the subject and the situation (showed confidence)    0 1 2 3 4 5

Method of performing the skill allowed the tester the ability to determine:
severity, proper progression, and the *fit* in the overall picture (Oral)    0 1 2 3 4 5

In order for a grade of *minimum standard* to be given, the total must be ≥11    **TOTAL =**

I_____I_____I

**Not Acceptable**          **Meets Minimum Standards**          **Exceeds Minimum Standards**

**L:** Laboratory/Classroom Testing
**C:** Clinical/Field Testing
**P:** Practicum Testing
**A:** Assessment/Mock Exam Testing
**S:** Self-Reporting

**Positive Finding:** Tightness and/or pain
**Involved Structure:** Piriformis/sciatic nerve
**Special Considerations:** N/A
**Reference(s):** Konin et al; Magee
**Supplies Needed:** Table

# SPECIAL TESTS
# (ST-L-Test 28)

Skill Acquisition: _____     Practice Opportunities: _____

*This problem allows you the opportunity to demonstrate the* **90/90 Straight Leg Raise Test (Hamstrings Contracture, Method 3)**. *You have 2 minutes to complete this task.*

| Tester places athlete and limb in appropriate position | YES | NO |
|---|---|---|
| Supine | ○○○ | ○○○ |
| Hips flexed to 90 degrees (supported by the athlete) | ○○○ | ○○○ |
| Knees flexed to 90 degrees | ○○○ | ○○○ |
| **Tester placed in proper position** | **YES** | **NO** |
| Standing to the side of the athlete (observing only) | ○○○ | ○○○ |
| **Tester performs test according to accepted guidelines** | **YES** | **NO** |
| Instructs athlete to actively extend knee | ○○○ | ○○○ |
| Performs assessment bilaterally | ○○○ | ○○○ |

| | |
|---|---|
| The psychomotor skill was performed completely and in the appropriate order | 0  1  2  3  4  5 |
| The tester had control of the subject and the situation (showed confidence) | 0  1  2  3  4  5 |
| Method of performing the skill allowed the tester the ability to determine: severity, proper progression, and the *fit* in the overall picture (Oral) | 0  1  2  3  4  5 |

In order for a grade of *minimum standard* to be given, the total must be ≥11          TOTAL =

I_____I_____I

**Not Acceptable**          **Meets Minimum Standards**          **Exceeds Minimum Standards**

**L:** Laboratory/Classroom Testing
**C:** Clinical/Field Testing
**P:** Practicum Testing
**A:** Assessment/Mock Exam Testing
**S:** Self-Reporting

**Positive Finding:** Not able to extend to 20 degrees
**Involved Structure:** Hamstrings
**Special Considerations:** N/A
**Reference(s):** Konin et al; Magee
**Supplies Needed:** Table

## SPECIAL TESTS
# (ST-L-Test 29)

Peer Review _____  Peer Review _____

Skill Acquisition: _____  Practice Opportunities: _____

*This problem allows you the opportunity to demonstrate the special test known as the* **Gillet's Test (Sacral Fixation Test)**. *You have 2 minutes to complete this task.*

| | YES | NO |
|---|---|---|
| **Tester places athlete and limb in appropriate position** | YES | NO |
| Standing | ○○○ | ○○○ |
| **Tester placed in proper position** | YES | NO |
| Standing behind the athlete | ○○○ | ○○○ |
| Hands palpating the PSIS (monitor movement of the PSIS) | ○○○ | ○○○ |
| **Tester performs test according to accepted guidelines** | YES | NO |
| Instructs the athlete to actively flex the knee and hip while balancing on one leg (pulling toward the chest) | ○○○ | ○○○ |
| Performs assessment bilaterally | ○○○ | ○○○ |

The psychomotor skill was performed completely and in the appropriate order     **0  1  2  3  4  5**

The tester had control of the subject and the situation (showed confidence)     **0  1  2  3  4  5**

Method of performing the skill allowed the tester the ability to determine:
severity, proper progression, and the *fit* in the overall picture (Oral)     **0  1  2  3  4  5**

In order for a grade of *minimum standard* to be given, the total must be ≥11     **TOTAL =**

I_____I_____I
**Not Acceptable**          **Meets Minimum Standards**          **Exceeds Minimum Standards**

**Positive Finding:** Flexed side moves upward hypomobility

**L:** Laboratory/Classroom Testing
**C:** Clinical/Field Testing
**P:** Practicum Testing
**A:** Assessment/Mock Exam Testing
**S:** Self-Reporting

**Involved Structure:** Sacroiliac
**Special Considerations:** Normal movement should be downward (inferiorly)
**Reference(s):** Magee
**Supplies Needed:** N/A

## Special Tests
# (ST-L-Test 30)

Peer Review _____ Peer Review _____

Skill Acquisition: _____     Practice Opportunities: _____

*This problem allows you the opportunity to demonstrate the special test known as the **Squish Test**. You have 2 minutes to complete this task.*

| Tester places athlete and limb in appropriate position | YES | NO |
|---|---|---|
| Supine | OOO | OOO |
| **Tester placed in proper position** | **YES** | **NO** |
| Stands behind the athlete | OOO | OOO |
| Places hands over the ASIS/iliac crest | OOO | OOO |
| **Tester performs test according to accepted guidelines** | **YES** | **NO** |
| Passively push down and in (45 degree angle) | OOO | OOO |
| Maintains relaxation of the limb | OOO | OOO |

The psychomotor skill was performed completely and in the appropriate order    0 1 2 3 4 5

The tester had control of the subject and the situation (showed confidence)    0 1 2 3 4 5

Method of performing the skill allowed the tester the ability to determine:
severity, proper progression, and the *fit* in the overall picture (Oral)    0 1 2 3 4 5

In order for a grade of *minimum standard* to be given, the total must be ≥11    TOTAL =

I_____I_____I

**Not Acceptable**    **Meets Minimum Standards**    **Exceeds Minimum Standards**

**L:** Laboratory/Classroom Testing
**C:** Clinical/Field Testing
**P:** Practicum Testing
**A:** Assessment/Mock Exam Testing
**S:** Self-Reporting

**Positive Finding:** Pain
**Involved Structure:** Posterior sacroiliac ligament
**Special Considerations:** N/A
**Reference(s):** Magee
**Supplies Needed:** Table

## SPECIAL TESTS
# (ST-L-Test 31)

Peer Review _____ Peer Review _____

Skill Acquisition: _____    Practice Opportunities: _____

*This problem allows you the opportunity to demonstrate the special test known as the* **Long Sit Test (Supine-to-Sit Test)**. *You have 2 minutes to perform this task.*

| Tester places athlete and limb in appropriate position | YES | NO |
|---|---|---|
| Supine | ○○○ | ○○○ |
| Heels off the table (both medial malleoli should be even with each other) | ○○○ | ○○○ |
| **Tester placed in proper position** | **YES** | **NO** |
| Stands at the athlete's feet | ○○○ | ○○○ |
| Places hands/thumbs over the medial malleoli | ○○○ | ○○○ |
| **Tester performs test according to accepted guidelines** | **YES** | **NO** |
| Instructs the athlete to actively sit up (supine to sitting) | ○○○ | ○○○ |
| Repeat (confirm the results) | ○○○ | ○○○ |

The psychomotor skill was performed completely and in the appropriate order    **0 1 2 3 4 5**

The tester had control of the subject and the situation (showed confidence)    **0 1 2 3 4 5**

Method of performing the skill allowed the tester the ability to determine:
severity, proper progression, and the *fit* in the overall picture (Oral)    **0 1 2 3 4 5**

In order for a grade of *minimum standard* to be given, the total must be ≥11    **TOTAL =**

I_____I_____I

**Not Acceptable**      **Meets Minimum Standards**      **Exceeds Minimum Standards**

**L:** Laboratory/Classroom Testing
**C:** Clinical/Field Testing
**P:** Practicum Testing
**A:** Assessment/Mock Exam Testing
**S:** Self-Reporting

**Positive Finding:** One leg moves further than the other (medial malleoli)
**Involved Structure:** Ilium (rotation/functional)
**Special Considerations:** N/A
**Reference(s):** Magee; Starkey et al
**Supplies Needed:** Table

## SPECIAL TESTS
# (ST-L-Test 32)

Peer Review _____ Peer Review _____

Skill Acquisition: _____     Practice Opportunities: _____

*This problem allows you the opportunity to demonstrate the **Slump Test**. You have 2 minutes to complete this task.*

| Tester places athlete and limb in appropriate position | YES | NO |
|---|---|---|
| Seated (knees off the edge of the table at 90 degrees) | ○○○ | ○○○ |
| Hands positioned behind the back | ○○○ | ○○○ |
| **Tester placed in proper position** | **YES** | **NO** |
| Stands to the side of the athlete | ○○○ | ○○○ |
| Hand position changes throughout the assessment | ○○○ | ○○○ |
| **Tester performs test according to accepted guidelines** | **YES** | **NO** |
| Instructs the athlete to actively flex the thoracic and lumbar area (head remains neutral) | ○○○ | ○○○ |
| Passively applies overpressure to maintain flexion of the thoracic and lumbar areas | ○○○ | ○○○ |
| Instructs the athlete to actively flex the head (chin to chest) | ○○○ | ○○○ |
| Passively applies overpressure to maintain flexion of the head | ○○○ | ○○○ |
| Passively dorsiflexes the foot (maintains) | ○○○ | ○○○ |
| Instructs the athlete to actively extend the knee | ○○○ | ○○○ |
| Performs assessment bilaterally | ○○○ | ○○○ |

The psychomotor skill was performed completely and in the appropriate order    **0 1 2 3 4 5**

The tester had control of the subject and the situation (showed confidence)    **0 1 2 3 4 5**

Method of performing the skill allowed the tester the ability to determine: severity, proper progression, and the *fit* in the overall picture (Oral)    **0 1 2 3 4 5**

In order for a grade of *minimum standard* to be given, the total must be ≥11    **TOTAL =**

I_____I_____I

**Not Acceptable**     **Meets Minimum Standards**     **Exceeds Minimum Standards**

**L:** Laboratory/Classroom Testing
**C:** Clinical/Field Testing
**P:** Practicum Testing
**A:** Assessment/Mock Exam Testing
**S:** Self-Reporting

**Positive Finding:** Pain/neurological symptoms
**Involved Structure:** Nerve root; neurological structures
**Special Considerations:** Do not continue to next stage if pain occurs
**Reference(s):** Magee; Starkey et al
**Supplies Needed:** Table

## SPECIAL TESTS
# (ST-L-Test 33)

Peer Review _____ Peer Review _____

Skill Acquisition: _____    Practice Opportunities: _____

*This problem allows you the opportunity to demonstrate the special test known as the **Straight Leg Raise Test** (**Unilateral Straight Leg Raise/Lasegue Test**). You have 2 minutes to complete this task.*

| | YES | NO |
|---|---|---|
| **Tester places athlete and limb in appropriate position** | | |
| Supine | OOO | OOO |
| Hip slightly adducted and medially rotated | OOO | OOO |
| **Tester placed in proper position** | YES | NO |
| Stands to the side of the athlete (may kneel on the table) | OOO | OOO |
| Places one hand on the anterior thigh (maintains knee extension) | OOO | OOO |
| Places the other hand around the foot | OOO | OOO |
| **Tester performs test according to accepted guidelines** | YES | NO |
| Passively flexes the hip (until painful) | OOO | OOO |
| Slowly lowers the limb until pain dissipates | OOO | OOO |
| Passively dorsiflexes the foot | OOO | OOO |
| Instructs the athlete to actively flex the head (chin to chest) | OOO | OOO |
| Maintains relaxation of the limb | OOO | OOO |
| Performs assessment bilaterally | OOO | OOO |

The psychomotor skill was performed completely and in the appropriate order     0  1  2  3  4  5

The tester had control of the subject and the situation (showed confidence)     0  1  2  3  4  5

Method of performing the skill allowed the tester the ability to determine:
severity, proper progression, and the *fit* in the overall picture (Oral)     0  1  2  3  4  5

In order for a grade of *minimum standard* to be given, the total must be ≥11     **TOTAL =**

I_____I_____I

**Not Acceptable**         **Meets Minimum Standards**         **Exceeds Minimum Standards**

**L:** Laboratory/Classroom Testing
**C:** Clinical/Field Testing
**P:** Practicum Testing
**A:** Assessment/Mock Exam Testing
**S:** Self-Reporting

**Positive Finding:** Increased pain with dorsiflexion and/or flexion of the head
**Involved Structure:** Dural involvement
**Special Considerations:** Must rule out hamstrings
**Reference(s):** Konin et al; Magee; Starkey et al
**Supplies Needed:** Table

## SPECIAL TESTS
# (ST-L-Test 34)

Peer Review _____ Peer Review _____

Skill Acquisition: _____   Practice Opportunities: _____

*This problem allows you the opportunity to demonstrate the special test known as the* **Well Straight Leg Raise Test (Well Straight Leg Raise Test of Fajersztajn/Lhermitt's Test/Crossover Sign)**. *You have 2 minutes to complete this task.*

| Tester places athlete and limb in appropriate position | YES | NO |
|---|---|---|
| Supine | ○○○ | ○○○ |
| **Tester placed in proper position** | **YES** | **NO** |
| Stands to the side of the athlete (may kneel on the table) | ○○○ | ○○○ |
| Places one hand on anterior thigh (maintain knee extension) | ○○○ | ○○○ |
| Place the other hand around the foot | ○○○ | ○○○ |
| **Tester performs test according to accepted guidelines** | **YES** | **NO** |
| Passively flexes the hip (until painful at opposite side) | ○○○ | ○○○ |
| Maintains relaxation of the limb | ○○○ | ○○○ |
| Performs assessment bilaterally | ○○○ | ○○○ |

| | |
|---|---|
| The psychomotor skill was performed completely and in the appropriate order | 0  1  2  3  4  5 |
| The tester had control of the subject and the situation (showed confidence) | 0  1  2  3  4  5 |
| Method of performing the skill allowed the tester the ability to determine: severity, proper progression, and the *fit* in the overall picture (Oral) | 0  1  2  3  4  5 |

In order for a grade of *minimum standard* to be given, the total must be ≥11    **TOTAL =**

I_____I_____I
**Not Acceptable**      **Meets Minimum Standards**      **Exceeds Minimum Standards**

**L:** Laboratory/Classroom Testing
**C:** Clinical/Field Testing
**P:** Practicum Testing
**A:** Assessment/Mock Exam Testing
**S:** Self-Reporting

**Positive Finding:** Pain on opposite side
**Involved Structure:** Space-occupying lesion
**Special Considerations:** N/A
**Reference(s):** Konin et al; Starkey et al; Magee
**Supplies Needed:** Table

## SPECIAL TESTS
# (ST-L-Test 35)

Peer Review _____ Peer Review _____

Skill Acquisition: _____    Practice Opportunities: _____

*This problem allows you the opportunity to demonstrate the special test known as the* **Kernig's Sign\***. *You have 2 minutes to complete this task.*

| Tester places athlete and limb in appropriate position | YES | NO |
|---|---|---|
| Supine | OOO | OOO |
| **Tester placed in proper position** | **YES** | **NO** |
| Stands to the side of the athlete (observes only) | OOO | OOO |
| **Tester performs test according to accepted guidelines** | **YES** | **NO** |
| Instructs the athlete to actively flex the hip until painful (maintain knee extension) | OOO | OOO |
| Instructs the athlete to slowly flex the knee until pain dissipates | OOO | OOO |
| Performs assessment bilaterally | OOO | OOO |

*Adding head flexion: Kernig-Brudzinski Test

The psychomotor skill was performed completely and in the appropriate order     0  1  2  3  4  5

The tester had control of the subject and the situation (showed confidence)     0  1  2  3  4  5

Method of performing the skill allowed the tester the ability to determine:
severity, proper progression, and the *fit* in the overall picture (Oral)     0  1  2  3  4  5

In order for a grade of *minimum standard* to be given, the total must be ≥11     TOTAL =

I_____I_____I

**Not Acceptable**          **Meets Minimum Standards**     **Exceeds Minimum Standards**

**L:** Laboratory/Classroom Testing
**C:** Clinical/Field Testing
**P:** Practicum Testing
**A:** Assessment/Mock Exam Testing
**S:** Self-Reporting

**Positive Finding:** Pain is relieved with flexion of the knee
**Involved Structure:** Nerve root (impingement)
**Special Considerations:** N/A
**Reference(s):** Starkey et al; Konin et al
**Supplies Needed:** Table

## SPECIAL TESTS
# (ST-L-Test 36)

Peer Review _____ Peer Review _____

Skill Acquisition: _____    Practice Opportunities: _____

*This problem allows you the opportunity to demonstrate the special test known as the* **Brudzinski's Sign**. *You have 2 minutes to complete this task.*

| Tester places athlete and limb in appropriate position | YES | NO |
|---|---|---|
| Supine | ○○○ | ○○○ |
| Cupped hands behind the neck | ○○○ | ○○○ |
| **Tester placed in proper position** | **YES** | **NO** |
| Stands to the side of the athlete | ○○○ | ○○○ |
| **Tester performs test according to accepted guidelines** | **YES** | **NO** |
| Instructs the athlete to actively flex the head (chin to chest) | ○○○ | ○○○ |
| May flex the head passively (overpressure) | ○○○ | ○○○ |

| | |
|---|---|
| The psychomotor skill was performed completely and in the appropriate order | 0  1  2  3  4  5 |
| The tester had control of the subject and the situation (showed confidence) | 0  1  2  3  4  5 |
| Method of performing the skill allowed the tester the ability to determine: severity, proper progression, and the *fit* in the overall picture (Oral) | 0  1  2  3  4  5 |

In order for a grade of *minimum standard* to be given, the total must be ≥11        **TOTAL =**

I_____I_____I
**Not Acceptable**          **Meets Minimum Standards**     **Exceeds Minimum Standards**

**L:** Laboratory/Classroom Testing
**C:** Clinical/Field Testing
**P:** Practicum Testing
**A:** Assessment/Mock Exam Testing
**S:** Self-Reporting

**Positive Finding:** Pain; involuntarily flexes knee(s)
**Involved Structure:** Nerve root
**Special Considerations:** N/A
**Reference(s):** Starkey et al; Konin et al; Magee
**Supplies Needed:** Table

## Special Tests
# (ST-L-Test 37)

Peer Review _____ Peer Review _____

Skill Acquisition: _____    Practice Opportunities: _____

*This problem allows you the opportunity to demonstrate the* **Bowstring Test (Cram Test/Popliteal Pressure Sign)** *in order to help rule out pressure on the sciatic nerve. You have 2 minutes to complete this task.*

| Tester places athlete and limb in appropriate position | YES | NO |
|---|---|---|
| Supine | OOO | OOO |
| Hip slightly adducted and medially rotated | OOO | OOO |
| **Tester placed in proper position** | **YES** | **NO** |
| Stands to the side of the athlete (may kneel on the table) | OOO | OOO |
| Places one hand on the anterior thigh (maintains knee extension) | OOO | OOO |
| Places the other hand around the foot | OOO | OOO |
| **Tester performs test according to accepted guidelines** | **YES** | **NO** |
| Passively flexes the hip (until painful) | OOO | OOO |
| Slowly flexes the knee about 20 degrees | OOO | OOO |
| Applies pressure into the popliteal space | OOO | OOO |
| Maintains relaxation of the limb | OOO | OOO |
| Performs assessment bilaterally | OOO | OOO |

The psychomotor skill was performed completely and in the appropriate order    **0  1  2  3  4  5**

The tester had control of the subject and the situation (showed confidence)    **0  1  2  3  4  5**

Method of performing the skill allowed the tester the ability to determine:
severity, proper progression, and the *fit* in the overall picture (Oral)    **0  1  2  3  4  5**

In order for a grade of *minimum standard* to be given, the total must be ≥11    **TOTAL =**

I_____I_____I

**Not Acceptable**        **Meets Minimum Standards**    **Exceeds Minimum Standards**

**L:** Laboratory/Classroom Testing    **Positive Finding:** Pain (with pressure)
**C:** Clinical/Field Testing    **Involved Structure:** Sciatic nerve
**P:** Practicum Testing    **Special Considerations:** N/A
**A:** Assessment/Mock Exam Testing    **Reference(s):** Konin et al; Magee
**S:** Self-Reporting    **Supplies Needed:** Table

# SPECIAL TESTS
# (ST-L-Test 38)

Peer Review _____ Peer Review _____

Skill Acquisition: _____    Practice Opportunities: _____

*This problem allows you the opportunity to demonstrate the special test known as the **Hoover's Sign**. You have 2 minutes to complete this task.*

| Tester places athlete and limb in appropriate position | YES | NO |
|---|---|---|
| Supine (heels completely on the table) | OOO | OOO |
| **Tester placed in proper position** | **YES** | **NO** |
| Stands at the athlete's feet | OOO | OOO |
| Places the palms of the hands under the heels (calcaneus) | OOO | OOO |
| **Tester performs test according to accepted guidelines** | **YES** | **NO** |
| Instructs the athlete to actively flex the hip | OOO | OOO |
| Instructs the athlete to actively flex the other hip | OOO | OOO |

| | |
|---|---|
| The psychomotor skill was performed completely and in the appropriate order | 0  1  2  3  4  5 |
| The tester had control of the subject and the situation (showed confidence) | 0  1  2  3  4  5 |
| Method of performing the skill allowed the tester the ability to determine: severity, proper progression, and the *fit* in the overall picture (Oral) | 0  1  2  3  4  5 |

In order for a grade of *minimum standard* to be given, the total must be ≥11          **TOTAL =**

I_____I_____I

**Not Acceptable**          **Meets Minimum Standards**          **Exceeds Minimum Standards**

**L:** Laboratory/Classroom Testing
**C:** Clinical/Field Testing
**P:** Practicum Testing
**A:** Assessment/Mock Exam Testing
**S:** Self-Reporting

**Positive Finding:** No downward pressure by the opposite leg
**Involved Structure:** Neuromuscular weakness or lack of effort by the subject
**Special Considerations:** N/A
**Reference(s):** Konin et al; Magee
**Supplies Needed:** Table

## SPECIAL TESTS
# (ST-L-Test 39)

Skill Acquisition: _____    Practice Opportunities: _____

*This problem allows you the opportunity to demonstrate the special test known as the* **Stork Standing Test (One Leg Standing Lumbar Extension Test)**. *You have 2 minutes to complete this task.*

| Tester places athlete and limb in appropriate position | YES | NO |
|---|---|---|
| Standing | OOO | OOO |
| **Tester placed in proper position** | **YES** | **NO** |
| Stands behind the athlete (observe only) | OOO | OOO |
| **Tester performs test according to accepted guidelines** | **YES** | **NO** |
| Instructs the athlete to balance on one leg | OOO | OOO |
| Instructs the athlete to hyperextend the trunk (maintain balance) | OOO | OOO |
| Repeat test on opposite leg | OOO | OOO |

| | |
|---|---|
| The psychomotor skill was performed completely and in the appropriate order | 0  1  2  3  4  5 |
| The tester had control of the subject and the situation (showed confidence) | 0  1  2  3  4  5 |
| Method of performing the skill allowed the tester the ability to determine: severity, proper progression, and the *fit* in the overall picture (Oral) | 0  1  2  3  4  5 |

In order for a grade of *minimum standard* to be given, the total must be ≥11          TOTAL =

I_____I_____I
**Not Acceptable**          **Meets Minimum Standards**          **Exceeds Minimum Standards**

**L:** Laboratory/Classroom Testing
**C:** Clinical/Field Testing
**P:** Practicum Testing
**A:** Assessment/Mock Exam Testing
**S:** Self-Reporting

**Positive Finding:** Pain
**Involved Structure:** Pars interarticularis (lumbar area)
**Special Considerations:** N/A
**Reference(s):** Magee
**Supplies Needed:** N/A

# SPECIAL TESTS
# (ST-L-Test 40)

Peer Review _____ Peer Review _____

Skill Acquisition: _____    Practice Opportunities: _____

*This problem allows you the opportunity to demonstrate the **Spring Test** to help rule out problems with hypo-mobility of the vertebrae. You have 2 minutes to complete this task.*

| Tester places athlete and limb in appropriate position | YES | NO |
|---|---|---|
| Prone | OOO | OOO |
| **Tester placed in proper position** | **YES** | **NO** |
| Stands to the side of the athlete | OOO | OOO |
| Places thumbs (or hypothenar eminence) over the spinous process | OOO | OOO |
| **Tester performs test according to accepted guidelines** | **YES** | **NO** |
| Applies pressure downward (P-A motion through the spinous process toward the table) | OOO | OOO |
| Repeats downward pressure (each lumbar vertebra) | OOO | OOO |

The psychomotor skill was performed completely and in the appropriate order    **0  1  2  3  4  5**

The tester had control of the subject and the situation (showed confidence)    **0  1  2  3  4  5**

Method of performing the skill allowed the tester the ability to determine:
severity, proper progression, and the *fit* in the overall picture (Oral)    **0  1  2  3  4  5**

In order for a grade of *minimum standard* to be given, the total must be ≥11    **TOTAL =**

I_____I_____I

**Not Acceptable**          **Meets Minimum Standards**          **Exceeds Minimum Standards**

**L:** Laboratory/Classroom Testing
**C:** Clinical/Field Testing
**P:** Practicum Testing
**A:** Assessment/Mock Exam Testing
**S:** Self-Reporting

**Positive Finding:** Lack of movement; pain
**Involved Structure:** Facet joints (lumbar)
**Special Considerations:** N/A
**Reference(s):** Konin et al; Starkey et al
**Supplies Needed:** Table

## SPECIAL TESTS
# (ST-L-Test 41)

Peer Review _____ Peer Review _____

Skill Acquisition: _____    Practice Opportunities: _____

*This problem allows you the opportunity to demonstrate the special test known as the* **Yeoman's Test**. *You have 2 minutes to complete this task.*

| Tester places athlete and limb in appropriate position | YES | NO |
|---|---|---|
| Prone | ○○○ | ○○○ |
| Knee flexed to 90 degrees | ○○○ | ○○○ |
| **Tester placed in proper position** | **YES** | **NO** |
| Stands to the side of the athlete | ○○○ | ○○○ |
| Places one hand under the knee (anterior thigh) | ○○○ | ○○○ |
| Places the other hand at the pelvis (stabilizes) | ○○○ | ○○○ |
| **Tester performs test according to accepted guidelines** | **YES** | **NO** |
| Maintains knee flexion | ○○○ | ○○○ |
| Passively hyperextends the hip | ○○○ | ○○○ |
| Maintains relaxation of the limb | ○○○ | ○○○ |
| Performs assessment bilaterally | ○○○ | ○○○ |

The psychomotor skill was performed completely and in the appropriate order      **0  1  2  3  4  5**

The tester had control of the subject and the situation (showed confidence)      **0  1  2  3  4  5**

Method of performing the skill allowed the tester the ability to determine:
severity, proper progression, and the *fit* in the overall picture (Oral)      **0  1  2  3  4  5**

In order for a grade of *minimum standard* to be given, the total must be ≥11      **TOTAL =**

I_____I_____I

**Not Acceptable**          **Meets Minimum Standards**          **Exceeds Minimum Standards**

**L:** Laboratory/Classroom Testing
**C:** Clinical/Field Testing
**P:** Practicum Testing
**A:** Assessment/Mock Exam Testing
**S:** Self-Reporting

**Positive Finding:** Pain
**Involved Structure:** Sacroiliac joint, lumbar joints, femoral nerve
**Special Considerations:** N/A
**Reference(s):** Magee
**Supplies Needed:** Table

*Chapter*

# TAPING/WRAPPING

# Taping/Wrapping
## (TW-U-Test 1)

Peer Review _____ Peer Review _____

Skill Acquisition: _____     Practice Opportunities: _____

*This problem allows you the opportunity to demonstrate a* **taping technique to prevent hyperextension of the elbow**. *You have 3 minutes to complete this task.*

| Tester places athlete and limb in appropriate position | YES | NO |
|---|---|---|
| Seated or standing | ○○○ | ○○○ |
| Extends elbow to the point of pain (backs off approximately 10 to 20 degrees) | ○○○ | ○○○ |
| Contracts biceps and forearm | ○○○ | ○○○ |
| **Taping technique** | **YES** | **NO** |
| Applies tape adhesive/applies underwrap (optional) | ○○○ | ○○○ |
| Applies anchor(s) to skin, mid-to-upper humerus | ○○○ | ○○○ |
| Applies anchor(s) to skin, mid-to-lower forearm | ○○○ | ○○○ |
| Applies longitudinal fan to anterior surface of the elbow (approximately five strips) | ○○○ | ○○○ |
| Reinforces the center of the fan | ○○○ | ○○○ |
| Secures fan at proximal and distal ends | ○○○ | ○○○ |
| Applies closures to secure holes and loose ends | ○○○ | ○○○ |
| Closes with stretch tape or elastic compression wrap | ○○○ | ○○○ |
| **Support and neatness** | **YES** | **NO** |
| Prevents elbow from moving into full extension | ○○○ | ○○○ |
| Maintains good circulation to the hand | ○○○ | ○○○ |
| No holes and/or loose ends | ○○○ | ○○○ |

The psychomotor skill was performed completely and in the appropriate order     **0  1  2  3  4  5**

The tester had control of the subject and the situation (showed confidence)     **0  1  2  3  4  5**

Method of performing the skill allowed the tester the ability to determine:
severity, proper progression, and the *fit* in the overall picture (Oral)     **0  1  2  3  4  5**

In order for a grade of *minimum standard* to be given, the total must be ≥11     **TOTAL =**

I_____I_____I
**Not Acceptable**          **Meets Minimum Standards**          **Exceeds Minimum Standards**

**L:** Laboratory/Classroom Testing
**C:** Clinical/Field Testing
**P:** Practicum Testing
**A:** Assessment/Mock Exam Testing
**S:** Self-Reporting

**Positive Finding:** Prevent hyperextension
**Involved Structure:** Elbow
**Special Considerations:** N/A
**Reference(s):** Wright et al; Perrin
**Supplies Needed:** 1.5-inch white tape, stretch tape or elastic wrap, prewrap

**TAPING/WRAPPING**
# (TW-U-Test 2)

Peer Review _____ Peer Review _____

Skill Acquisition: _____    Practice Opportunities: _____

*Please demonstrate how you would perform a **shoulder spica taping** of the **glenohumeral joint** to help prevent external rotation. You have 3 minutes to complete this task.*

| Tester places athlete and limb in appropriate position | YES | NO |
|---|---|---|
| Standing | ○○○ | ○○○ |
| Shoulder abducted with the hand resting on the low back (elbow flexed) | ○○○ | ○○○ |
| Contracts biceps | | |
|   For a male athlete, cover both nipples with either gauze or band-aids | ○○○ | ○○○ |
|   For a female athlete, tape over a sports bra | ○○○ | ○○○ |
| **Taping technique** | **YES** | **NO** |
| Taping begins at the distal portion of the affected upper arm and moves anteriorly, encircling the affected arm | ○○○ | ○○○ |
| Continues the tape across the anterior portion of the chest, under the opposite arm, and across the back | ○○○ | ○○○ |
| Repeats the above procedure a second time, ending by encircling the affected upper arm | ○○○ | ○○○ |
| Places a check rein between the upper arm and the torso (optional) | ○○○ | ○○○ |
| **Support and neatness** | **YES** | **NO** |
| Prevents abduction and external rotation of the shoulder | ○○○ | ○○○ |
| Maintains good circulation to the hands and finger | ○○○ | ○○○ |
| No holes and/or loose ends | ○○○ | ○○○ |

The psychomotor skill was performed completely and in the appropriate order    0  1  2  3  4  5

The tester had control of the subject and the situation (showed confidence)    0  1  2  3  4  5

Method of performing the skill allowed the tester the ability to determine: severity, proper progression, and the *fit* in the overall picture (Oral)    0  1  2  3  4  5

In order for a grade of *minimum standard* to be given, the total must be ≥11    **TOTAL =**

I_____I_____I

**Not Acceptable**　　**Meets Minimum Standards**　　**Exceeds Minimum Standards**

**L:** Laboratory/Classroom Testing
**C:** Clinical/Field Testing
**P:** Practicum Testing
**A:** Assessment/Mock Exam Testing
**S:** Self-Reporting

**Positive Finding:** Restrict abduction/external rotation
**Involved Structure:** Glenohumeral joint
**Special Considerations:** May practice with ACE wrap
**Reference(s):** Wright et al
**Supplies Needed:** Elastic tape, 1.5-inch white tape, gauze/band-aids, prewrap

# TAPING/WRAPPING
## (TW-U-Test 3)

Peer Review _____ Peer Review _____

Skill Acquisition: _____    Practice Opportunities: _____

*Please demonstrate how you would perform a **shoulder spica elastic wrap** in order to help support the **gleno-humeral joint**. You have 3 minutes to complete this task.*

| Tester places athlete and limb in appropriate position | YES | NO |
|---|---|---|
| Standing | ○○○ | ○○○ |
| Shoulder abducted with hand resting on low back (elbow flexed) | ○○○ | ○○○ |
| Contracts biceps | ○○○ | ○○○ |
| Instructs the athlete to breathe deeply (expand the chest) | ○○○ | ○○○ |
| **Taping technique** | **YES** | **NO** |
| Using 6-inch elastic (double) wrap, begins at the distal aspect of the biceps muscle and encircles the arm, pulling the wrap from posterior to anterior | ○○○ | ○○○ |
| Continues the wrap across the chest, beneath the opposite arm, around the back, and encircles the upper arm | ○○○ | ○○○ |
| Repeats the above steps until the wrap runs out | ○○○ | ○○○ |
| Secures the wrap with elastic tape and adhesive tape | ○○○ | ○○○ |
| **Support and neatness** | **YES** | **NO** |
| Provides support to the glenohumeral joint | ○○○ | ○○○ |
| Maintains good circulation to the hand and fingers | ○○○ | ○○○ |
| No gaps and/or loose ends | ○○○ | ○○○ |

| | |
|---|---|
| The psychomotor skill was performed completely and in the appropriate order | 0  1  2  3  4  5 |
| The tester had control of the subject and the situation (showed confidence) | 0  1  2  3  4  5 |
| Method of performing the skill allowed the tester the ability to determine: severity, proper progression, and the *fit* in the overall picture (Oral) | 0  1  2  3  4  5 |

In order for a grade of *minimum standard* to be given, the total must be ≥11        **TOTAL =**

I_____I_____I
**Not Acceptable**        **Meets Minimum Standards**        **Exceeds Minimum Standards**

**L:** Laboratory/Classroom Testing
**C:** Clinical/Field Testing
**P:** Practicum Testing
**A:** Assessment/Mock Exam Testing
**S:** Self-Reporting

**Positive Finding:** Support/stabilize
**Involved Structure:** Glenohumeral joint
**Special Considerations:** N/A
**Reference(s):** Wright et al; Perrin
**Supplies Needed:** 6- to 4-inch double elastic wrap, 1.5-inch white tape

# TAPING/WRAPPING
## (TW-U-Test 4)

Peer Review _____ Peer Review _____

Skill Acquisition: _____     Practice Opportunities: _____

*Please demonstrate how you would perform a **shoulder spica taping** for injury to the **acromioclavicular joint**. You have 3 minutes to complete this task.*

| Tester places athlete and limb in appropriate position | YES | NO |
|---|---|---|
| Standing | ○○○ | ○○○ |
| Shoulder abducted with hand resting on low back (elbow flexed) | ○○○ | ○○○ |
| Contracts biceps | | |
|    For a male athlete, cover both nipples with either gauze or band-aids | ○○○ | ○○○ |
|    For a female athlete, tape over a sports bra | ○○○ | ○○○ |

| Taping technique | YES | NO |
|---|---|---|
| Places a horizontal anchor from the anterior to posterior midline of the body, covering the mid-to-lower portion of the ribs (note: on a female athlete, all strips should end above the breast) | ○○○ | ○○○ |
| Applies strips of tape over the AC joint by placing the middle of the strip over the AC joint and applying equal tension toward both the anterior and posterior ends, attaching the tape to the midline anchor | ○○○ | ○○○ |
| Repeats the above step three more times (overlap) | ○○○ | ○○○ |
| Applies another anchor that encircles the entire torso, securing the strips | ○○○ | ○○○ |

| Support and neatness | YES | NO |
|---|---|---|
| Provides proper support to the AC joint | ○○○ | ○○○ |
| Maintains good circulation to hands and fingers | ○○○ | ○○○ |
| Should not hinder movement or breathing | ○○○ | ○○○ |
| No holes and/or loose ends | ○○○ | ○○○ |

The psychomotor skill was performed completely and in the appropriate order   **0  1  2  3  4  5**

The tester had control of the subject and the situation (showed confidence)   **0  1  2  3  4  5**

Method of performing the skill allowed the tester the ability to determine: severity, proper progression, and the *fit* in the overall picture (Oral)   **0  1  2  3  4  5**

In order for a grade of *minimum standard* to be given, the total must be ≥11   **TOTAL =**

I_____I_____I

**Not Acceptable**    **Meets Minimum Standards**    **Exceeds Minimum Standards**

**L:** Laboratory/Classroom Testing
**C:** Clinical/Field Testing
**P:** Practicum Testing
**A:** Assessment/Mock Exam Testing
**S:** Self-Reporting

**Positive Finding:** Support
**Involved Structure:** AC joint
**Special Considerations:** N/A
**Reference(s):** Wright et al; Perrin
**Supplies Needed:** 2-inch elastic tape, 1.5-inch white tape, gauze/band-aids

## TAPING/WRAPPING
# (TW-U-Test 5)

Peer Review _____ Peer Review _____

Skill Acquisition: _____    Practice Opportunities: _____

*Please demonstrate how you would perform a **shoulder spica elastic wrap** to secure a doughnut pad over the* **acromioclavicular joint**. *You have 3 minutes to complete this task.*

| Tester places athlete and limb in appropriate position | YES | NO |
|---|---|---|
| Standing | OOO | OOO |
| Shoulder abducted with hand resting on low back (elbow flexed) | OOO | OOO |
| Contracts biceps | OOO | OOO |
| Instructs the athlete to breathe deeply (expand the chest) | OOO | OOO |
| **Taping technique** | **YES** | **NO** |
| Places the doughnut pad over the AC joint | OOO | OOO |
| Using 6-inch elastic wrap, begins at the distal aspect of the biceps muscle and encircles the arm, pulling the wrap from posterior to anterior | OOO | OOO |
| Continues the wrap across the chest, beneath the opposite arm, around the back, and encircle the upper arm | OOO | OOO |
| Repeats the above steps until you run out of wrap | OOO | OOO |
| Secures the wrap with elastic tape and adhesive tape | OOO | OOO |
| **Support and neatness** | **YES** | **NO** |
| Holds pad over the AC joint | OOO | OOO |
| Maintains good circulation to hand and fingers | OOO | OOO |
| No gaps and/or loose ends | OOO | OOO |

The psychomotor skill was performed completely and in the appropriate order   **0 1 2 3 4 5**

The tester had control of the subject and the situation (showed confidence)   **0 1 2 3 4 5**

Method of performing the skill allowed the tester the ability to determine:
severity, proper progression, and the *fit* in the overall picture (Oral)   **0 1 2 3 4 5**

In order for a grade of *minimum standard* to be given, the total must be ≥11      **TOTAL =**

I_____I_____I
**Not Acceptable**      **Meets Minimum Standards**   **Exceeds Minimum Standards**

**L:** Laboratory/Classroom Testing
**C:** Clinical/Field Testing
**P:** Practicum Testing
**A:** Assessment/Mock Exam Testing
**S:** Self-Reporting

**Positive Finding:** Secure pad
**Involved Structure:** AC joint
**Special Considerations:** N/A
**Reference(s):** Perrin
**Supplies Needed:** 6- to 4-inch double elastic wrap, 1.5-inch white tape, AC pad

# Taping/Wrapping
# (TW-U-Test 6)

Peer Review _____  Peer Review _____

Skill Acquisition: _____   Practice Opportunities: _____

*Please demonstrate how you would perform* **wrist taping neutralization** *to prevent flexion and extension. You have 3 minutes to complete this task.*

| Tester places athlete and limb in appropriate position | YES | NO |
|---|---|---|
| Seated or standing | OOO | OOO |
| Wrist position into neutral (0 degrees) | OOO | OOO |
| **Taping technique** | **YES** | **NO** |
| Applies a 2-inch anchor around the distal forearm | OOO | OOO |
| Applies a smaller anchor around the hand (second to fifth metacarpal heads) | OOO | OOO |
| Constructs a fan of tape ("X-shaped"), extending from proximal to distal anchors (fan placed on dorsal side to prevent hyperflexion and on palmar side to prevent hyperextension) | OOO | OOO |
| Applies a second set of anchors (holding the fan down) | OOO | OOO |
| Applies tape in a figure-eight pattern, encircling the wrist | OOO | OOO |
| Closes with a spiral taping from proximal anchor to distal anchor | OOO | OOO |
| **Support and neatness** | **YES** | **NO** |
| Prevents hyperextension and flexion of the wrist (good support) | OOO | OOO |
| Maintains good circulation to hand and fingers | OOO | OOO |
| No holes and/or loose ends | OOO | OOO |

The psychomotor skill was performed completely and in the appropriate order     0  1  2  3  4  5

The tester had control of the subject and the situation (showed confidence)     0  1  2  3  4  5

Method of performing the skill allowed the tester the ability to determine:
severity, proper progression, and the *fit* in the overall picture (Oral)     0  1  2  3  4  5

In order for a grade of *minimum standard* to be given, the total must be ≥11          **TOTAL =** _____

I_____I_____I

**Not Acceptable**          **Meets Minimum Standards**          **Exceeds Minimum Standards**

**L:** Laboratory/Classroom Testing
**C:** Clinical/Field Testing
**P:** Practicum Testing
**A:** Assessment/Mock Exam Testing
**S:** Self-Reporting

**Positive Finding:** Neutralize the wrist (flexion/extension)
**Involved Structure:** Wrist
**Special Considerations:** N/A
**Reference(s):** Wright et al; Perrin
**Supplies Needed:** 1.5-inch white tape/prewrap

## TAPING/WRAPPING
# (TW-U-Test 7)

Peer Review _____ Peer Review _____

Skill Acquisition: _____     Practice Opportunities: _____

*Please demonstrate how you would perform a **thumb spica taping** in order to support the first metacarpopha-langeal joint of the hand. You have 3 minutes to complete this task.*

| Tester places athlete and limb in appropriate position | YES | NO |
|---|---|---|
| Standing or seated | OOO | OOO |
| Hand pronated and slightly extended | OOO | OOO |
| Thumb slightly flexed/fingers abducted | OOO | OOO |
| **Taping technique** | YES | NO |
| Applies an anchor around the distal forearm just above the ulnar condyle | OOO | OOO |
| Applies a figure-eight around the thumb, starting at the ulnar condyle, across the dorsal aspect of the hand, around the thumb, across the palmar aspect of the hand, and back to the ulnar condyle | OOO | OOO |
| Repeats the above step one to two more times | OOO | OOO |
| Secures tape with a second anchor around the wrist | OOO | OOO |
| **Support and neatness** | YES | NO |
| Provides support and stability to the MP joint | OOO | OOO |
| Maintains good circulation to the hand and thumb (check capillary refill) | OOO | OOO |
| No holes and/or loose ends | OOO | OOO |

The psychomotor skill was performed completely and in the appropriate order    0 1 2 3 4 5

The tester had control of the subject and the situation (showed confidence)    0 1 2 3 4 5

Method of performing the skill allowed the tester the ability to determine: severity, proper progression, and the *fit* in the overall picture (Oral)    0 1 2 3 4 5

In order for a grade of *minimum standard* to be given, the total must be ≥11    TOTAL =

I_____I_____I
**Not Acceptable**    **Meets Minimum Standards**    **Exceeds Minimum Standards**

**L:** Laboratory/Classroom Testing
**C:** Clinical/Field Testing
**P:** Practicum Testing
**A:** Assessment/Mock Exam Testing
**S:** Self-Reporting

**Positive Finding:** Support and stabilize
**Involved Structure:** MP joint (thumb) and wrist
**Special Considerations:** N/A
**Reference(s):** Wright et al; Perrin
**Supplies Needed:** 1.5-inch white tape/prewrap

## TAPING/WRAPPING
# (TW-U-Test 8)

Peer Review _____  Peer Review _____

Skill Acquisition: _____  Practice Opportunities: _____

*Please demonstrate how you would perform a* **collateral interphalangeal joint taping** *of the fourth finger. You have 2 minutes to complete this task.*

| Tester places athlete and limb in appropriate position | YES | NO |
|---|---|---|
| Standing or seated | OOO | OOO |
| Finger slightly flexed (PIP joint) | OOO | OOO |
| Fingers abducted (spread apart) | OOO | OOO |
| **Taping technique** | **YES** | **NO** |
| Applies anchor strips around the proximal and distal aspects of the finger | OOO | OOO |
| Applies a strip of tape, beginning on the anterior proximal anchor, crossing the medial joint line, under the finger, and ending on the posterior distal anchor | OOO | OOO |
| Applies a strip of tape from the anterior distal anchor, across the medial joint line, under the finger, and ending on the posterior proximal anchor | OOO | OOO |
| Repeats the above two steps, crossing on the lateral joint line | OOO | OOO |
| Secures the tape with a second set of proximal and distal anchors | OOO | OOO |
| **Support and neatness** | **YES** | **NO** |
| Prevents valgus and varus stress on the PIP joint | OOO | OOO |
| Maintains good circulation to the finger (check capillary refill) | OOO | OOO |
| No holes and/or loose ends | OOO | OOO |

The psychomotor skill was performed completely and in the appropriate order      **0  1  2  3  4  5**

The tester had control of the subject and the situation (showed confidence)      **0  1  2  3  4  5**

Method of performing the skill allowed the tester the ability to determine:
severity, proper progression, and the *fit* in the overall picture (Oral)      **0  1  2  3  4  5**

In order for a grade of *minimum standard* to be given, the total must be ≥11      **TOTAL =**

I_____I_____I

**Not Acceptable**          **Meets Minimum Standards**          **Exceeds Minimum Standards**

**L:** Laboratory/Classroom Testing
**C:** Clinical/Field Testing
**P:** Practicum Testing
**A:** Assessment/Mock Exam Testing
**S:** Self-Reporting

**Positive Finding:** Supports/prevents motion
**Involved Structure:** PIP joint
**Special Considerations:** N/A
**Reference(s):** Wright et al; Perrin
**Supplies Needed:** 1.5-inch white tape/prewrap

## Taping/Wrapping
# (TW-L-Test 1)

Peer Review _____    Peer Review _____

Skill Acquisition: _____    Practice Opportunities: _____

*Please demonstrate how you would perform a **hip spica wrap (hip flexor wrap)** for an injury to the hip flexors. You have 3 minutes to complete this task.*

| Tester places athlete and limb in appropriate position | YES | NO |
|---|---|---|
| Standing | OOO | OOO |
| Hip in slight flexion (heel may be propped up on a small block) | OOO | OOO |
| Foot/lower leg in a neutral position (quadriceps contracted) | OOO | OOO |
| **Taping technique** | **YES** | **NO** |
| Beginning at the proximal end of the thigh, wraps a 6-inch elastic wrap down to the distal lateral aspect of the quadriceps (pulls down and out) | OOO | OOO |
| Spirals back up the thigh (pulls up and out), overlapping each layer by half the wrap's width | OOO | OOO |
| At the proximal end up the thigh, continues the wrap around the waist, across the back, around the torso, and back to the proximal hip | OOO | OOO |
| Repeats the above steps until the wrap in gone (start and finish on the thigh) | OOO | OOO |
| Secures the wrap with elastic and white adhesive tape | OOO | OOO |
| **Support and neatness** | **YES** | **NO** |
| Provides support and stability | OOO | OOO |
| Good circulation to the lower leg and foot | OOO | OOO |
| No gaps and/or loose ends | OOO | OOO |

The psychomotor skill was performed completely and in the appropriate order     **0  1  2  3  4  5**

The tester had control of the subject and the situation (showed confidence)     **0  1  2  3  4  5**

Method of performing the skill allowed the tester the ability to determine:
severity, proper progression, and the *fit* in the overall picture (Oral)     **0  1  2  3  4  5**

In order for a grade of *minimum standard* to be given, the total must be ≥11     **TOTAL =**

I_____I_____I

**Not Acceptable**          **Meets Minimum Standards**          **Exceeds Minimum Standards**

**Positive Finding:** Support
**Involved Structure:** Hip flexors
**Special Considerations:** Adductors (pull inward)
**Reference(s):** Wright et al; Perrin
**Supplies Needed:** 6-inch double elastic wrap; elastic tape; 1.5-inch white adhesive tape

**L:** Laboratory/Classroom Testing
**C:** Clinical/Field Testing
**P:** Practicum Testing
**A:** Assessment/Mock Exam Testing
**S:** Self-Reporting

# TAPING/WRAPPING
# (TW-L-Test 2)

Peer Review _____ Peer Review _____

Skill Acquisition: _____    Practice Opportunities: _____

*Please demonstrate how you would perform a* **hip spica wrap (hip adductor wrap)** *for an injury to the groin area. You have 3 minutes to complete this task.*

| Tester places athlete and limb in appropriate position | YES | NO |
|---|---|---|
| Standing | OOO | OOO |
| Hip in slight flexion (heel may be propped up on a small block) | OOO | OOO |
| Foot/lower leg in slight internal rotation (quadriceps contracted) | OOO | OOO |
| **Taping technique** | **YES** | **NO** |
| Beginning at the proximal end of the thigh, wrap a 6-inch (double) elastic wrap down to the distal medial aspect of the quadriceps, pulling the wrap down and in | OOO | OOO |
| Spirals back up, overlapping each layer by half the wrap's width | OOO | OOO |
| At the proximal end of the thigh, continue the wrap around the waist, pulling across the abdomen, around the torso, and back to the proximal hip | OOO | OOO |
| Repeats the above steps until the wrap is gone (start and finish on the thigh) | OOO | OOO |
| Secures the ends with elastic and white adhesive tape | OOO | OOO |
| **Support and neatness** | **YES** | **NO** |
| Provides support and stability | OOO | OOO |
| Good circulation to the lower leg and foot | OOO | OOO |
| No gaps and/or loose ends | OOO | OOO |

The psychomotor skill was performed completely and in the appropriate order     **0  1  2  3  4  5**

The tester had control of the subject and the situation (showed confidence)     **0  1  2  3  4  5**

Method of performing the skill allowed the tester the ability to determine:
severity, proper progression, and the *fit* in the overall picture (Oral)     **0  1  2  3  4  5**

In order for a grade of *minimum standard* to be given, the total must be ≥11          **TOTAL =**

I_____I_____I

**Not Acceptable**          **Meets Minimum Standards**          **Exceeds Minimum Standards**

**Positive Finding:** Support
**Involved Structure:** Adductors

**L:** Laboratory/Classroom Testing          **Special Considerations:** Hip flexors (pull outward)
**C:** Clinical/Field Testing                      **Reference(s):** Wright et al; Perrin
**P:** Practicum Testing                          **Supplies Needed:** 6-inch double elastic wrap; elas-
**A:** Assessment/Mock Exam Testing                    tic tape; 1.5-inch white adhesive
**S:** Self-Reporting                                              tape

# TAPING/WRAPPING
# (TW-L-Test 3)

Peer Review _____  Peer Review _____

Skill Acquisition: _____  Practice Opportunities: _____

*Please demonstrate how you would perform a **knee compression wrap** to secure an ice bag over the medial pole of the patella. You have 2 minutes to complete this task.*

| Tester places athlete and limb in appropriate position | YES | NO |
|---|---|---|
| Supine | ○○○ | ○○○ |
| Knee slightly flexed | ○○○ | ○○○ |
| Place ice bag in appropriate area | ○○○ | ○○○ |
| **Taping technique** | YES | NO |
| Begin wrapping the leg with a 6-inch elastic wrap, beginning about 6 inches below the knee | ○○○ | ○○○ |
| Spirals up the leg, overlapping each layer by half the wrap's width | ○○○ | ○○○ |
| Wraps should end above the knee at approximately mid-quadriceps | ○○○ | ○○○ |
| Secures the wrap with white adhesive tape | ○○○ | ○○○ |
| **Support and neatness** | YES | NO |
| Provides compression to the knee (holds ice bag in place) | ○○○ | ○○○ |
| Maintains good circulation to the foot | ○○○ | ○○○ |
| No gaps and/or loose ends | ○○○ | ○○○ |

The psychomotor skill was performed completely and in the appropriate order    0 1 2 3 4 5

The tester had control of the subject and the situation (showed confidence)    0 1 2 3 4 5

Method of performing the skill allowed the tester the ability to determine: severity, proper progression, and the fit in the overall picture (Oral)    0 1 2 3 4 5

In order for a grade of minimum standard to be given, the total must be >11    TOTAL =

I_____I_____I
**Not Acceptable**    **Meets Minimum Standards**    **Exceeds Minimum Standards**

**L:** Laboratory/Classroom Testing
**C:** Clinical/Field Testing
**P:** Practicum Testing
**A:** Assessment/Mock Exam Testing
**S:** Self-Reporting

**Positive Finding:** Compression/holds bag in place
**Involved Structure:** Knee
**Special Considerations:** N/A
**Reference(s):** Wright et al
**Supplies Needed:** 6-inch elastic wrap, white adhesive tape, ice bag

## TAPING/WRAPPING
# (TW-L-Test 4)

Peer Review _____ Peer Review _____

Skill Acquisition: _____     Practice Opportunities: _____

*Please demonstrate how you would perform a **patellar check strap** in order help reduce symptoms of patella tendonitis. You have 2 minutes to complete this task.*

| Tester places athlete and limb in appropriate position | YES | NO |
|---|---|---|
| Standing | OOO | OOO |
| Knee slightly flexed (lower leg muscles relaxed) | OOO | OOO |
| **Taping technique** | **YES** | **NO** |
| Applies a strip of tape between the distal patella and superior tibial tuberosity, applying direct pressure on the patellar tendon. | OOO | OOO |
| Applies tape in a circling motion from lateral to medial across the tendon | OOO | OOO |
| Repeats above steps (two to three times) | OOO | OOO |
| **Support and neatness** | **YES** | **NO** |
| Reduces stress on the patellar tendon | OOO | OOO |
| Good circulation to the lower leg, no numbness or tingling | OOO | OOO |
| No holes and/or loose ends | OOO | OOO |

The psychomotor skill was performed completely and in the appropriate order    0  1  2  3  4  5

The tester had control of the subject and the situation (showed confidence)    0  1  2  3  4  5

Method of performing the skill allowed the tester the ability to determine: severity, proper progression, and the *fit* in the overall picture (Oral)    0  1  2  3  4  5

In order for a grade of *minimum standard* to be given, the total must be ≥11    TOTAL =

I_____I_____I

**Not Acceptable**        **Meets Minimum Standards**        **Exceeds Minimum Standards**

**L:** Laboratory/Classroom Testing
**C:** Clinical/Field Testing
**P:** Practicum Testing
**A:** Assessment/Mock Exam Testing
**S:** Self-Reporting

**Positive Finding:** Apply pressure
**Involved Structure:** Patella tendon
**Special Considerations:** N/A
**Reference(s):** Wright et al
**Supplies Needed:** Prewrap, white adhesive tape

**TAPING/WRAPPING**

# (TW-L-Test 5)

Peer Review _____ Peer Review _____

Skill Acquisition: _____    Practice Opportunities: _____

*Please demonstrate how you would perform a* **closed basketweave taping** *to prevent excessive inversion of the ankle. You have 2 minutes to complete this task.*

| Tester places athlete and limb in appropriate position | YES | NO |
|---|---|---|
| Seated (leg supported in full extension) | ○○○ | ○○○ |
| Ankle/foot dorsiflexed to 0 degrees (maintained throughout) | ○○○ | ○○○ |
| **Taping technique** | **YES** | **NO** |
| Places heel/lace pads to dorsal ankle joint line (distal Achilles' tendon [optional]) | ○○○ | ○○○ |
| Secures pads with a layer of prewrap | ○○○ | ○○○ |
| Places two anchors around the lower leg at the base of the gastrocnemius muscle | ○○○ | ○○○ |
| Places a second anchor around the instep,proximal to the base of the fifth metatarsal | ○○○ | ○○○ |
| Applies a stirrup (medial to lateral) | ○○○ | ○○○ |
| Places a horseshoe around the foot just below the malleoli | ○○○ | ○○○ |
| Repeats the above two steps two additional times | ○○○ | ○○○ |
| Applies a figure-eight, starting at the dorsal aspect of the ankle, followed by heel-locks (repeat) | ○○○ | ○○○ |
| Closes taping with horseshoes, overlapping by half the tape width, from distal to proximal | ○○○ | ○○○ |
| Places a final anchor around the instep, proximal to the base of the fifth metatarsal | ○○○ | ○○○ |
| **Support and neatness** | **YES** | **NO** |
| Limits excessive inversion | ○○○ | ○○○ |
| Maintains good circulation to the foot and toes | ○○○ | ○○○ |
| No holes and/or loose ends | ○○○ | ○○○ |

The psychomotor skill was performed completely and in the appropriate order    0  1  2  3  4  5

The tester had control of the subject and the situation (showed confidence)    0  1  2  3  4  5

Method of performing the skill allowed the tester the ability to determine:
severity, proper progression, and the *fit* in the overall picture (Oral)    0  1  2  3  4  5

In order for a grade of *minimum standard* to be given, the total must be ≥11    **TOTAL =**

I_____I_____I
**Not Acceptable**       **Meets Minimum Standards**   **Exceeds Minimum Standards**

**L:** Laboratory/Classroom Testing
**C:** Clinical/Field Testing
**P:** Practicum Testing
**A:** Assessment/Mock Exam Testing
**S:** Self-Reporting

**Positive Finding:** Prevent excessive inversion
**Involved Structure:** Subtalar joint (ankle)
**Special Considerations:** N/A
**Reference(s):** Wright et al; Perrin
**Supplies Needed:** 1.5-inch white adhesive tape, prewrap

## TAPING/WRAPPING
# (TW-L-Test 6)

Peer Review _____ Peer Review _____

Skill Acquisition: _____     Practice Opportunities: _____

*Please demonstrate how you would perform an* **Achilles' tendon taping** *in order to prevent dorsiflexion of the ankle. You have 3 minutes to complete this task.*

| Tester places athlete and limb in appropriate position | YES | NO |
|---|---|---|
| Seated (leg supported in full extension) | OOO | OOO |
| Ankle/foot plantar flexed (approximately 25 degrees) | OOO | OOO |
| **Taping technique** | **YES** | **NO** |
| Places heel/lace pad over the dorsal ankle joint (distal Achilles' tendon) | OOO | OOO |
| Places anchor around the proximal gastrocnemius and around the instep of the foot | OOO | OOO |
| Measures a strip of elastic tape slightly longer than the distance between the two anchors and cuts both ends of the strip about 1 inch longitudinally | OOO | OOO |
| With one end of the strip, wraps the split under the plantar side of the foot to anchor the strip to the foot | OOO | OOO |
| Pulls the strip up, pulling the foot into plantar flexion and attaches it to the proximal anchor by wrapping the split ends of the strip around the gastrocnemius (Note: the above three steps may be repeated for added support) | OOO | OOO |
| Secures both ends of the elastic strip with adhesive tape anchors | OOO | OOO |
| Closes the tape job with either elastic or adhesive tape from distal to proximal | OOO | OOO |
| **Support and neatness** | **YES** | **NO** |
| Limits excessive dorsiflexion | OOO | OOO |
| Good circulation to the foot | OOO | OOO |
| No holes and/or loose ends | OOO | OOO |

The psychomotor skill was performed completely and in the appropriate order  **0  1  2  3  4  5**

The tester had control of the subject and the situation (showed confidence)  **0  1  2  3  4  5**

Method of performing the skill allowed the tester the ability to determine:
severity, proper progression, and the *fit* in the overall picture (Oral)  **0  1  2  3  4  5**

In order for a grade of *minimum standard* to be given, the total must be ≥11     **TOTAL =**

I_____I_____I

**Not Acceptable**          **Meets Minimum Standards**     **Exceeds Minimum Standards**

**Positive Finding:** Reduce stress to tendon; prevent dorsiflexion

**L:** Laboratory/Classroom Testing
**C:** Clinical/Field Testing
**P:** Practicum Testing
**A:** Assessment/Mock Exam Testing
**S:** Self-Reporting

**Involved Structure:** Achilles' tendon, talocrural joint
**Special Considerations:** N/A
**Reference(s):** Wright et al
**Supplies Needed:** Elastic tape, white adhesive tape, heel/lace pads

## TAPING/WRAPPING
# (TW-L-Test 7)

Peer Review _____ Peer Review _____

Skill Acquisition: _____    Practice Opportunities: _____

*Please demonstrate how you would tape the **longitudinal arch** to give added support to the involved bones, ligaments, and muscles. You have 3 minutes to complete this task.*

| Tester places athlete and limb in appropriate position | YES | NO |
|---|---|---|
| Seated (leg supported in full extension) | OOO | OOO |
| Ankle/foot slightly plantar flexed | OOO | OOO |
| **Taping technique** | **YES** | **NO** |
| Place an anchor at the head of the metatarsals | OOO | OOO |
| Begins at the medial head (first metatarsal); attaches a strip of tape, bringing the tape along the medial foot from anterior-posterior, around the heel, and diagonally along the plantar side of the foot, back to the medial head of the first metatarsal | OOO | OOO |
| Repeats above step | OOO | OOO |
| Makes a teardrop beginning on the plantar side of the third metatarsal head, back around the heel, and returns to the starting point | OOO | OOO |
| Repeats above step | OOO | OOO |
| Places the tape on the plantar side of the fifth metatarsal head and draws the tape diagonally across the foot to the medial side of the heel, around the heel, and back to the lateral head of the fifth metatarsal | OOO | OOO |
| Repeats above step | OOO | OOO |
| Places tape strips along the plantar surface of the foot, pulling the tape from lateral to medial, beginning distally and moving proximally; each strip should overlap by half the width of the tape | OOO | OOO |
| Places tape around the heads of the metatarsals to anchor | OOO | OOO |
| **Support and neatness** | **YES** | **NO** |
| Provides support to the longitudinal arch | OOO | OOO |
| Maintains good circulation throughout the foot | OOO | OOO |
| No holes and/or loose ends | OOO | OOO |

The psychomotor skill was performed completely and in the appropriate order    0 1 2 3 4 5

The tester had control of the subject and the situation (showed confidence)    0 1 2 3 4 5

Method of performing the skill allowed the tester the ability to determine: severity, proper progression, and the *fit* in the overall picture (Oral)    0 1 2 3 4 5

In order for a grade of *minimum standard* to be given, the total must be ≥11    **TOTAL =**

**Not Acceptable**        **Meets Minimum Standards**        **Exceeds Minimum Standards**

**L:** Laboratory/Classroom Testing
**C:** Clinical/Field Testing
**P:** Practicum Testing
**A:** Assessment/Mock Exam Testing
**S:** Self-Reporting

**Positive Finding:** Support longitudinal arch
**Involved Structure:** Plantar surface of the foot
**Special Considerations:** N/A
**Reference(s):** Wright et al; Perrin
**Supplies Needed:** White adhesive tape

# TAPING/WRAPPING
## (TW-L-Test 8)

Peer Review _____ Peer Review _____

Skill Acquisition: _____    Practice Opportunities: _____

*Please demonstrate* **great toe taping** *in order to neutralize the first metatarsophalangeal joint. You have 3 minutes to complete this task.*

| Tester places athlete and limb in appropriate position | YES | NO |
|---|---|---|
| Seated (leg supported in full extension) | OOO | OOO |
| First metatarsal placed in a neutral position | OOO | OOO |
| **Taping technique** | **YES** | **NO** |
| Places 2 inches elastic anchor around midfoot (lateral to medial), 1-inch adhesive tape anchor around the distal great toe | OOO | OOO |
| A fan of four to six strips of adhesive tape should be placed on the dorsal side of the foot, beginning on the distal anchor and attaching on the proximal anchor | OOO | OOO |
| A fan of four to six strips of adhesive tape should be placed on the planter side of the foot, beginning on the distal anchor and attaching on the proximal anchor | OOO | OOO |
| Using a continuous strip of elastic tape, make a figure-eight around the great toe and midfoot, aiding the abduction of the first metatarsal joint | OOO | OOO |
| Secure the figure-eight with adhesive tape | OOO | OOO |
| **Support and neatness** | **YES** | **NO** |
| Limits excessive motion of the first MP joint (flexion/extension) | OOO | OOO |
| Maintains good circulation to the great toe (check capillary refill) | OOO | OOO |
| No holes and/or loose ends | OOO | OOO |

The psychomotor skill was performed completely and in the appropriate order    **0  1  2  3  4  5**

The tester had control of the subject and the situation (showed confidence)    **0  1  2  3  4  5**

Method of performing the skill allowed the tester the ability to determine:
severity, proper progression, and the *fit* in the overall picture (Oral)    **0  1  2  3  4  5**

In order for a grade of *minimum standard* to be given, the total must be ≥11    **TOTAL =**

I_____I_____I

**Not Acceptable**    **Meets Minimum Standards**    **Exceeds Minimum Standards**

**L:** Laboratory/Classroom Testing
**C:** Clinical/Field Testing
**P:** Practicum Testing
**A:** Assessment/Mock Exam Testing
**S:** Self-Reporting

**Positive Finding:** Limits flexion and extension
**Involved Structure:** First MP joint
**Special Considerations:** N/A
**Reference(s):** Wright et al; Perrin
**Supplies Needed:** Elastic tape; white adhesive tape

# Chapter 10

# PROTECTIVE DEVICE CONSTRUCTION

# PROTECTIVE DEVICE CONSTRUCTION
# (PDC-U-Test 1)

Peer Review _____ Peer Review _____

Skill Acquisition: _____     Practice Opportunities: _____

*This situation allows you to demonstrate your proficiency in properly* **fitting a football helmet**. *You have 3 minutes to complete this task.*

| Tester places athlete and limb in appropriate position | YES | NO |
|---|---|---|
| Standing | ○○○ | ○○○ |
| Head looking forward (neutral position) | ○○○ | ○○○ |
| **Tester placed in proper position** | **YES** | **NO** |
| Standing (facing the athlete) | ○○○ | ○○○ |
| **Tester performs test according to accepted guidelines** | **YES** | **NO** |
| Inspects the helmet (no visual damage and NOCSAE [National Operating Committee on Standards for Athletic Equipment] sticker is in place) | ○○○ | ○○○ |
| Helmet pads cover the base of the skull (occipital) | ○○○ | ○○○ |
| Space between helmet pad and eyebrows should be .75 inch (two fingers' width) | ○○○ | ○○○ |
| Ear holes of the helmet should match the helmet holes | ○○○ | ○○○ |
| Space between the facemask and nose should be 2 inches (three fingers' width) | ○○○ | ○○○ |
| Chin strap should be centered (four-point attachment) | ○○○ | ○○○ |
| Helmet should fit snugly around all parts of the athlete's head grabs facemask (manual pressure), asks athlete to look upward and downward | ○○○ | ○○○ |
| Helmet should fit snugly around all parts of the athlete's head grabs facemask (manual pressure), asks athlete to rotate head left and right | ○○○ | ○○○ |

The psychomotor skill was performed completely and in the appropriate order     0  1  2  3  4  5

The tester had control of the subject and the situation (showed confidence)     0  1  2  3  4  5

Method of performing the skill allowed the tester the ability to determine:
severity, proper progression, and the *fit* in the overall picture (Oral)     0  1  2  3  4  5

In order for a grade of *minimum standard* to be given, the total must be ≥11     TOTAL =

I_____I_____I

**Not Acceptable**          **Meets Minimum Standards**          **Exceeds Minimum Standards**

**L:** Laboratory/Classroom Testing
**C:** Clinical/Field Testing
**P:** Practicum Testing
**A:** Assessment/Mock Exam Testing
**S:** Self-Reporting

**Special Considerations:** May want to wet the hair first
**Reference(s):** Arnheim et al
**Supplies Needed:** Football helmet, chin strap, cheek pads, air pump for helmet

# PROTECTIVE DEVICE CONSTRUCTION
## (PDC-U-Test 2)

Peer Review _____ Peer Review _____

Skill Acquisition: _____     Practice Opportunities: _____

*This problem allows you the opportunity to demonstrate the application of a cervical arm **sling and swath** to immobilize the upper extremity. You have 3 minutes to complete this task.*

| Tester places athlete and limb in appropriate position | YES | NO |
|---|---|---|
| Standing | ○○○ | ○○○ |
| Elbow flexed to approximately 70 degrees | ○○○ | ○○○ |
| **Tester applies protective device to injured area** | **YES** | **NO** |
| Slides sling underneath injured extremity with apex facing the elbow | ○○○ | ○○○ |
| Drapes end of bandage closest to body over the injured shoulder | ○○○ | ○○○ |
| Pulls other end of bandage over the opposite shoulder | ○○○ | ○○○ |
| Secures sling with square knot behind the neck | ○○○ | ○○○ |
| Fastens apex of the bandage at elbow with a safety pin | ○○○ | ○○○ |
| Secures sling to body by applying swath around the trunk | ○○○ | ○○○ |
| **Tester evaluates injured area after device application** | **YES** | **NO** |
| Checks distal pulse | ○○○ | ○○○ |
| Checks distal sensation and capillary refill | ○○○ | ○○○ |

| | |
|---|---|
| The psychomotor skill was performed completely and in the appropriate order | 0  1  2  3  4  5 |
| The tester had control of the subject and the situation (showed confidence) | 0  1  2  3  4  5 |
| Method of performing the skill allowed the tester the ability to determine: severity, proper progression, and the *fit* in the overall picture (Oral) | 0  1  2  3  4  5 |

In order for a grade of *minimum standard* to be given, the total must be ≥11          **TOTAL =**

I_____I_____I

**Not Acceptable**          **Meets Minimum Standards**          **Exceeds Minimum Standards**

**L:** Laboratory/Classroom Testing
**C:** Clinical/Field Testing
**P:** Practicum Testing
**A:** Assessment/Mock Exam Testing
**S:** Self-Reporting

**Special Considerations:** N/A
**Reference(s):** Arnheim et al
**Supplies Needed:** Triangular bandage, swath, safety pin

# PROTECTIVE DEVICE CONSTRUCTION
## (PDC-U-Test 3)

Peer Review _____    Peer Review _____

Skill Acquisition: _____    Practice Opportunities: _____

*This problem allows you the opportunity to demonstrate the application of a **finger splint** to immobilize the PIP joint of the middle finger. You have 2 minutes to complete this task.*

| Tester places athlete and limb in appropriate position | YES | NO |
|---|---|---|
| Seated | OOO | OOO |
| Places hand in position of function | OOO | OOO |
| Moves injured area as little as possible | OOO | OOO |
| **Tester applies protective device to injured area** | **YES** | **NO** |
| Slides splint under the affected finger | OOO | OOO |
| Adjusts splint to cover one joint above and below the fracture site | OOO | OOO |
| Secures splint to affected finger with white tape | OOO | OOO |
| **Tester evaluates injured area after device application** | **YES** | **NO** |
| Checks distal pulse | OOO | OOO |
| Checks distal sensation and capillary refill | OOO | OOO |

| | |
|---|---|
| The psychomotor skill was performed completely and in the appropriate order | 0  1  2  3  4  5 |
| The tester had control of the subject and the situation (showed confidence) | 0  1  2  3  4  5 |
| Method of performing the skill allowed the tester the ability to determine: severity, proper progression, and the *fit* in the overall picture (Oral) | 0  1  2  3  4  5 |

In order for a grade of *minimum standard* to be given, the total must be $\geq 11$    TOTAL =

I_____I_____I

**Not Acceptable**          **Meets Minimum Standards**          **Exceeds Minimum Standards**

**L:** Laboratory/Classroom Testing
**C:** Clinical/Field Testing
**P:** Practicum Testing
**A:** Assessment/Mock Exam Testing
**S:** Self-Reporting

**Special Considerations:** Do not reduce deformity
**Reference(s):** Street
**Supplies Needed:** Finger splint, white tape

## Protective Device Construction
# (PDC-U-Test 4)

Peer Review _____ Peer Review _____

Skill Acquisition: _____    Practice Opportunities: _____

*This problem allows you the opportunity to demonstrate the construction of a **hardshell doughnut pad** to protect the **acromioclavicular joint**. You have 4 minutes to complete this task.*

| Tester places athlete and limb in appropriate position | YES | NO |
|---|---|---|
| Cuts foam to create doughnut pad | ○○○ | ○○○ |
| Cuts hole in pad to fit around AC joint | ○○○ | ○○○ |
| Cuts thermomoldable material to same size as doughnut pad | ○○○ | ○○○ |
| Heats thermomoldable material until pliable | ○○○ | ○○○ |
| Molds a convex dome in thermomoldable material | ○○○ | ○○○ |
| Secures thermomoldable to doughnut pad with elastic tape | ○○○ | ○○○ |
| **Tester applies protective device to injured area** | **YES** | **NO** |
| Secures finished pad over the AC joint (optional) | ○○○ | ○○○ |

The psychomotor skill was performed completely and in the appropriate order　0 1 2 3 4 5

The tester had control of the subject and the situation (showed confidence)　0 1 2 3 4 5

Method of performing the skill allowed the tester the ability to determine:
severity, proper progression, and the *fit* in the overall picture (Oral)　0 1 2 3 4 5

In order for a grade of *minimum standard* to be given, the total must be ≥11　　TOTAL =

I_____I_____I

**Not Acceptable**　　**Meets Minimum Standards**　　**Exceeds Minimum Standards**

**L:** Laboratory/Classroom Testing
**C:** Clinical/Field Testing
**P:** Practicum Testing
**A:** Assessment/Mock Exam Testing
**S:** Self-Reporting

**Special Considerations:** N/A
**Reference(s):** Arnheim et al; Perrin
**Supplies Needed:** Thermomoldable material, heating source, foam/felt, elastic tape, white tape, scissors

# PROTECTIVE DEVICE CONSTRUCTION
# (PDC-L-Test 1)

Peer Review _____ Peer Review _____

Skill Acquisition: _____     Practice Opportunities: _____

*This problem allows you the opportunity to demonstrate the application of an **adjustable SAM splint (ladder splint)** to immobilize the ankle joint. You have 4 minutes to complete this task.*

| Tester places athlete and limb in appropriate position | YES | NO |
|---|---|---|
| Maintains injured body part in position it was found | ○○○ | ○○○ |
| Limits movement of injured area as much as possible | ○○○ | ○○○ |
| **Tester selects appropriate device and applies to injured area** | **YES** | **NO** |
| Positions splint in horseshoe shape around the foot and ankle (forms around deformity and does not relocate) | ○○○ | ○○○ |
| Applies compression wrap distal to proximal | ○○○ | ○○○ |
| Secures splint, stabilizing the bones above and below the ankle joint | ○○○ | ○○○ |
| **Tester evaluates injured area after device application** | **YES** | **NO** |
| Checks distal pulse | ○○○ | ○○○ |
| Checks distal sensation and capillary refill | ○○○ | ○○○ |

The psychomotor skill was performed completely and in the appropriate order      0  1  2  3  4  5

The tester had control of the subject and the situation (showed confidence)      0  1  2  3  4  5

Method of performing the skill allowed the tester the ability to determine:
severity, proper progression, and the *fit* in the overall picture (Oral)      0  1  2  3  4  5

In order for a grade of *minimum standard* to be given, the total must be ≥11          **TOTAL =**

I_____I_____I

**Not Acceptable**          **Meets Minimum Standards**          **Exceeds Minimum Standards**

**L:** Laboratory/Classroom Testing
**C:** Clinical/Field Testing
**P:** Practicum Testing
**A:** Assessment/Mock Exam Testing
**S:** Self-Reporting

**Special Considerations:** N/A
**Reference(s):** Manufacturer's recommendations
**Supplies Needed:** SAM splint/ladder splint, white tape, compression wrap, neuro pinwheel

## PROTECTIVE DEVICE CONSTRUCTION
# (PDC-L-Test 2)

Peer Review _____ Peer Review _____

Skill Acquisition: _____    Practice Opportunities: _____

*This problem allows you the opportunity to demonstrate the application of a* **knee immobilizer**. *You have 2 minutes to complete this task.*

| Tester places athlete and limb in appropriate position | YES | NO |
|---|---|---|
| Knee extended | OOO | OOO |
| Limits movement of injured area as much as possible | OOO | OOO |
| **Tester selects appropriate device and applies to injured area** | **YES** | **NO** |
| Obtains appropriate size immobilizer | OOO | OOO |
| Slides immobilizer under affected limb | OOO | OOO |
| Secures straps near joint first | OOO | OOO |
| Follows by securing proximal and distal straps | OOO | OOO |
| Verifies that device is snug but comfortable | OOO | OOO |
| **Tester evaluates injured area after device application** | **YES** | **NO** |
| Checks distal pulse | OOO | OOO |
| Checks distal sensation and capillary refill | OOO | OOO |

The psychomotor skill was performed completely and in the appropriate order    **0  1  2  3  4  5**

The tester had control of the subject and the situation (showed confidence)    **0  1  2  3  4  5**

Method of performing the skill allowed the tester the ability to determine:
severity, proper progression, and the *fit* in the overall picture (Oral)    **0  1  2  3  4  5**

In order for a grade of *minimum standard* to be given, the total must be ≥11    **TOTAL =**

I_____I_____I

**Not Acceptable**        **Meets Minimum Standards**        **Exceeds Minimum Standards**

**L:** Laboratory/Classroom Testing
**C:** Clinical/Field Testing
**P:** Practicum Testing
**A:** Assessment/Mock Exam Testing
**S:** Self-Reporting

**Special Considerations:** N/A
**Reference(s):** Perrin
**Supplies Needed:** Various-sized knee immobilizers, neuro pinwheel

# PROTECTIVE DEVICE CONSTRUCTION
## (PDC-L-Test 3)

Peer Review _____  Peer Review _____

Skill Acquisition: _____    Practice Opportunities: _____

*This problem allows you the opportunity to demonstrate the application of a* **ankle horseshoe pad and compression wrap** *to prevent swelling. You have 3 minutes to complete this task.*

| Tester places athlete and limb in appropriate position | YES | NO |
|---|---|---|
| Seated with foot extended over the table | OOO | OOO |
| Ankle dorsiflexed at 90 degrees (if possible) | OOO | OOO |
| **Tester selects appropriate device and applies to injured area** | **YES** | **NO** |
| Applies horseshoe pad to lateral malleolus | OOO | OOO |
| Applies compression wrap just proximal to toes | OOO | OOO |
| Applies compression wrap proximally to lower third of the calf | OOO | OOO |
| Secures compression wrap with tape | OOO | OOO |
| **Tester evaluates injured area after device application** | **YES** | **NO** |
| Checks distal pulse | OOO | OOO |
| Checks distal sensation and capillary refill | OOO | OOO |

| | |
|---|---|
| The psychomotor skill was performed completely and in the appropriate order | **0  1  2  3  4  5** |
| The tester had control of the subject and the situation (showed confidence) | **0  1  2  3  4  5** |
| Method of performing the skill allowed the tester the ability to determine: severity, proper progression, and the *fit* in the overall picture (Oral) | **0  1  2  3  4  5** |

In order for a grade of *minimum standard* to be given, the total must be ≥11        **TOTAL =**

I_____I_____I

**Not Acceptable**      **Meets Minimum Standards**      **Exceeds Minimum Standards**

**L:** Laboratory/Classroom Testing
**C:** Clinical/Field Testing
**P:** Practicum Testing
**A:** Assessment/Mock Exam Testing
**S:** Self-Reporting

**Special Considerations:** N/A
**Reference(s):** Arnheim et al
**Supplies Needed:** Horseshoe pad, white tape, compression wrap, neuro pinwheel

## PROTECTIVE DEVICE CONSTRUCTION
# (PDC-L-Test 4)

Peer Review _____ Peer Review _____

Skill Acquisition: _____     Practice Opportunities: _____

*This problem allows you the opportunity to demonstrate the application of a **vacuum splint for a tibia fracture**. You have 3 minutes to complete this task.*

| Tester places athlete and limb in appropriate position | YES | NO |
|---|---|---|
| Seated or supine | ООО | ООО |
| Maintains injured body part in position it was found | ООО | ООО |
| **Tester selects appropriate device and applies to injured area** | **YES** | **NO** |
| Slides splint under affected limb | ООО | ООО |
| Adjusts splint to cover one joint above and below fracture site | ООО | ООО |
| Secures splint to affected limb | ООО | ООО |
| Removes residual air from splint | ООО | ООО |
| **Tester evaluates injured area after device application** | **YES** | **NO** |
| Checks distal pulse | ООО | ООО |
| Checks distal sensation and capillary refill | ООО | ООО |

The psychomotor skill was performed completely and in the appropriate order     **0  1  2  3  4  5**

The tester had control of the subject and the situation (showed confidence)     **0  1  2  3  4  5**

Method of performing the skill allowed the tester the ability to determine:
severity, proper progression, and the *fit* in the overall picture (Oral)     **0  1  2  3  4  5**

In order for a grade of *minimum standard* to be given, the total must be ≥11     **TOTAL =**

I_____I_____I
**Not Acceptable**          **Meets Minimum Standards**     **Exceeds Minimum Standards**

**L:** Laboratory/Classroom Testing
**C:** Clinical/Field Testing
**P:** Practicum Testing     **Special Considerations:** N/A
**A:** Assessment/Mock Exam Testing     **Reference(s):** Manufacturer's recommendations
**S:** Self-Reporting     **Supplies Needed:** Vacuum splint, neuro pinwheel

# VITAL SIGNS/
# GENERAL MEDICAL EXAMINATION

# VITAL SIGNS
## (VS-Test 1)

Peer Review _____    Peer Review _____

Skill Acquisition: _____    Practice Opportunities: _____

*This problem allows you the opportunity to demonstrate assessment of the **radial pulse** for an athlete. You have 2 minutes to complete this task.*

| Tester places athlete and limb in appropriate position | YES | NO |
|---|---|---|
| Supine | ○○○ | ○○○ |
| **Tester placed in proper position** | **YES** | **NO** |
| Stands to the side to the athlete | ○○○ | ○○○ |
| Locates the radial pulse using the index and middle fingers | ○○○ | ○○○ |
| **Tester performs test according to accepted guidelines** | **YES** | **NO** |
| Counts the number of beats/minute (Note: 10 seconds x 6 or 15 seconds x 4) | ○○○ | ○○○ |
| Assesses rhythm (good, irregular, etc) | ○○○ | ○○○ |
| Assesses strength (strong, weak) | ○○○ | ○○○ |
| Records and rechecks at regular intervals | ○○○ | ○○○ |

The psychomotor skill was performed completely and in the appropriate order    **0  1  2  3  4  5**

The tester had control of the subject and the situation (showed confidence)    **0  1  2  3  4  5**

Method of performing the skill allowed the tester the ability to determine:
severity, proper progression, and the *fit* in the overall picture (Oral)    **0  1  2  3  4  5**

In order for a grade of *minimum standard* to be given, the total must be ≥11    **TOTAL =**

I_____I_____I
**Not Acceptable**        **Meets Minimum Standards**    **Exceeds Minimum Standards**

**L:** Laboratory/Classroom Testing
**C:** Clinical/Field Testing
**P:** Practicum Testing
**A:** Assessment/Mock Exam Testing
**S:** Self-Reporting

**Positive Finding:** Improper rate, rhythm, strength
**Involved Structure:** Cardiovascular system
**Special Considerations:** N/A
**Reference(s):** Starkey et al; Bickley
**Supplies Needed:** Watch (with a second hand), pencil/paper

# VITAL SIGNS
## (VS-Test 2)

Peer Review _____ Peer Review _____

Skill Acquisition: _____    Practice Opportunities: _____

*This problem allows you the opportunity to demonstrate assessment of the **carotid pulse** of an athlete. You have 2 minutes to complete this task.*

| Tester places athlete and limb in appropriate position | YES | NO |
|---|---|---|
| Seated or supine | ○○○ | ○○○ |
| **Tester placed in proper position** | **YES** | **NO** |
| Stands to the side of the athlete | ○○○ | ○○○ |
| Locates the carotid pulse (using index and middle fingers) | ○○○ | ○○○ |
| **Tester performs test according to accepted guidelines** | **YES** | **NO** |
| Counts the number beats/minute (Note: 10 seconds x 6 or 15 seconds x 4) | ○○○ | ○○○ |
| Assesses rhythm (good, irregular, etc) | ○○○ | ○○○ |
| Assesses strength (strong, weak) | ○○○ | ○○○ |
| Records and rechecks at regular intervals | ○○○ | ○○○ |

The psychomotor skill was performed completely and in the appropriate order        0  1  2  3  4  5

The tester had control of the subject and the situation (showed confidence)        0  1  2  3  4  5

Method of performing the skill allowed the tester the ability to determine:
severity, proper progression, and the *fit* in the overall picture (Oral)        0  1  2  3  4  5

In order for a grade of *minimum standard* to be given, the total must be ≥11        **TOTAL =**

I_____I_____I
**Not Acceptable**        **Meets Minimum Standards**        **Exceeds Minimum Standards**

**L:** Laboratory/Classroom Testing
**C:** Clinical/Field Testing
**P:** Practicum Testing
**A:** Assessment/Mock Exam Testing
**S:** Self-Reporting

**Positive Finding:** Improper rate, rhythm, and/or strength
**Involved Structure:** Cardiovascular system
**Special Considerations:** N/A
**Reference(s):** Starkey et al; Bickley
**Supplies Needed:** Watch (with a second hand), pencil/paper

# VITAL SIGNS
## (VS-Test 3)

Peer Review _____ Peer Review _____

Skill Acquisition: _____    Practice Opportunities: _____

*This problem allows you the opportunity to demonstrate* **blood pressure assessment** *for an athlete. You have 2 minutes to complete this task.*

| | YES | NO |
|---|---|---|
| **Tester places athlete and limb in appropriate position** | YES | NO |
| Supine or seated | OOO | OOO |
| **Tester placed in proper position** | YES | NO |
| Stands to the side of the athlete (in position to read BP cuff) | OOO | OOO |
| **Tester performs test according to accepted guidelines** | YES | NO |
| Determines the appropriate size BP cuff | OOO | OOO |
| Positions the brachial artery at approximately heart level | OOO | OOO |
| Centers BP cuff (inflatable bladder) over the upper arm (secures the cuff snugly) | OOO | OOO |
| Positions the bell of the stethoscope over the brachial artery | OOO | OOO |
| Inflates the cuff to about 200 mmHg of pressure or about 30 mmHg over the predicted systolic value | OOO | OOO |
| Releases the air in the cuff slowly at about 2 to 3 mmHg per second (Note: when the first sound is heard and the last pulse is heard) | OOO | OOO |
| Records and rechecks at regular intervals (5 to 10 mmHg difference may occur in opposite arms) | OOO | OOO |

| | |
|---|---|
| The psychomotor skill was performed completely and in the appropriate order | 0  1  2  3  4  5 |
| The tester had control of the subject and the situation (showed confidence) | 0  1  2  3  4  5 |
| Method of performing the skill allowed the tester the ability to determine: severity, proper progression, and the *fit* in the overall picture (Oral) | 0  1  2  3  4  5 |

In order for a grade of *minimum standard* to be given, the total must be ≥11        **TOTAL =**

I_____I_____I
**Not Acceptable**         **Meets Minimum Standards**     **Exceeds Minimum Standards**

**L:** Laboratory/Classroom Testing
**C:** Clinical/Field Testing
**P:** Practicum Testing
**A:** Assessment/Mock Exam Testing
**S:** Self-Reporting

**Positive Finding:** High or low blood pressure
**Involved Structure:** Cardiovascular system
**Special Considerations:** Ideally the athlete should be at rest for about 5 minutes prior to taking BP
**Reference(s):** Starkey et al; Bickley
**Supplies Needed:** BP cuff, stethoscope

# VITAL SIGNS
# (VS-Test 4)

Peer Review _____ Peer Review _____

Skill Acquisition: _____     Practice Opportunities: _____

*This problem allows you the opportunity to perform* **cardiac auscultation** *to help identify abnormal heart sounds. You have 3 minutes to complete this task.*

| Tester places athlete and limb in appropriate position | YES | NO |
|---|---|---|
| Supine | ○○○ | ○○○ |
| Instructs the athlete to properly disrobe | ○○○ | ○○○ |
| **Tester placed in proper position** | **YES** | **NO** |
| Stands to the side of the athlete | ○○○ | ○○○ |
| Places the stethoscope properly into his or her ears | ○○○ | ○○○ |
| **Tester performs test according to accepted guidelines** | **YES** | **NO** |
| Instructs the athlete to breathe normally | ○○○ | ○○○ |
| Places the diaphragm of the stethoscope in the appropriate locations: | ○○○ | ○○○ |
| Mitral valve (apex of the heart-fifth intercostal space/about 1 to 2 inches left of the inferior sternum) | ○○○ | ○○○ |
| Tricuspid valve (inferior right sternal border at fifth intercostal space) | ○○○ | ○○○ |
| Aortic valve (superior right sternal border at second intercostal space) | ○○○ | ○○○ |
| Pulmonary valve (superior left sternal border at second intercostal space) | ○○○ | ○○○ |
| Listens at each location during several contraction cycles | ○○○ | ○○○ |
| Notes and records any findings | ○○○ | ○○○ |

| | |
|---|---|
| The psychomotor skill was performed completely and in the appropriate order | **0  1  2  3  4  5** |
| The tester had control of the subject and the situation (showed confidence) | **0  1  2  3  4  5** |
| Method of performing the skill allowed the tester the ability to determine: severity, proper progression, and the *fit* in the overall picture (Oral) | **0  1  2  3  4  5** |

In order for a grade of *minimum standard* to be given, the total must be ≥11          **TOTAL =**

I_____I_____I

**Not Acceptable**          **Meets Minimum Standards**          **Exceeds Minimum Standards**

**L:** Laboratory/Classroom Testing
**C:** Clinical/Field Testing
**P:** Practicum Testing
**A:** Assessment/Mock Exam Testing
**S:** Self-Reporting

**Positive Finding:** Abnormal sounds
**Involved Structure:** Cardiovascular system
**Special Considerations:** May repeat, turning subject on left side
**Reference(s):** O'Connor
**Supplies Needed:** Stethoscope, table, paper/pencil

## Vital Signs
# (VS-Test 5)

Peer Review _____ Peer Review _____

Skill Acquisition: _____    Practice Opportunities: _____

*This problem allows you the opportunity to perform* **pulmonary auscultation** *to help identify abnormal breath sounds. You have 3 minutes to complete this task.*

| Tester places athlete and limb in appropriate position | YES | NO |
|---|---|---|
| Supine | ○○○ | ○○○ |
| Instructs the athlete to properly disrobe | ○○○ | ○○○ |
| **Tester placed in proper position** | **YES** | **NO** |
| Stands to the side of the athlete | ○○○ | ○○○ |
| Places the stethoscope properly into his or her ears | ○○○ | ○○○ |
| **Tester performs test according to accepted guidelines** | **YES** | **NO** |
| Instructs the athlete to take a full, deep breath and let it out slowly (with each placement) | ○○○ | ○○○ |
| Places the diaphragm of the stethoscope in the appropriate locations: Anterior thorax, posterior thorax | ○○○ | ○○○ |
| Right     Left | | |
| 1         1  Just below the clavicle—first intercostal space | ○○○ | ○○○ |
| 2         2  Medial—third intercostal space | ○○○ | ○○○ |
| 3         3  Lateral—third intercostal space | ○○○ | ○○○ |
| 4         4  Medial—fourth intercostal space | ○○○ | ○○○ |
| 5         5  Lateral—fourth intercostal space | ○○○ | ○○○ |
| 6         6  Just below the xiphoid process (eighth intercostal space) | ○○○ | ○○○ |
| Assesses sounds at each location upon both inspiration and expiration | ○○○ | ○○○ |
| Notes and records any findings | ○○○ | ○○○ |

The psychomotor skill was performed completely and in the appropriate order    **0  1  2  3  4  5**

The tester had control of the subject and the situation (showed confidence)    **0  1  2  3  4  5**

Method of performing the skill allowed the tester the ability to determine:
severity, proper progression, and the *fit* in the overall picture (Oral)    **0  1  2  3  4  5**

In order for a grade of *minimum standard* to be given, the total must be ≥11    **TOTAL =**

I_____I_____I

**Not Acceptable**         **Meets Minimum Standards**         **Exceeds Minimum Standards**

**L:** Laboratory/Classroom Testing
**C:** Clinical/Field Testing
**P:** Practicum Testing
**A:** Assessment/Mock Exam Testing
**S:** Self-Reporting

**Positive Finding:** Abnormal sounds
**Involved Structure:** Respiratory system
**Special Considerations:** May repeat having the athlete speak (whisper) "a"/"e" sounds
**Reference(s):** O'Connor
**Supplies Needed:** Stethoscope, pencil/paper

# VITAL SIGNS
# (VS-Test 6)

Skill Acquisition: _____    Practice Opportunities: _____

*This problem allows you the opportunity to demonstrate the proper method for administering medicine through the use of an **asthma inhaler**. You have 2 minutes to complete this task.*

| | YES | NO |
|---|---|---|
| **Tester places athlete and limb in appropriate position** | | |
| Standing or seated | OOO | OOO |
| **Tester placed in proper position** | YES | NO |
| Stands in front of or to the side of the athlete | OOO | OOO |
| **Tester performs test according to accepted guidelines** | YES | NO |
| Shakes the inhaler (prior to the first puff) | OOO | OOO |
| Attaches a 2- to 4-inch spacer to the inhaler (inhaler mouthpiece) | OOO | OOO |
| Instructs the athlete to take slow, deep breaths (3 to 5 seconds) while administering the medication (sprays only one puff at a time) | OOO | OOO |
| Instructs the athlete to hold the breath in for about 10 seconds | OOO | OOO |
| Repeats (wait at least 30 seconds between puffs or longer depending on the medication) | OOO | OOO |

The psychomotor skill was performed completely and in the appropriate order    0 1 2 3 4 5

The tester had control of the subject and the situation (showed confidence)    0 1 2 3 4 5

Method of performing the skill allowed the tester the ability to determine: severity, proper progression, and the *fit* in the overall picture (Oral)    0 1 2 3 4 5

In order for a grade of *minimum standard* to be given, the total must be ≥11    **TOTAL =**

I_____I_____I

**Not Acceptable**          **Meets Minimum Standards**          **Exceeds Minimum Standards**

**L:** Laboratory/Classroom Testing
**C:** Clinical/Field Testing
**P:** Practicum Testing
**A:** Assessment/Mock Exam Testing
**S:** Self-Reporting

**Positive Finding:** N/A
**Involved Structure:** Respiratory system
**Special Considerations:** N/A
**Reference(s):** *Physician's Desk Reference;* Goldman et al
**Supplies Needed:** Empty inhaler, spacer

# VITAL SIGNS
# (VS-Test 7)

Peer Review _____ Peer Review _____

Skill Acquisition: _____   Practice Opportunities: _____

*In determining whether or not the vital signs of an athlete are normal, this problem allows you the opportunity to perform* **respiration assessment***. You have 2 minutes to complete this task.*

| Tester places athlete and limb in appropriate position | YES | NO |
|---|---|---|
| Supine | OOO | OOO |
| **Tester placed in proper position** | **YES** | **NO** |
| Stands or kneels to the side of the athlete | OOO | OOO |
| Positions to observe the rising and falling of the chest (look, listen, and/or feel) | OOO | OOO |
| **Tester performs test according to accepted guidelines** | **YES** | **NO** |
| Assesses rate of breath: Counts the number of breaths/minute. (Note: 12 to 20) | OOO | OOO |
| Assesses depth/character of breath. (Note: Shallow, rapid, left/right side the same, etc) | OOO | OOO |
| Assesses length of inspiration and expiration (Note: 1:1) | OOO | OOO |
| Records and rechecks at regular intervals | OOO | OOO |

The psychomotor skill was performed completely and in the appropriate order   **0 1 2 3 4 5**

The tester had control of the subject and the situation (showed confidence)   **0 1 2 3 4 5**

Method of performing the skill allowed the tester the ability to determine:
severity, proper progression, and the *fit* in the overall picture (Oral)   **0 1 2 3 4 5**

In order for a grade of *minimum standard* to be given, the total must be ≥11   **TOTAL =**

I_____I_____I
**Not Acceptable**      **Meets Minimum Standards**   **Exceeds Minimum Standards**

**L:** Laboratory/Classroom Testing
**C:** Clinical/Field Testing
**P:** Practicum Testing
**A:** Assessment/Mock Exam Testing
**S:** Self-Reporting

**Positive Finding:** Improper rate and/or depth
**Involved Structure:** Respiratory system
**Special Considerations:** N/A
**Reference(s):** Starkey et al; O'Connor
**Supplies Needed:** Watch (with a second hand), paper/pencil

# VITAL SIGNS
# (VS-Test 8)

Peer Review _____ Peer Review _____

Skill Acquisition: _____     Practice Opportunities: _____

*This problem allows you the opportunity to demonstrate the proper method for administering a* **peak flow meter** *on an athlete suspected of exercise-induced asthma. You have 2 minutes to complete this task.*

| Tester places athlete and limb in appropriate position | YES | NO |
|---|---|---|
| Standing | ООО | ООО |
| **Tester placed in proper position** | **YES** | **NO** |
| Stands in front of the athlete | ООО | ООО |
| **Tester performs test according to accepted guidelines** | **YES** | **NO** |
| Instructs the athlete to take a deep breath | ООО | ООО |
| Instructs the athlete to place the mouthpiece of the peak flow meter into his or her mouth | ООО | ООО |
| Instructs the athlete to blow as hard and fast as possible into the peak flow meter | ООО | ООО |
| Repeats steps | ООО | ООО |

The psychomotor skill was performed completely and in the appropriate order     0 1 2 3 4 5

The tester had control of the subject and the situation (showed confidence)     0 1 2 3 4 5

Method of performing the skill allowed the tester the ability to determine: severity, proper progression, and the *fit* in the overall picture (Oral)     0 1 2 3 4 5

In order for a grade of *minimum standard* to be given, the total must be ≥11     **TOTAL =**

I_____I_____I

**Not Acceptable**     **Meets Minimum Standards**     **Exceeds Minimum Standards**

**L:** Laboratory/Classroom Testing
**C:** Clinical/Field Testing
**P:** Practicum Testing
**A:** Assessment/Mock Exam Testing
**S:** Self-Reporting

**Positive Finding:** Air not moving out of the lungs
**Involved Structure:** Respiratory system
**Special Considerations:** Do not allow the tongue to impede air flow
**Reference(s):** Starkey et al
**Supplies Needed:** Peak flow meter, mouthpiece

# VITAL SIGNS
# (VS-Test 9)

Peer Review _____ Peer Review _____

Skill Acquisition: _____    Practice Opportunities: _____

*This problem allows you the opportunity to inspect the ear canal and ear drum of an athlete by using an **oto-scope**. You have 2 minutes to complete this task.*

| Tester places athlete and limb in appropriate position | YES | NO |
|---|---|---|
| Seated | ○○○ | ○○○ |
| Position the athlete's head so that the tester can see comfortably through the otoscope | ○○○ | ○○○ |
| **Tester placed in proper position** | YES | NO |
| Stands or sits to the side of the athlete | ○○○ | ○○○ |
| Grasps the auricle and pulls in an upward/backward direction | ○○○ | ○○○ |
| **Tester performs test according to accepted guidelines** | YES | NO |
| Holds the otoscope properly. (Note: Hand rests against the athlete's face) | ○○○ | ○○○ |
| Inserts the otoscope (speculum) gently into the ear canal (Note: Uses the largest ear speculum that fits into the canal) | ○○○ | ○○○ |
| Turns on the light | ○○○ | ○○○ |
| Gently moves the speculum in multiple directions | ○○○ | ○○○ |

The psychomotor skill was performed completely and in the appropriate order    0 1 2 3 4 5

The tester had control of the subject and the situation (showed confidence)    0 1 2 3 4 5

Method of performing the skill allowed the tester the ability to determine: severity, proper progression, and the *fit* in the overall picture (Oral)    0 1 2 3 4 5

In order for a grade of *minimum standard* to be given, the total must be ≥11    **TOTAL =**

I_____I_____I

**Not Acceptable**    **Meets Minimum Standards**    **Exceeds Minimum Standards**

**L:** Laboratory/Classroom Testing
**C:** Clinical/Field Testing
**P:** Practicum Testing
**A:** Assessment/Mock Exam Testing
**S:** Self-Reporting

**Positive Finding:** Abnormal structures and/or redness
**Involved Structure:** Ear drum/canal
**Special Considerations:** N/A
**Reference(s):** Bickley
**Supplies Needed:** Otoscope, chair

# VITAL SIGNS
# (VS-Test 10)

Peer Review _____ Peer Review _____

Skill Acquisition: _____    Practice Opportunities: _____

*This problem allows you the opportunity to check the core temperature of an athlete using a **tympanic thermometer**. You have 2 minutes to complete this task.*

| | YES | NO |
|---|---|---|
| **Tester places athlete and limb in appropriate position** | YES | NO |
| Seated | ○○○ | ○○○ |
| **Tester placed in proper position** | YES | NO |
| Stands to the side of the athlete | ○○○ | ○○○ |
| **Tester performs test according to accepted guidelines** | YES | NO |
| Inserts the thermometer in the ear canal | ○○○ | ○○○ |
| Holds the thermometer in this position for about 3 seconds (until the digital reading appears) | ○○○ | ○○○ |
| Accurately reads and records the temperature | ○○○ | ○○○ |

The psychomotor skill was performed completely and in the appropriate order    **0  1  2  3  4  5**

The tester had control of the subject and the situation (showed confidence)    **0  1  2  3  4  5**

Method of performing the skill allowed the tester the ability to determine: severity, proper progression, and the *fit* in the overall picture (Oral)    **0  1  2  3  4  5**

In order for a grade of *minimum standard* to be given, the total must be ≥11    **TOTAL =**

I_____I_____I

**Not Acceptable**        **Meets Minimum Standards**    **Exceeds Minimum Standards**

**L:** Laboratory/Classroom Testing
**C:** Clinical/Field Testing
**P:** Practicum Testing
**A:** Assessment/Mock Exam Testing
**S:** Self-Reporting

**Positive Finding:** Abnormal reading
**Involved Structure:** Body temperature
**Special Considerations:** Reading will be a little higher than using an oral thermometer (about 1.4°F higher)
**Reference(s):** Bickley
**Supplies Needed:** Tympanic thermometer, chair, pencil/paper

## VITAL SIGNS
# (VS-Test 11)

Peer Review _____ Peer Review _____

Skill Acquisition: _____    Practice Opportunities: _____

*This problem allows you the opportunity to check the internal body temperature of an athlete using a standard* **oral thermometer**. *You have 2 minutes to complete this task.*

| **Tester places athlete and limb in appropriate position** |
|---|
| Seated |
| **Tester placed in proper position** |
| Stands in front of the athlete |
| **Tester performs test according to accepted guidelines** |
| Sterilizes the thermometer |
| Shakes the thermometer mercury down (Note: To about 96°F) |
| Inserts the thermometer under the athlete's tongue |
| Instructs the athlete to close both lips and hold the thermometer under the tongue |
| Maintains this position for 3 minutes |
| Removes the thermometer from the athlete's mouth |
| Accurately reads and records the temperature |

The psychomotor skill was performed completely and in the appropriate order       0  1  2  3  4  5

The tester had control of the subject and the situation (showed confidence)       0  1  2  3  4  5

Method of performing the skill allowed the tester the ability to determine:
severity, proper progression, and the *fit* in the overall picture (Oral)       0  1  2  3  4  5

In order for a grade of *minimum standard* to be given, the total must be ≥11       **TOTAL =**

I_____I_____I

**Not Acceptable**        **Meets Minimum Standards**        **Exceeds Minimum Standards**

**L:** Laboratory/Classroom Testing
**C:** Clinical/Field Testing
**P:** Practicum Testing
**A:** Assessment/Mock Exam Testing
**S:** Self-Reporting

**Positive Finding:** Abnormal reading
**Involved Structure:** Body temperature
**Special Considerations:** N/A
**Reference(s):** Bickley
**Supplies Needed:** Glass oral thermometer, alcohol
wipe, chair, paper/pencil

# VITAL SIGNS
# (VS-Test 12)

Peer Review _____ Peer Review _____

Skill Acquisition: _____    Practice Opportunities: _____

*This problem allows you the opportunity to inspect the posterior structures of the retinal surface of an athlete's eye by using an* **ophthalmoscope**. *You have 3 minutes to complete this task.*

| Tester places athlete and limb in appropriate position | YES | NO |
|---|---|---|
| Seated or standing | OOO | OOO |
| Head placed in a neutral, upright position | OOO | OOO |
| **Tester placed in proper position** | **YES** | **NO** |
| Stands in front of the athlete | OOO | OOO |
| Holds the ophthalmoscope in the right hand to evaluate the subject's right eye (switch left-to-left) | OOO | OOO |
| Holds ophthalmoscope firmly under the medial aspect of the bony orbit (handle tilted laterally about 20 degrees) | OOO | OOO |
| **Tester performs test according to accepted guidelines** | **YES** | **NO** |
| Darkens the lights in the room | OOO | OOO |
| Turns on the ophthalmoscope light (adjusts the light to a large, round beam of white light) | OOO | OOO |
| Sets ophthalmoscope lens disk at 0 diopters (keeps index finger on lens disk in order to focus) | OOO | OOO |
| Instructs the athlete to look over the tester's shoulder and gaze at a specific point on the wall | OOO | OOO |
| Positions the ophthalmoscope about 15 inches away from the athlete | OOO | OOO |
| Shines the light on the pupil (focuses the light on the red reflex) | OOO | OOO |
| Moves the ophthalmoscope slowly toward the eye (almost touching the lashes) | OOO | OOO |
| Notes and records any findings | OOO | OOO |

| | | |
|---|---|---|
| The psychomotor skill was performed completely and in the appropriate order | | 0  1  2  3  4  5 |
| The tester had control of the subject and the situation (showed confidence) | | 0  1  2  3  4  5 |
| Method of performing the skill allowed the tester the ability to determine: severity, proper progression, and the *fit* in the overall picture (Oral) | | 0  1  2  3  4  5 |

In order for a grade of *minimum standard* to be given, the total must be ≥11          **TOTAL =**

I_____I_____I

**Not Acceptable**          **Meets Minimum Standards**          **Exceeds Minimum Standards**

**L:** Laboratory/Classroom Testing
**C:** Clinical/Field Testing
**P:** Practicum Testing
**A:** Assessment/Mock Exam Testing
**S:** Self-Reporting

**Positive Finding:** Abnormal structures/swelling
**Involved Structure:** Eye
**Special Considerations:** Do not dilate subject's pupils
**Reference(s):** Bickley
**Supplies Needed:** Ophthalmoscope, paper/pencil

# Vital Signs
## (VS-Test 13)

*This problem allows you the opportunity to check the eyes for a normal reflex to light using the* **Consensual Reaction Test (Pupillary Reflex Test)**. *You have 2 minutes to complete this task.*

| Tester places athlete and limb in appropriate position | YES | NO |
|---|---|---|
| Standing or seated | ○○○ | ○○○ |
| **Tester placed in proper position** | YES | NO |
| Stands in front of the athlete | ○○○ | ○○○ |
| **Tester performs test according to accepted guidelines** | YES | NO |
| Instructs the athlete to keep both eyes open | ○○○ | ○○○ |
| Shines the light into the pupil of one eye for about 1 second and observes for constriction of the opposite pupil | ○○○ | ○○○ |
| Removes the light and observes for dilation of the opposite pupil | ○○○ | ○○○ |
| Repeats above scenario using the other eye | ○○○ | ○○○ |

The psychomotor skill was performed completely and in the appropriate order        0  1  2  3  4  5

The tester had control of the subject and the situation (showed confidence)        0  1  2  3  4  5

Method of performing the skill allowed the tester the ability to determine:
severity, proper progression, and the *fit* in the overall picture (Oral)        0  1  2  3  4  5

In order for a grade of *minimum standard* to be given, the total must be ≥11        **TOTAL =**

I_____I_____I
**Not Acceptable**         **Meets Minimum Standards**      **Exceeds Minimum Standards**

**L:** Laboratory/Classroom Testing
**C:** Clinical/Field Testing
**P:** Practicum Testing
**A:** Assessment/Mock Exam Testing
**S:** Self-Reporting

**Positive Finding:** Inappropriate or no movement of the pupil
**Involved Structure:** Neurological
**Special Considerations:** Room should be darkened
**Reference(s):** Bickley
**Supplies Needed:** Penlight

# VITAL SIGNS
# (VS-Test 14)

Peer Review _____ Peer Review _____

Skill Acquisition: _____    Practice Opportunities: _____

*This problem allows you the opportunity to check the eyes for normal reaction to light (constriction/dilation) by using the **pupillary reaction test**. You have 2 minutes to complete this task.*

| Tester places athlete and limb in appropriate position | YES | NO |
|---|---|---|
| Standing or seated | ○○○ | ○○○ |
| **Tester placed in proper position** | **YES** | **NO** |
| Stands in front of the athlete | ○○○ | ○○○ |
| **Tester performs test according to accepted guidelines** | **YES** | **NO** |
| Instructs athlete to cover one eye (may use hand or an eye patch/card) | ○○○ | ○○○ |
| Instructs athlete to keep the uncovered eye open (Note: looking at a distant point) | ○○○ | ○○○ |
| Shines the light from a penlight into the pupil of the open eye for about 1 second and observes for constriction of the eye | ○○○ | ○○○ |
| Removes the light and checks for dilation of the pupil | ○○○ | ○○○ |
| Repeats above scenario on other eye on lower leg | ○○○ | ○○○ |
| Performs assessment bilaterally | ○○○ | ○○○ |

The psychomotor skill was performed completely and in the appropriate order    0 1 2 3 4 5

The tester had control of the subject and the situation (showed confidence)    0 1 2 3 4 5

Method of performing the skill allowed the tester the ability to determine:
severity, proper progression, and the *fit* in the overall picture (Oral)    0 1 2 3 4 5

In order for a grade of *minimum standard* to be given, the total must be ≥11    **TOTAL =**

I_____I_____I

**Not Acceptable**        **Meets Minimum Standards**    **Exceeds Minimum Standards**

**L:** Laboratory/Classroom Testing
**C:** Clinical/Field Testing
**P:** Practicum Testing
**A:** Assessment/Mock Exam Testing
**S:** Self-Reporting

**Positive Finding:** Inappropriate or no movement of the pupil
**Involved Structure:** Iris
**Special Considerations:** Room should be darkened
**Reference(s):** Starkey et al; Bickley
**Supplies Needed:** Pen light, eye patch/card

## VITAL SIGNS
# (VS-Test 15)

Peer Review _____ Peer Review _____

Skill Acquisition: _____    Practice Opportunities: _____

*This problem allows you the opportunity to check the field of gaze for eye motility using the* **Test for Eye Motility (tracking)**. *You have 2 minutes to complete this task.*

| Tester places athlete and limb in appropriate position | YES | NO |
|---|---|---|
| Standing or seated | OOO | OOO |
| **Tester placed in proper position** | **YES** | **NO** |
| Stands in front of the athlete | OOO | OOO |
| Holds a pencil or index finger approximately 2 feet from the athlete's nose | OOO | OOO |
| **Tester performs test according to accepted guidelines** | **YES** | **NO** |
| Instructs the athlete to focus on the object (moving eyes only, not the head) | OOO | OOO |
| Moves the object through the field of gaze—12,6,3,9 o'clock and 2,7,10,5 o'clock (Note: Smooth, symmetrical movement; equal distance traveled by both eyes) | OOO | OOO |

The psychomotor skill was performed completely and in the appropriate order    **0  1  2  3  4  5**

The tester had control of the subject and the situation (showed confidence)    **0  1  2  3  4  5**

Method of performing the skill allowed the tester the ability to determine: severity, proper progression, and the *fit* in the overall picture (Oral)    **0  1  2  3  4  5**

In order for a grade of *minimum standard* to be given, the total must be ≥11    **TOTAL =**

I_____I_____I

**Not Acceptable          Meets Minimum Standards          Exceeds Minimum Standards**

**L:** Laboratory/Classroom Testing
**C:** Clinical/Field Testing
**P:** Practicum Testing
**A:** Assessment/Mock Exam Testing
**S:** Self-Reporting

**Positive Finding:** Asymmetrical movement
**Involved Structure:** Eye
**Special Considerations:** N/A
**Reference(s):** Starkey et al
**Supplies Needed:** Pencil/paper; pen light

## VITAL SIGNS
# (VS-Test 16)

Peer Review _____ Peer Review _____

Skill Acquisition: _____    Practice Opportunities: _____

*This problem allows you the opportunity to assess corrected visual acuity using a **Snellen Eye Chart**. You have 2 minutes to complete this task.*

| Tester places athlete and limb in appropriate position | YES | NO |
|---|---|---|
| Standing | ○○○ | ○○○ |
| Instructs the athlete to stand 20 feet away from the eye chart | ○○○ | ○○○ |
| Instructs the athlete to leave corrective eyewear (glasses/contacts) in place | ○○○ | ○○○ |
| **Tester placed in proper position** | YES | NO |
| Stands in position to read the eye chart | ○○○ | ○○○ |
| **Tester performs test according to accepted guidelines** | YES | NO |
| Instructs the athlete to cover one eye (may use hand or an eye patch/card) | ○○○ | ○○○ |
| Instructs the athlete to read each line (starting at the top) | ○○○ | ○○○ |
| Instructs the athlete to cover the other eye and read each line | ○○○ | ○○○ |
| Records the information | ○○○ | ○○○ |

The psychomotor skill was performed completely and in the appropriate order    0 1 2 3 4 5

The tester had control of the subject and the situation (showed confidence)    0 1 2 3 4 5

Method of performing the skill allowed the tester the ability to determine: severity, proper progression, and the *fit* in the overall picture (Oral)    0 1 2 3 4 5

In order for a grade of *minimum standard* to be given, the total must be ≥11    **TOTAL =**

I_____I_____I

**Not Acceptable**    **Meets Minimum Standards**    **Exceeds Minimum Standards**

**L:** Laboratory/Classroom Testing
**C:** Clinical/Field Testing
**P:** Practicum Testing
**A:** Assessment/Mock Exam Testing
**S:** Self-Reporting

**Positive Finding:** Inability to read the appropriate letters
**Involved Structure:** Eye
**Special Considerations:** Area should be well-lit
**Reference(s):** Starkey et al; Bickley; Hillman
**Supplies Needed:** Snellen Eye Chart, 20-foot tape measure, pencil/paper

# VITAL SIGNS
# (VS-Test 17)

Skill Acquisition: _____    Practice Opportunities: _____

*This problem allows you the opportunity to administer a* **"clean catch" dipstick urinalysis** *in order to rule out hematuria. You have 2 minutes to complete this task.*

| Tester places athlete and limb in appropriate position | YES | NO |
|---|---|---|
| Instructions are given to the athlete | OOO | OOO |
| **Tester performs test according to accepted guidelines** | **YES** | **NO** |
| Instructs athlete to discards the initial flow of urine into a toilet bowl | OOO | OOO |
| Delivers a "clean catch" specimen into a specimen cup | OOO | OOO |
| Collects about 2 oz of urine | OOO | OOO |
| Immerses dipstick into the specimen cup for the recommended time (see manufacturer's recommendations) | OOO | OOO |
| Records the results (matches the proper colors of the dipstick to the values provided by themanufacturer) | OOO | OOO |

The psychomotor skill was performed completely and in the appropriate order        **0  1  2  3  4  5**

The tester had control of the subject and the situation (showed confidence)        **0  1  2  3  4  5**

Method of performing the skill allowed the tester the ability to determine:
severity, proper progression, and the *fit* in the overall picture (Oral)        **0  1  2  3  4  5**

In order for a grade of *minimum standard* to be given, the total must be ≥11        **TOTAL =**

I_____I_____I
**Not Acceptable**          **Meets Minimum Standards**          **Exceeds Minimum Standards**

**L:** Laboratory/Classroom Testing
**C:** Clinical/Field Testing
**P:** Practicum Testing
**A:** Assessment/Mock Exam Testing
**S:** Self-Reporting

**Positive Finding:** Results outside the norm
**Involved Structure:** N/A
**Special Considerations:** N/A
**Reference(s):** Starkey et al
**Supplies Needed:** Clean specimen cup, dipstick, manufacturer's recommendations for time and interpretation

# OTHER TESTS

## OTHER TESTS
# (O-Test 1)

Peer Review _____ Peer Review _____

Skill Acquisition: _____    Practice Opportunities: _____

*Please demonstrate the proper use of a* **goniometer** *for measuring an athlete's* **ankle** *active range of motion for* **inversion/eversion** *at the subtalar joint. You have 3 minutes to complete this task.*

| Tester places athlete and limb in appropriate position | YES | NO |
|---|---|---|
| Prone | ○○○ | ○○○ |
| Foot place over the edge of the table | ○○○ | ○○○ |
| **Tester provides appropriate stabilization** | **YES** | **NO** |
| Tibia and fibula | ○○○ | ○○○ |
| **Tester places goniometer in appropriate position** | **YES** | **NO** |
| Fulcrum: Posterior aspect, midway between the malleoli | ○○○ | ○○○ |
| Stationary arm: Midline of the lower leg | ○○○ | ○○○ |
| Moving arm: Posterior midline of the calcaneus | ○○○ | ○○○ |
| **Tester performs test according to accepted guidelines** | **YES** | **NO** |
| Correct reading: Inversion/eversion | ○○○ | ○○○ |
| Performs assessment bilaterally | ○○○ | ○○○ |

The psychomotor skill was performed completely and in the appropriate order    **0  1  2  3  4  5**

The tester had control of the subject and the situation (showed confidence)    **0  1  2  3  4  5**

Method of performing the skill allowed the tester the ability to determine:
severity, proper progression, and the *fit* in the overall picture (Oral)    **0  1  2  3  4  5**

In order for a grade of *minimum standard* to be given, the total must be ≥11    **TOTAL =**

I_____I_____I

**Not Acceptable        Meets Minimum Standards        Exceeds Minimum Standards**

**L:** Laboratory/Classroom Testing
**C:** Clinical/Field Testing
**P:** Practicum Testing
**A:** Assessment/Mock Exam Testing
**S:** Self-Reporting

**Positive Finding:** Range of motion
**Involved Structure:** Subtalar joint
**Special Considerations:** N/A
**Reference(s):** Norkin et al
**Supplies Needed:** Goniometer, dots/markers

# OTHER TESTS
# (O-Test 2)

Peer Review _____ Peer Review _____

Skill Acquisition: _____          Practice Opportunities: _____

*Please demonstrate the proper use of a **goniometer** for measuring an athlete's **shoulder** active range of motion for **flexion** at the glenohumeral joint. You have 3 minutes to complete this task.*

| Tester places athlete and limb in appropriate position | YES | NO |
|---|---|---|
| Supine | ○○○ | ○○○ |
| Knee flexed to 90 degrees | ○○○ | ○○○ |
| Shoulder adducted to 0 degrees | ○○○ | ○○○ |
| Palm against the body | ○○○ | ○○○ |
| **Tester provides appropriate stabilization** | **YES** | **NO** |
| Scapula | ○○○ | ○○○ |
| **Tester places goniometer in appropriate position** | **YES** | **NO** |
| Fulcrum: Acromial process | ○○○ | ○○○ |
| Stationary arm: Midaxillary line of the thorax | ○○○ | ○○○ |
| Moving arm: Lateral midline of the humerus (lateral epicondyle) | ○○○ | ○○○ |
| **Tester performs test according to accepted guidelines** | **YES** | **NO** |
| Correct reading: Flexion | ○○○ | ○○○ |
| Performs assessment bilaterally | ○○○ | ○○○ |

The psychomotor skill was performed completely and in the appropriate order    0  1  2  3  4  5

The tester had control of the subject and the situation (showed confidence)    0  1  2  3  4  5

Method of performing the skill allowed the tester the ability to determine:
severity, proper progression, and the *fit* in the overall picture (Oral)    0  1  2  3  4  5

In order for a grade of *minimum standard* to be given, the total must be ≥11          TOTAL =

I_____I_____I
**Not Acceptable**          **Meets Minimum Standards**          **Exceeds Minimum Standards**

**L:** Laboratory/Classroom Testing
**C:** Clinical/Field Testing
**P:** Practicum Testing
**A:** Assessment/Mock Exam Testing
**S:** Self-Reporting

**Positive Finding:** Range of motion
**Involved Structure:** Glenohumeral joint
**Special Considerations:** N/A
**Reference(s):** Norkin et al
**Supplies Needed:** Goniometer, dots/markers

## OTHER TESTS
# (O-Test 3)

Skill Acquisition: _____    Practice Opportunities: _____

*Please demonstrate the proper use of a **goniometer** for measuring an athlete's **shoulder** active range of motion for **internal/external rotation** at the glenohumeral joint. You have 3 minutes to complete this task.*

| Tester places athlete and limb in appropriate position | YES | NO |
|---|---|---|
| Supine | ○○○ | ○○○ |
| Shoulder abducted to 90 degrees | ○○○ | ○○○ |
| Forearm maintained at 0 degrees | ○○○ | ○○○ |
| Pad/towel under humerus | ○○○ | ○○○ |
| **Tester provides appropriate stabilization** | **YES** | **NO** |
| Distal end of humerus (beginning of motion) | ○○○ | ○○○ |
| Scapula (end of motion) | ○○○ | ○○○ |
| **Tester places goniometer in appropriate position** | **YES** | **NO** |
| Fulcrum: Olecranon process | ○○○ | ○○○ |
| Stationary Arm: Parallel or perpendicular to the floor | ○○○ | ○○○ |
| Moving Arm: Align with the ulna; ulnar styloid | ○○○ | ○○○ |
| **Tester performs test according to accepted guidelines** | **YES** | **NO** |
| Correct reading: Internal/external rotation | ○○○ | ○○○ |
| Performs assessment bilaterally | ○○○ | ○○○ |

The psychomotor skill was performed completely and in the appropriate order    0 1 2 3 4 5

The tester had control of the subject and the situation (showed confidence)    0 1 2 3 4 5

Method of performing the skill allowed the tester the ability to determine:
severity, proper progression, and the *fit* in the overall picture (Oral)    0 1 2 3 4 5

In order for a grade of *minimum standard* to be given, the total must be ≥11    **TOTAL =**

I_____I_____I
**Not Acceptable**      **Meets Minimum Standards**      **Exceeds Minimum Standards**

**L:** Laboratory/Classroom Testing
**C:** Clinical/Field Testing
**P:** Practicum Testing
**A:** Assessment/Mock Exam Testing
**S:** Self-Reporting

**Positive Finding:** Range of motion
**Involved Structure:** Glenohumeral joint
**Special Considerations:** N/A
**Reference(s):** Norkin et al
**Supplies Needed:** Goniometer, dots/markers, towel/pad

# OTHER TESTS
# (O-Test 4)

Peer Review _____ Peer Review _____

Skill Acquisition: _____    Practice Opportunities: _____

*Please demonstrate the proper use of a* **goniometer** *for measuring an athlete's* **elbow** *active range of motion for* **flexion/extension** *at the humeroulnar joint. You have 3 minutes to complete this task.*

| | YES | NO |
|---|---|---|
| **Tester places athlete and limb in appropriate position** | **YES** | **NO** |
| Supine | ○○○ | ○○○ |
| Anatomical position | ○○○ | ○○○ |
| Pad/towel under the distal end of the humerus | ○○○ | ○○○ |
| **Tester provides appropriate stabilization** | **YES** | **NO** |
| Distal end of the humerus | ○○○ | ○○○ |
| **Tester places goniometer in appropriate position** | **YES** | **NO** |
| Fulcrum: Lateral epicondyle of humerus | ○○○ | ○○○ |
| Stationary arm: Lateral midline of the humerus | ○○○ | ○○○ |
| Moving arm: Lateral midline of the radius (radial head) | ○○○ | ○○○ |
| **Tester performs test according to accepted guidelines** | **YES** | **NO** |
| Correct reading: Flexion/extension | ○○○ | ○○○ |
| Performs assessment bilaterally | ○○○ | ○○○ |

The psychomotor skill was performed completely and in the appropriate order    **0  1  2  3  4  5**

The tester had control of the subject and the situation (showed confidence)    **0  1  2  3  4  5**

Method of performing the skill allowed the tester the ability to determine:
severity, proper progression, and the *fit* in the overall picture (Oral)    **0  1  2  3  4  5**

In order for a grade of *minimum standard* to be given, the total must be ≥11    **TOTAL =**

I_____I_____I

**Not Acceptable          Meets Minimum Standards    Exceeds Minimum Standards**

**L:** Laboratory/Classroom Testing
**C:** Clinical/Field Testing
**P:** Practicum Testing
**A:** Assessment/Mock Exam Testing
**S:** Self-Reporting

**Positive Finding:** Range of motion
**Involved Structure:** Humeroradial joint, humeroulnar joint
**Special Considerations:** N/A
**Reference(s):** Norkin et al
**Supplies Needed:** Goniometer, dots/markers, towel, table

# OTHER TESTS
# (O-Test 5)

Peer Review _____   Peer Review _____

Skill Acquisition: _____   Practice Opportunities: _____

*Please demonstrate the proper use of a **goniometer** for measuring an athlete's **elbow** (forearm) active range of motion for **pronation** at the radioulnar joint. You have 3 minutes to complete this task.*

| Tester places athlete and limb in appropriate position | YES | NO |
|---|---|---|
| Sitting | ○○○ | ○○○ |
| Shoulder adducted to 0 degrees | ○○○ | ○○○ |
| Elbow flexed to 90 degrees | ○○○ | ○○○ |
| Forearm supinated to 0 degrees (thumb pointing up) | ○○○ | ○○○ |
| **Tester provides appropriate stabilization** | **YES** | **NO** |
| Distal end of the humerus | ○○○ | ○○○ |
| **Tester places goniometer in appropriate position** | **YES** | **NO** |
| Fulcrum: Lateral to the ulnar styloid process | ○○○ | ○○○ |
| Stationary arm: Parallel to the anterior midline of the humerus | ○○○ | ○○○ |
| Moving arm: Across the dorsal aspect of the forearm | ○○○ | ○○○ |
| **Tester performs test according to accepted guidelines** | **YES** | **NO** |
| Correct reading: Pronation | ○○○ | ○○○ |
| Performs assessment bilaterally | ○○○ | ○○○ |

| | |
|---|---|
| The psychomotor skill was performed completely and in the appropriate order | **0  1  2  3  4  5** |
| The tester had control of the subject and the situation (showed confidence) | **0  1  2  3  4  5** |
| Method of performing the skill allowed the tester the ability to determine: severity, proper progression, and the *fit* in the overall picture (Oral) | **0  1  2  3  4  5** |

In order for a grade of *minimum standard* to be given, the total must be ≥11      **TOTAL =**

I_____I_____I
**Not Acceptable**       **Meets Minimum Standards**       **Exceeds Minimum Standards**

**L:** Laboratory/Classroom Testing
**C:** Clinical/Field Testing
**P:** Practicum Testing
**A:** Assessment/Mock Exam Testing
**S:** Self-Reporting

**Positive Finding:** Range of motion
**Involved Structure:** Superior radioulnar joint, inferior radioulnar joint
**Special Considerations:** N/A
**Reference(s):** Norkin et al
**Supplies Needed:** Goniometer, dots/markers

# OTHER TESTS
# (O-Test 6)

Peer Review _____ Peer Review _____

Skill Acquisition: _____    Practice Opportunities: _____

*Please demonstrate the proper use of a* **goniometer** *for measuring an athlete's* **wrist** *active range of motion for* **flexion/extension** *at the midcarpal joints. You have 3 minutes to complete this task.*

| Tester places athlete and limb in appropriate position | YES | NO |
|---|---|---|
| Sitting next to a supporting surface | ○○○ | ○○○ |
| Shoulder abducted to 90 degrees/elbow flexed to 90 degrees | ○○○ | ○○○ |
| Forearm supinated to 0 degrees (palm facing down, hanging off the table) | ○○○ | ○○○ |
| **Tester provides appropriate stabilization** | **YES** | **NO** |
| Radius and ulna | ○○○ | ○○○ |
| **Tester places goniometer in appropriate position** | **YES** | **NO** |
| Fulcrum: Lateral aspect of the wrist (triquetrum) | ○○○ | ○○○ |
| Stationary arm: Lateral midline of the ulna | ○○○ | ○○○ |
| Moving arm: Lateral midline of the fifth metacarpal | ○○○ | ○○○ |
| **Tester performs test according to accepted guidelines** | **YES** | **NO** |
| Correct reading: Flexion/extension | ○○○ | ○○○ |
| Performs assessment bilaterally | ○○○ | ○○○ |

| | |
|---|---|
| The psychomotor skill was performed completely and in the appropriate order | 0  1  2  3  4  5 |
| The tester had control of the subject and the situation (showed confidence) | 0  1  2  3  4  5 |
| Method of performing the skill allowed the tester the ability to determine: severity, proper progression, and the *fit* in the overall picture (Oral) | 0  1  2  3  4  5 |

In order for a grade of *minimum standard* to be given, the total must be $\geq 11$     **TOTAL =**

I_____I_____I

**Not Acceptable**        **Meets Minimum Standards**        **Exceeds Minimum Standards**

**L:** Laboratory/Classroom Testing
**C:** Clinical/Field Testing
**P:** Practicum Testing
**A:** Assessment/Mock Exam Testing
**S:** Self-Reporting

**Positive Finding:** Range of motion
**Involved Structure:** Wrist
**Special Considerations:** N/A
**Reference(s):** Norkin et al
**Supplies Needed:** Goniometer, dots/markers, chair, table

# OTHER TESTS
# (O-Test 7)

Skill Acquisition: _____    Practice Opportunities: _____

*Please demonstrate the proper use of a* **goniometer** *for measuring an athlete's* **wrist** *active range of motion for* **radial deviation** *at the radiocarpal joint. You have 3 minutes to complete this task.*

| Tester places athlete and limb in appropriate position | YES | NO |
|---|---|---|
| Sitting next to a supporting surface | ○○○ | ○○○ |
| Shoulder abducted to 90 degrees/elbow flexed to 90 degrees | ○○○ | ○○○ |
| Forearm supinated to 0 degrees (palm facing down, supported by the table) | ○○○ | ○○○ |
| **Tester provides appropriate stabilization** | **YES** | **NO** |
| Distal end of the radius and ulna | ○○○ | ○○○ |
| **Tester places goniometer in appropriate position** | **YES** | **NO** |
| Fulcrum: Dorsal aspect of the wrist (capitate) | ○○○ | ○○○ |
| Stationary arm: Dorsal midline of the forearm | ○○○ | ○○○ |
| Moving arm: Dorsal midline of the third metacarpal | ○○○ | ○○○ |
| **Tester performs test according to accepted guidelines** | **YES** | **NO** |
| Correct reading: Radial deviation | ○○○ | ○○○ |
| Performs assessment bilaterally | ○○○ | ○○○ |

| | |
|---|---|
| The psychomotor skill was performed completely and in the appropriate order | 0  1  2  3  4  5 |
| The tester had control of the subject and the situation (showed confidence) | 0  1  2  3  4  5 |
| Method of performing the skill allowed the tester the ability to determine: severity, proper progression, and the *fit* in the overall picture (Oral) | 0  1  2  3  4  5 |

In order for a grade of *minimum standard* to be given, the total must be ≥11          **TOTAL =**

I_____I_____I
**Not Acceptable**       **Meets Minimum Standards**       **Exceeds Minimum Standards**

**L:** Laboratory/Classroom Testing
**C:** Clinical/Field Testing
**P:** Practicum Testing
**A:** Assessment/Mock Exam Testing
**S:** Self-Reporting

**Positive Finding:** Range of motion
**Involved Structure:** Radiocarpal joint
**Special Considerations:** N/A
**Reference(s):** Norkin et al
**Supplies Needed:** Goniometer, dots/markers, chair, table

# OTHER TESTS
# (O-Test 8)

Peer Review _____ Peer Review _____

Skill Acquisition: _____    Practice Opportunities: _____

*Please demonstrate the proper use of a **goniometer** for measuring an athlete's **hip** active range of motion for **abduction** at the iliofemoral joint. You have 3 minutes to complete this task.*

| Tester places athlete and limb in appropriate position | YES | NO |
|---|---|---|
| Supine | OOO | OOO |
| Hip/knee in anatomical position | OOO | OOO |
| **Tester provides appropriate stabilization** | **YES** | **NO** |
| Pelvis | OOO | OOO |
| **Tester places goniometer in appropriate postion** | **YES** | **NO** |
| Fulcrum: ASIS of extremity being tested | OOO | OOO |
| Stationary arm: ASIS of extremity not being tested | OOO | OOO |
| Moving arm: Anterior midline of the femur (reference patella) | OOO | OOO |
| **Tester performs test according to accepted guidelines** | **YES** | **NO** |
| Correct reading: Abduction | OOO | OOO |
| Performs assessment bilaterally | OOO | OOO |

The psychomotor skill was performed completely and in the appropriate order    0 1 2 3 4 5

The tester had control of the subject and the situation (showed confidence)    0 1 2 3 4 5

Method of performing the skill allowed the tester the ability to determine:
severity, proper progression, and the *fit* in the overall picture (Oral)    0 1 2 3 4 5

In order for a grade of *minimum standard* to be given, the total must be ≥11    TOTAL =

I_____I_____I

**Not Acceptable**    **Meets Minimum Standards**    **Exceeds Minimum Standards**

**L:** Laboratory/Classroom Testing
**C:** Clinical/Field Testing
**P:** Practicum Testing
**A:** Assessment/Mock Exam Testing
**S:** Self-Reporting

**Positive Finding:** Range of motion
**Involved Structure:** Iliofemoral joint (hip)
**Special Considerations:** N/A
**Reference(s):** Norkin et al
**Supplies Needed:** Goniometer, dots/markers, table

# OTHER TESTS
## (O-Test 9)

Peer Review _____ Peer Review _____

Skill Acquisition: _____     Practice Opportunities: _____

*Please demonstrate the proper use of a **goniometer** for measuring an athlete's **hip** active range of motion for **lateral (external) rotation** at the iliofemoral joint. You have 3 minutes to complete this task.*

| Tester places athlete and limb in appropriate position | YES | NO |
|---|---|---|
| Seated (knee flexed to 90 degrees) | OOO | OOO |
| Hip in anatomical position | OOO | OOO |
| Towel roll under distal end of femur | OOO | OOO |
| **Tester provides appropriate stabilization** | YES | NO |
| Distal end of femur | OOO | OOO |
| **Tester places goniometer in appropriate position** | YES | NO |
| Fulcrum: Anterior aspect of the patella | OOO | OOO |
| Stationary arm: Perpendicular to or parallel to the floor | OOO | OOO |
| Moving arm: Anterior midline of lower leg | OOO | OOO |
| **Tester performs test according to accepted guidelines** | YES | NO |
| Correct reading: Lateral/external rotation | OOO | OOO |
| Performs assessment bilaterally | OOO | OOO |

The psychomotor skill was performed completely and in the appropriate order    0 1 2 3 4 5

The tester had control of the subject and the situation (showed confidence)    0 1 2 3 4 5

Method of performing the skill allowed the tester the ability to determine:
severity, proper progression, and the *fit* in the overall picture (Oral)    0 1 2 3 4 5

In order for a grade of *minimum standard* to be given, the total must be ≥11    **TOTAL =**

I_____I_____I
**Not Acceptable**    **Meets Minimum Standards**    **Exceeds Minimum Standards**

**L:** Laboratory/Classroom Testing
**C:** Clinical/Field Testing
**P:** Practicum Testing
**A:** Assessment/Mock Exam Testing
**S:** Self-Reporting

**Positive Finding:** Range of motion
**Involved Structure:** Iliofemoral joint
**Special Considerations:** N/A
**Reference(s):** Norkin et al
**Supplies Needed:** Goniometer, dots/markers, towel roll, table

# OTHER TESTS
# (O-Test 10)

Peer Review _____ Peer Review _____

Skill Acquisition: _____    Practice Opportunities: _____

*Please demonstrate the proper use of a **goniometer** for measuring an athlete's **knee** active range of motion for **flexion** at the tibiofemoral joint. You have 3 minutes to complete this task.*

| | YES | NO |
|---|---|---|
| **Tester places athlete and limb in appropriate position** | **YES** | **NO** |
| Supine | ○○○ | ○○○ |
| Hip/knee in anatomical position | ○○○ | ○○○ |
| **Tester provides appropriate stabilization** | **YES** | **NO** |
| Femur | ○○○ | ○○○ |
| **Tester places goniometer in appropriate position** | **YES** | **NO** |
| Fulcrum: Lateral epicondyle of the femur | ○○○ | ○○○ |
| Stationary arm: Lateral midline of the femur (reference greater trochanter) | ○○○ | ○○○ |
| Moving arm: Lateral midline of the fibula (reference lateral malleolus) | ○○○ | ○○○ |
| **Tester performs test according to accepted guidelines** | **YES** | **NO** |
| Correct reading: Flexion | ○○○ | ○○○ |
| Performs assessment bilaterally | ○○○ | ○○○ |

| | |
|---|---|
| The psychomotor skill was performed completely and in the appropriate order | 0  1  2  3  4  5 |
| The tester had control of the subject and the situation (showed confidence) | 0  1  2  3  4  5 |
| Method of performing the skill allowed the tester the ability to determine: severity, proper progression, and the *fit* in the overall picture (Oral) | 0  1  2  3  4  5 |

In order for a grade of *minimum standard* to be given, the total must be ≥11        TOTAL =

I_____I_____I

**Not Acceptable**        **Meets Minimum Standards**        **Exceeds Minimum Standards**

**L:** Laboratory/Classroom Testing
**C:** Clinical/Field Testing
**P:** Practicum Testing
**A:** Assessment/Mock Exam Testing
**S:** Self-Reporting

**Positive Finding:** Range of motion
**Involved Structure:** Tibiofemoral joint (knee)
**Special Considerations:** N/A
**Reference(s):** Norkin et al
**Supplies Needed:** Goniometer, dots/markers, table

# OTHER TESTS
# (O-Test 11)

Peer Review _____    Peer Review _____

Skill Acquisition: _____    Practice Opportunities: _____

*Please demonstrate the proper use of a* **goniometer** *for measuring an athlete's* **ankle** *active range of motion for* **dorsiflexion** *at the talocrural joint. You have 2 minutes to complete this task.*

| | YES | NO |
|---|---|---|
| **Tester places athlete and limb in appropriate position** | **YES** | **NO** |
| Supine or seated | ○○○ | ○○○ |
| Knee flexed to 90 degrees | ○○○ | ○○○ |
| Foot dorsiflexed to 0 degrees | ○○○ | ○○○ |
| **Tester provides appropriate stabilization** | **YES** | **NO** |
| Tibia and fibula | ○○○ | ○○○ |
| **Tester places goniometer in appropriate position** | **YES** | **NO** |
| Fulcrum: Lateral malleolus | ○○○ | ○○○ |
| Stationary arm: Lateral midline of the fibula (reference head of the fibula) | ○○○ | ○○○ |
| Moving arm: Parallel to the lateral aspect of the fifth metatarsal | ○○○ | ○○○ |
| **Tester performs test according to accepted guidelines** | **YES** | **NO** |
| Correct reading: Dorsiflexion | ○○○ | ○○○ |
| Performs assessment bilaterally | ○○○ | ○○○ |

| | |
|---|---|
| The psychomotor skill was performed completely and in the appropriate order | **0  1  2  3  4  5** |
| The tester had control of the subject and the situation (showed confidence) | **0  1  2  3  4  5** |
| Method of performing the skill allowed the tester the ability to determine: severity, proper progression, and the *fit* in the overall picture (Oral) | **0  1  2  3  4  5** |

In order for a grade of *minimum standard* to be given, the total must be ≥11    **TOTAL =**

I_____I_____I

**Not Acceptable**    **Meets Minimum Standards**    **Exceeds Minimum Standards**

**L:** Laboratory/Classroom Testing
**C:** Clinical/Field Testing
**P:** Practicum Testing
**A:** Assessment/Mock Exam Testing
**S:** Self-Reporting

**Positive Finding:** Range of motion
**Involved Structure:** Talocrural joint
**Special Considerations:** N/A
**Reference(s):** Norkin et al
**Supplies Needed:** Goniometer, dots/markers, table

# OTHER TESTS
# (O-Test 12)

Peer Review _____ Peer Review _____

Skill Acquisition: _____    Practice Opportunities: _____

*Please demonstrate the proper use of a **goniometer** for measuring an athlete's **trunk** active range of motion for **lateral rotation to the left**. You have 3 minutes to complete this task.*

| | YES | NO |
|---|---|---|
| **Tester places athlete and limb in appropriate position** | | |
| Seated on a stool with feet on the ground | ○○○ | ○○○ |
| Cervical/thoracic/lumbar spine in anatomical position | ○○○ | ○○○ |
| **Tester provides appropriate stabilization** | **YES** | **NO** |
| Pelvis | ○○○ | ○○○ |
| **Tester places goniometer in appropriate position** | **YES** | **NO** |
| Fulcrum: Over the center of the cranial aspect of the head | ○○○ | ○○○ |
| Stationary arm: Parallel to the line between the two prominent tubercles on the iliac crest | ○○○ | ○○○ |
| Moving arm: Distal with a line between the two acromial processes | ○○○ | ○○○ |
| **Tester performs test according to accepted guidelines** | **YES** | **NO** |
| Correct reading: Lateral rotation left | ○○○ | ○○○ |
| Performs assessment bilaterally | ○○○ | ○○○ |

The psychomotor skill was performed completely and in the appropriate order    0  1  2  3  4  5

The tester had control of the subject and the situation (showed confidence)    0  1  2  3  4  5

Method of performing the skill allowed the tester the ability to determine:
severity, proper progression, and the *fit* in the overall picture (Oral)    0  1  2  3  4  5

In order for a grade of *minimum standard* to be given, the total must be ≥11    **TOTAL =**

I_____I_____I

**Not Acceptable**        **Meets Minimum Standards**        **Exceeds Minimum Standards**

**L:** Laboratory/Classroom Testing
**C:** Clinical/Field Testing
**P:** Practicum Testing
**A:** Assessment/Mock Exam Testing
**S:** Self-Reporting

**Positive Finding:** Range of motion
**Involved Structure:** Trunk
**Special Considerations:** N/A
**Reference(s):** Norkin et al
**Supplies Needed:** Goniometer, dots/markers, stationary stool

# OTHER TESTS
# (O-Test 13)

Skill Acquisition: _____    Practice Opportunities: _____

*This problem allows you the opportunity to demonstrate the proper technique for performing a* **supine straight leg raise**, *incorporating a 5-lb cuff weight as fixed resistance. You have 2 minutes to complete this task.*

| Tester places athlete and limb in appropriate position | YES | NO |
|---|---|---|
| Supine | ○○○ | ○○○ |
| Hip/knee in anatomical position (heels on the table) | ○○○ | ○○○ |
| Attaches cuff weight securely to the involved limb | ○○○ | ○○○ |
| **Tester performs test according to accepted guidelines** | **YES** | **NO** |
| Tightens involved quadriceps (hold) | ○○○ | ○○○ |
| Lifts involved limb off the table (6 to 8 inches) | ○○○ | ○○○ |
| Retightens involved quadriceps (hold) | ○○○ | ○○○ |
| Lowers involved limb slowly | ○○○ | ○○○ |
| Allows the calf (gastrocnemius) muscle to make contact with the table first, not the heel | ○○○ | ○○○ |

The psychomotor skill was performed completely and in the appropriate order    **0  1  2  3  4  5**

The tester had control of the subject and the situation (showed confidence)    **0  1  2  3  4  5**

Method of performing the skill allowed the tester the ability to determine:
severity, proper progression, and the *fit* in the overall picture (Oral)    **0  1  2  3  4  5**

In order for a grade of *minimum standard* to be given, the total must be ≥11    **TOTAL =**

I_____I_____I
**Not Acceptable**      **Meets Minimum Standards**    **Exceeds Minimum Standards**

**L:** Laboratory/Classroom Testing
**C:** Clinical/Field Testing
**P:** Practicum Testing
**A:** Assessment/Mock Exam Testing
**S:** Self-Reporting

**Positive Finding:** Muscle re-education
**Involved Structure:** Quadriceps
**Special Considerations:** N/A
**Reference(s):** Prentice
**Supplies Needed:** 5-lb cuff weight, table

# OTHER TESTS
## (O-Test 14)

Peer Review _____ Peer Review _____

Skill Acquisition: _____    Practice Opportunities: _____

*Using a broom handle, demonstrate the* **proper technique for performing a back squat** *exercise to parallel depth. You have 3 minutes to complete this task.*

| Tester places athlete and limb in appropriate position | YES | NO |
|---|---|---|
| Standing | OOO | OOO |
| Instructs the athlete to look toward the ceiling (head slightly extended) | OOO | OOO |
| **Tester performs test according to accepted guidelines** | **YES** | **NO** |
| Beginning position: | | |
| Grasps the bar with a closed, pronated grip (slightly wider than shoulder width) | OOO | OOO |
| Feet parallel to each other (shoulder width apart) | OOO | OOO |
| Places the bar across posterior deltoids/middle trapezius (balanced position) | OOO | OOO |
| Downward movement (descent): | | |
| Allows the hips and knees to slowly flex (minimal trunk flexion is acceptable) | OOO | OOO |
| Maintains flat back, elbows high, chest up and out | OOO | OOO |
| Keeps heels on the floor | OOO | OOO |
| Keeps knees over the feet | OOO | OOO |
| Continues downward movement until thighs are parallel to the floor | OOO | OOO |
| Upward movement (ascent): | | |
| Extends the hips and knees | OOO | OOO |
| Maintains flat back, elbows high, chest up and out | OOO | OOO |
| Keeps heels on the floor | OOO | OOO |
| Keeps knees over the feet | OOO | OOO |
| Continues upward movement (does not fully "lock out") | OOO | OOO |

The psychomotor skill was performed completely and in the appropriate order    0 1 2 3 4 5

The tester had control of the subject and the situation (showed confidence)    0 1 2 3 4 5

Method of performing the skill allowed the tester the ability to determine:
severity, proper progression, and the *fit* in the overall picture (Oral)    0 1 2 3 4 5

In order for a grade of *minimum standard* to be given, the total must be ≥11    **TOTAL =**

I_____I_____I
**Not Acceptable**    **Meets Minimum Standards**    **Exceeds Minimum Standards**

**L:** Laboratory/Classroom Testing
**C:** Clinical/Field Testing
**P:** Practicum Testing
**A:** Assessment/Mock Exam Testing
**S:** Self-Reporting

**Positive Finding:** Strength development
**Involved Structure:** Quadriceps
**Special Considerations:** N/A
**Reference(s):** Baechle et al
**Supplies Needed:** Broom handle

## OTHER TESTS
# (O-Test 15)

Peer Review _____  Peer Review _____

Skill Acquisition: _____        Practice Opportunities: _____

*This problem allows you the opportunity to demonstrate the proper* **spotting technique** *for an athlete who is performing a* **forward lunge**. *You have 3 minutes to complete this task.*

| Tester places athlete and limb in appropriate position | YES | NO |
|---|---|---|
| Standing behind the athlete | ○○○ | ○○○ |
| **Tester performs test according to accepted guidelines** | **YES** | **NO** |
| Beginning position (spotter): | | |
|   Positions hands near the athlete's hips/wrist | ○○○ | ○○○ |
|   Feet side-by-side (shoulder width apart) | ○○○ | ○○○ |
| Forward movement phase (spotter): | | |
|   Steps forward with the athlete (same foot as the athlete) | ○○○ | ○○○ |
|   Keeps the lead knee about 15 inches behind the athlete's foot | ○○○ | ○○○ |
|   Keeps hands near the athlete's torso | ○○○ | ○○○ |
| Backward movement phase (spotter): | | |
|   Pushes backward with the lead leg at the same time the athlete moves (returns to legs in side-by-side) | ○○○ | ○○○ |
|   Keeps hands near the athlete's torso | ○○○ | ○○○ |
| Repeat alternating lead leg | ○○○ | ○○○ |

The psychomotor skill was performed completely and in the appropriate order    **0  1  2  3  4  5**

The tester had control of the subject and the situation (showed confidence)    **0  1  2  3  4  5**

Method of performing the skill allowed the tester the ability to determine:
severity, proper progression, and the *fit* in the overall picture (Oral)    **0  1  2  3  4  5**

In order for a grade of *minimum standard* to be given, the total must be ≥11        **TOTAL =**

I_____I_____I
**Not Acceptable**        **Meets Minimum Standards**    **Exceeds Minimum Standards**

**L:** Laboratory/Classroom Testing
**C:** Clinical/Field Testing
**P:** Practicum Testing
**A:** Assessment/Mock Exam Testing
**S:** Self-Reporting

**Positive Finding:** Safety
**Involved Structure:** N/A
**Special Considerations:** N/A
**Reference(s):** Baechle et al
**Supplies Needed:** Broom handle or dumbbells

# OTHER TESTS
# (O-Test 16)

Peer Review _____ Peer Review _____

Skill Acquisition: _____    Practice Opportunities: _____

*Using a fully inflated basketball and a flat surface (eg, floor), develop a balance test that helps assess* **upper extremity proprioception**. *You have 3 minutes to develop and complete this task.*

| Tester places athlete and limb in appropriate position | YES | NO |
|---|---|---|
| Prone (push-up position) | OOO | OOO |
| **Tester performs test according to accepted guidelines** | **YES** | **NO** |
| Places the basketball under the athlete's uninvolved limb | OOO | OOO |
| Moves the opposite limb away from the floor | OOO | OOO |
| Instructs the athlete to balance on the uninvolved limb (as long possible or for a maximum of 1 minute) | OOO | OOO |
| Repeats the above three steps with the involved limb | OOO | OOO |
| Compares time in a balanced position (to determine deficit) | OOO | OOO |

| | |
|---|---|
| The psychomotor skill was performed completely and in the appropriate order | **0  1  2  3  4  5** |
| The tester had control of the subject and the situation (showed confidence) | **0  1  2  3  4  5** |
| Method of performing the skill allowed the tester the ability to determine: severity, proper progression, and the *fit* in the overall picture (Oral) | **0  1  2  3  4  5** |

In order for a grade of *minimum standard* to be given, the total must be ≥11    **TOTAL =**

I_____I_____I

**Not Acceptable**          **Meets Minimum Standards**          **Exceeds Minimum Standards**

**L:** Laboratory/Classroom Testing
**C:** Clinical/Field Testing
**P:** Practicum Testing
**A:** Assessment/Mock Exam Testing
**S:** Self-Reporting

**Positive Finding:** Proprioception development
**Involved Structure:** Muscle spindles, etc
**Special Considerations:** N/A
**Reference(s):** Prentice
**Supplies Needed:** Stop watch, fully inflated ball

## OTHER TESTS
# (O-Test 17)

Peer Review _____ Peer Review _____

Skill Acquisition: _____    Practice Opportunities: _____

*Using a partially deflated soccer ball, develop a balance test that helps assess* **lower extremity proprioception.**
*You have 3 minutes to develop and complete this task.*

| Tester places athlete and limb in appropriate position | YES | NO |
|---|---|---|
| Standing | ○○○ | ○○○ |
| **Tester performs test according to accepted guidelines** | **YES** | **NO** |
| Places a deflated soccer ball under the athlete's uninvolved limb | ○○○ | ○○○ |
| Removes the opposite limb away from the floor | ○○○ | ○○○ |
| Instructs the athlete to balance on the uninvolved limb (as long as possible or for a maximum of 1 minute) | ○○○ | ○○○ |
| Repeats the above three steps with the involved limb | ○○○ | ○○○ |
| Compares time in a balanced position (to determine deficit) | ○○○ | ○○○ |

The psychomotor skill was performed completely and in the appropriate order    0  1  2  3  4  5

The tester had control of the subject and the situation (showed confidence)    0  1  2  3  4  5

Method of performing the skill allowed the tester the ability to determine:
severity, proper progression, and the *fit* in the overall picture (Oral)    0  1  2  3  4  5

In order for a grade of *minimum standard* to be given, the total must be ≥11    **TOTAL =**

I_____I_____I
**Not Acceptable**      **Meets Minimum Standards**   **Exceeds Minimum Standards**

**L:** Laboratory/Classroom Testing
**C:** Clinical/Field Testing
**P:** Practicum Testing
**A:** Assessment/Mock Exam Testing
**S:** Self-Reporting

**Positive Finding:** Proprioception development
**Involved Structure:** Muscle spindles, etc
**Special Considerations:** N/A
**Reference(s):** Adapted from Prentice
**Supplies Needed:** Stop watch, deflated soccer ball

## OTHER TESTS
# (O-Test 18)

Peer Review _____ Peer Review _____

Skill Acquisition: _____        Practice Opportunities: _____

*Using a 10-lb dumbbell, develop an endurance-based* **strength test** *in order to determine the* **percent fatigue** *of the* **middle deltoid** *muscle. This type of testing is also known as a "% Fatigue Test." You have 3 minutes to develop and administer this test.*

| Tester places athlete and limb in appropriate position | YES | NO |
|---|---|---|
| Standing or seated | ○○○ | ○○○ |
| Arms hanging to the side | ○○○ | ○○○ |
| **Tester performs test according to accepted guidelines** | **YES** | **NO** |
| Instructs the athlete to hold a 10-lb dumbbell with the uninvolved limb Instructs the athlete to fully abduct the shoulder (slow, controlled pace) | ○○○ | ○○○ |
| Continues until the athlete cannot complete the next repetition or for 1 minute continuously (count the number of repetitions completed) | ○○○ | ○○○ |
| Repeats the above three steps with the involved limb | ○○○ | ○○○ |
| Compares the number of repetitions completed (determines deficit) | ○○○ | ○○○ |

The psychomotor skill was performed completely and in the appropriate order          **0  1  2  3  4  5**

The tester had control of the subject and the situation (showed confidence)          **0  1  2  3  4  5**

Method of performing the skill allowed the tester the ability to determine:
severity, proper progression, and the *fit* in the overall picture (Oral)          **0  1  2  3  4  5**

In order for a grade of *minimum standard* to be given, the total must be ≥11          **TOTAL =**

I_____I_____I

**Not Acceptable          Meets Minimum Standards          Exceeds Minimum Standards**

**L:** Laboratory/Classroom Testing
**C:** Clinical/Field Testing
**P:** Practicum Testing
**A:** Assessment/Mock Exam Testing
**S:** Self-Reporting

**Positive Finding:** Determine strength deficit
**Involved Structure:** Middle deltoid
**Special Considerations:** N/A
**Reference(s):** Adapted from Baechle et al
**Supplies Needed:** 10-lb dumbbell, stop watch

## OTHER TESTS
# (O-Test 19)

Peer Review _____ Peer Review _____

Skill Acquisition: _____    Practice Opportunities: _____

*Using an imaginary wall pulley ("lateral pulldown" machine), develop a **strength test** in order to determine a **10 RM** for an athlete's shoulder extensors. This type of testing is also known as "% 1 x 10 Test." You have 3 minutes to develop and administer this test.*

| Tester places athlete and limb in appropriate position | YES | NO |
|---|---|---|
| Seated or kneeling | OOO | OOO |
| **Tester performs test according to accepted guidelines** | **YES** | **NO** |
| Instructs the athlete to grip the wall pulley/lateral pulldown machine with the uninvolved limb | OOO | OOO |
| Instructs the athlete to fully adduct the shoulder and flex the elbow (slow, controlled pace) | OOO | OOO |
| Continues until the athlete cannot complete the 11th repetition (during this simulation, the amount of weight is only a guess; choose a weight that the uninvolved limb can only do 10 times) | OOO | OOO |
| Repeats the above three steps with the involved limb (using the same weight) | OOO | OOO |
| Compares the number repetitions completed (to determine deficit) | OOO | OOO |

The psychomotor skill was performed completely and in the appropriate order    0 1 2 3 4 5

The tester had control of the subject and the situation (showed confidence)    0 1 2 3 4 5

Method of performing the skill allowed the tester the ability to determine: severity, proper progression, and the *fit* in the overall picture (Oral)    0 1 2 3 4 5

In order for a grade of *minimum standard* to be given, the total must be ≥11    **TOTAL =**

I_____I_____I
**Not Acceptable**        **Meets Minimum Standards**    **Exceeds Minimum Standards**

**L:** Laboratory/Classroom Testing
**C:** Clinical/Field Testing
**P:** Practicum Testing
**A:** Assessment/Mock Exam Testing
**S:** Self-Reporting

**Positive Finding:** Determine strength deficit
**Involved Structure:** Latissimus dorsi, teres major
**Special Considerations:** N/A
**Reference(s):** Adapted from Baechle et al
**Supplies Needed:** Lateral pulldown machine (ideally)

# OTHER TESTS
# (O-Test 20)

Skill Acquisition: _____    Practice Opportunities: _____

*Using a dumbbell, develop a **strength test** in order to determine a **5 RM** for an athlete's **wrist flexors**. This type of testing is also known as a "% 1 x 5 Test." You have 3 minutes to develop and administer this test.*

| Tester places athlete and limb in appropriate position | YES | NO |
|---|---|---|
| Seated | OOO | OOO |
| Wrist support hanging off the edge of the table | OOO | OOO |
| Forearm supinated to 90 degrees | OOO | OOO |
| **Tester performs test according to accepted guidelines** | **YES** | **NO** |
| Instructs the athlete to hold the dumbbell with the uninvolved limb | OOO | OOO |
| Instructs the athlete to fully flex the wrist (slow, controlled pace) | OOO | OOO |
| Continues until the athlete cannot complete the sixth repetition (during this simulation the amount of weight is only a guess; choose a weight that the uninvolved limb can only do five times) | OOO | OOO |
| Repeats the above three steps with the involved limb (using the same weight) | OOO | OOO |
| Compares the number repetitions completed (determines deficit) | OOO | OOO |

| | |
|---|---|
| The psychomotor skill was performed completely and in the appropriate order | 0  1  2  3  4  5 |
| The tester had control of the subject and the situation (showed confidence) | 0  1  2  3  4  5 |
| Method of performing the skill allowed the tester the ability to determine: severity, proper progression, and the *fit* in the overall picture (Oral) | 0  1  2  3  4  5 |

In order for a grade of *minimum standard* to be given, the total must be ≥11     **TOTAL =**

I_____I_____I
**Not Acceptable**          **Meets Minimum Standards**    **Exceeds Minimum Standards**

**L:** Laboratory/Classroom Testing
**C:** Clinical/Field Testing
**P:** Practicum Testing
**A:** Assessment/Mock Exam Testing
**S:** Self-Reporting

**Positive Finding:** Determine strength deficit
**Involved Structure:** Wrist flexors
**Special Considerations:** N/A
**Reference(s):** Adapted from Baechle et al
**Supplies Needed:** Dumbbells

## OTHER TESTS
# (Os-Test 21)

Skill Acquisition: _____    Practice Opportunities: _____

*Using a 10-lb dumbbell, develop a **strength test** that will assess **power** bilaterally for the **triceps**. This type of testing is also known as a "% Power Test." You have 3 minutes to develop and administer this test.*

| Tester places athlete and limb in appropriate position | YES | NO |
|---|---|---|
| Supine or seated | OOO | OOO |
| **Tester performs test according to accepted guidelines** | **YES** | **NO** |
| Instructs the athlete to hold the 10-lb dumbbell with the uninvolved limb | OOO | OOO |
| Instructs the athlete to fully extend the elbow (as quickly as possible) | OOO | OOO |
| Continues contraction as quickly as possible for 20 seconds (during this simulation, the amount of time can vary; it is up to the tester to determine whether the time chosen is appropriate) | OOO | OOO |
| Repeats the above three steps with the involved limb (using the same weight and amount of time) | OOO | OOO |
| Compares the number repetitions completed (determines deficit) | OOO | OOO |

The psychomotor skill was performed completely and in the appropriate order    **0 1 2 3 4 5**

The tester had control of the subject and the situation (showed confidence)    **0 1 2 3 4 5**

Method of performing the skill allowed the tester the ability to determine:
severity, proper progression, and the *fit* in the overall picture (Oral)    **0 1 2 3 4 5**

In order for a grade of *minimum standard* to be given, the total must be ≥11    **TOTAL =**

I_____I_____I
**Not Acceptable**        **Meets Minimum Standards**    **Exceeds Minimum Standards**

**L:** Laboratory/Classroom Testing
**C:** Clinical/Field Testing
**P:** Practicum Testing
**A:** Assessment/Mock Exam Testing
**S:** Self-Reporting

**Positive Finding:** Determine strength deficit
**Involved Structure:** Triceps
**Special Considerations:** N/A
**Reference(s):** Adapted from Baechle et al
**Supplies Needed:** Dumbbell, stop watch

# OTHER TESTS
# (O-Test 22)

Peer Review _____ Peer Review _____

Skill Acquisition: _____    Practice Opportunities: _____

*Using a 10-lb cuff weight, develop an endurance-based* **strength test** *in order to determine the* **percent fatigue** *of the* **tibialis anterior**. *This type of testing is also known as a "% Fatigue Test." You have 3 minutes to develop and administer this test.*

| Tester places athlete and limb in appropriate position | YES | NO |
|---|---|---|
| Seated (leg off the table) | ooo | ooo |
| Knee flexed to 90 degrees | ooo | ooo |
| **Tester performs test according to accepted guidelines** | **YES** | **NO** |
| Fastens the 10-lb cuff weight around the foot of the uninvolved limb | ooo | ooo |
| Instructs the athlete to fully dorsiflex the ankle (slow, controlled pace) | ooo | ooo |
| Continues until the athlete cannot complete the next repetition or for 1 minute continuously (count the number of repetitions completed) | ooo | ooo |
| Repeats the above three steps with the involved limb | ooo | ooo |
| Compares the number of repetitions completed (to determine deficit) | ooo | ooo |

The psychomotor skill was performed completely and in the appropriate order    **0  1  2  3  4  5**

The tester had control of the subject and the situation (showed confidence)    **0  1  2  3  4  5**

Method of performing the skill allowed the tester the ability to determine:
severity, proper progression, and the *fit* in the overall picture (Oral)    **0  1  2  3  4  5**

In order for a grade of *minimum standard* to be given, the total must be ≥11    **TOTAL =**

I_____I_____I
**Not Acceptable            Meets Minimum Standards      Exceeds Minimum Standards**

**L:** Laboratory/Classroom Testing
**C:** Clinical/Field Testing
**P:** Practicum Testing
**A:** Assessment/Mock Exam Testing
**S:** Self-Reporting

**Positive Finding:** Determine strength deficit
**Involved Structure:** Tibialis anterior
**Special Considerations:** N/A
**Reference(s):** Adapted from Baechle et al
**Supplies Needed:** Cuff weight, stop watch

## OTHER TESTS
# (O-Test 23)

Skill Acquisition: _____    Practice Opportunities: _____

*Using an imaginary prone leg curl machine (knee curl), develop a **strength test** in order to determine a **10 RM** for an athlete's **hamstrings**. This type of testing is also known as "% 1 x 10 Test." You have 3 minutes to develop and administer this test.*

| Tester places athlete and limb in appropriate position | YES | NO |
|---|---|---|
| Prone | ○○○ | ○○○ |
| **Tester performs test according to accepted guidelines** | **YES** | **NO** |
| Selects the appropriate weight needed for the uninvolved limb | ○○○ | ○○○ |
| Instructs the athlete to fully flex the knee (slow, controlled pace) | ○○○ | ○○○ |
| Continues until the athlete cannot complete the 11th repetition (during this simulation, the amount of weight is only a guess; choose a weight that the uninvolved limb can only do 10 times) | ○○○ | ○○○ |
| Repeats the above three steps with the involved limb (using the same weight) | ○○○ | ○○○ |
| Compares the number of repetitions completed (to determine deficit) | ○○○ | ○○○ |

| | |
|---|---|
| The psychomotor skill was performed completely and in the appropriate order | **0  1  2  3  4  5** |
| The tester had control of the subject and the situation (showed confidence) | **0  1  2  3  4  5** |
| Method of performing the skill allowed the tester the ability to determine: severity, proper progression, and the *fit* in the overall picture (Oral) | **0  1  2  3  4  5** |

In order for a grade of *minimum standard* to be given, the total must be ≥11          **TOTAL =**

I_____I_____I

**Not Acceptable**          **Meets Minimum Standards**          **Exceeds Minimum Standards**

**L:** Laboratory/Classroom Testing
**C:** Clinical/Field Testing
**P:** Practicum Testing
**A:** Assessment/Mock Exam Testing
**S:** Self-Reporting

**Positive Finding:** Determine strength deficit
**Involved Structure:** Hamstrings
**Special Considerations:** N/A
**Reference(s):** Adapted from Baechle et al
**Supplies Needed:** Cuff weight, table (leg curl machine ideally)

# OTHER TESTS
# (O-Test 24)

Peer Review _____ Peer Review _____

Skill Acquisition: _____    Practice Opportunities: _____

*Using an* imaginary *leg press machine, develop a* **strength test** *in order to determine a* **5 RM** *for an athlete's* **ankle plantar flexors**. *This type of testing is also known as a "% 1 x 5 Test." You have 3 minutes to develop and administer this test.*

| Tester places athlete and limb in appropriate position | YES | NO |
|---|---|---|
| Seated | OOO | OOO |
| Knee extended to 0 degrees | OOO | OOO |

| Tester performs test according to accepted guidelines | YES | NO |
|---|---|---|
| Selects the appropriate weight needed for the uninvolved limb | OOO | OOO |
| Instructs the athlete to fully plantar flex the ankle (slow, controlled pace) | OOO | OOO |
| Continues until the athlete cannot complete the sixth repetition (during this simulation the amount of weight is only a guess; choose a weight that the uninvolved limb can only do five times) | OOO | OOO |
| Repeats the above three steps with the involved limb (using the same weight) | OOO | OOO |
| Compares the number of repetitions completed (to determine deficit) | OOO | OOO |

The psychomotor skill was performed completely and in the appropriate order     0 1 2 3 4 5

The tester had control of the subject and the situation (showed confidence)     0 1 2 3 4 5

Method of performing the skill allowed the tester the ability to determine:
severity, proper progression, and the *fit* in the overall picture (Oral)     0 1 2 3 4 5

In order for a grade of *minimum standard* to be given, the total must be ≥11     **TOTAL =**

I_____I_____I

**Not Acceptable        Meets Minimum Standards      Exceeds Minimum Standards**

**L:** Laboratory/Classroom Testing
**C:** Clinical/Field Testing
**P:** Practicum Testing
**A:** Assessment/Mock Exam Testing
**S:** Self-Reporting

**Positive Finding:** Determine strength deficit
**Involved Structure:** Gastrocnemius, soleus
**Special Considerations:** N/A
**Reference(s):** Adapted from Baechle et al
**Supplies Needed:** Leg press machine, ideally

## OTHER TESTS
# (O-Test 25)

Peer Review _____ Peer Review _____

Skill Acquisition: _____    Practice Opportunities: _____

*Using a 10-lb cuff weight, develop a* **strength test** *that will assess* **power** *bilaterally for the* **knee extensors**. *This type of testing is also known as a "% Power Test." You have 3 minutes to develop and administer this test.*

| Tester places athlete and limb in appropriate position | YES | NO |
|---|---|---|
| Seated (knee flexed) | OOO | OOO |

| Tester performs test according to accepted guidelines | YES | NO |
|---|---|---|
| Fastens the 10-lb cuff weight to the distal tibia/fibula of the uninvolved limb | OOO | OOO |
| Instructs the athlete to fully extend the knee (as quickly as possible) | OOO | OOO |
| Continues contractions as quickly as possible for 20 seconds (during this simulation, the amount time can vary; it is up to the tester to determine if the time chosen is appropriate) | OOO | OOO |
| Repeats the above three steps with the involved limb (using the same weight and amount of time) | OOO | OOO |
| Compares the number of repetitions completed (to determine deficit) | OOO | OOO |

The psychomotor skill was performed completely and in the appropriate order    **0  1  2  3  4  5**

The tester had control of the subject and the situation (showed confidence)    **0  1  2  3  4  5**

Method of performing the skill allowed the tester the ability to determine:
severity, proper progression, and the *fit* in the overall picture (Oral)    **0  1  2  3  4  5**

In order for a grade of *minimum standard* to be given, the total must be ≥11    **TOTAL =**

I_____I_____I
**Not Acceptable**          **Meets Minimum Standards**    **Exceeds Minimum Standards**

**L:** Laboratory/Classroom Testing
**C:** Clinical/Field Testing
**P:** Practicum Testing
**A:** Assessment/Mock Exam Testing
**S:** Self-Reporting

**Positive Finding:** Determine strength deficit
**Involved Structure:** Quadriceps
**Special Considerations:** N/A
**Reference(s):** Adapted from Baechle et al
**Supplies Needed:** Cuff weight, table, stop watch

## OTHER TESTS
# (O-Test 26)

Peer Review _____ Peer Review _____

Skill Acquisition: _____  Practice Opportunities: _____

*This problem allows you the opportunity to set up and assess an athlete using an **isokinetic device test**. This specific scenario requires you to set up the **shoulder** for abduction/adduction at 90, 180, and 270 degrees per second. You have 5 minutes to complete this task.*

| Tester places athlete and limb in appropriate position | YES | NO |
|---|---|---|
| Seated | ○○○ | ○○○ |

| Tester performs proper set-up of the Isokinetic Device | YES | NO |
|---|---|---|
| All components of the isokinetic device are in proper working order | ○○○ | ○○○ |
| Proper attachments are collected and secured to the isokinetic device | ○○○ | ○○○ |
| Shoulder joint is in line with the axis of the isokinetic dynamometer | ○○○ | ○○○ |
| Lever arm is adjusted to match the length of the involved limb | ○○○ | ○○○ |
| All straps are properly placed and secured (if appropriate) | ○○○ | ○○○ |

| Tester performs test according to accepted guidelines | YES | NO |
|---|---|---|
| Proper warm-up is provided | ○○○ | ○○○ |
| Proper instructions are given: | | |
|   Moves limb through full range of motion | ○○○ | ○○○ |
|   Generates maximal contraction for each repetition | ○○○ | ○○○ |
|   Moves limb as hard and as fast a possible | ○○○ | ○○○ |
| Velocities are preset at 90/180/270 degrees per second prior to the start of each set | ○○○ | ○○○ |
| Number of repetitions are given and explained to the athlete | ○○○ | ○○○ |
| Isokinetic test is administered and recorded/printed | ○○○ | ○○○ |

The psychomotor skill was performed completely and in the appropriate order    **0  1  2  3  4  5**

The tester had control of the subject and the situation (showed confidence)    **0  1  2  3  4  5**

Method of performing the skill allowed the tester the ability to determine:
severity, proper progression, and the *fit* in the overall picture (Oral)    **0  1  2  3  4  5**

In order for a grade of *minimum standard* to be given, the total must be ≥11    **TOTAL =**

I_____I_____I
**Not Acceptable**    **Meets Minimum Standards**    **Exceeds Minimum Standards**

**L:** Laboratory/Classroom Testing
**C:** Clinical/Field Testing
**P:** Practicum Testing
**A:** Assessment/Mock Exam Testing
**S:** Self-Reporting

**Positive Finding:** Isokinetic testing
**Involved Structure:** Abduction/adduction
**Special Considerations:** Print reports available from testing device
**Reference(s):** Adapted from Prentice
**Supplies Needed:** Isokinetic device

# OTHER TESTS
# (O-Test 27)

Peer Review _____ Peer Review _____

Skill Acquisition: _____     Practice Opportunities: _____

*This problem allows you the opportunity to set up and assess an athlete using an* **isokinetic device test**. *This specific scenario requires you to set up the* **knee** *for flexion/extension at 60, 120, and 210 degrees per second. You have 5 minutes to complete this task.*

| Tester places athlete and limb in appropriate position | YES | NO |
|---|---|---|
| Seated | ○○○ | ○○○ |
| **Tester performs proper set-up of the isokinetic device** | **YES** | **NO** |
| All components of the isokinetic device are in proper working order | ○○○ | ○○○ |
| Proper attachments are collected and secured to the isokinetic device | ○○○ | ○○○ |
| Knee joint is in line with the axis of the isokinetic dynamometer | ○○○ | ○○○ |
| Lever arm is adjusted to match the length of the involved limb | ○○○ | ○○○ |
| All straps are properly placed and secured (if appropriate) | ○○○ | ○○○ |
| **Tester performs test according to accepted guidelines** | **YES** | **NO** |
| Proper warm-up is provided | ○○○ | ○○○ |
| Proper instructions are given: | | |
|   Moves limb through full range of motion | ○○○ | ○○○ |
|   Generates maximal contraction for each repetition | ○○○ | ○○○ |
|   Moves limb as hard and as fast a possible | ○○○ | ○○○ |
| Velocities are preset at 60/120/210 degrees per second prior to the start of each set | ○○○ | ○○○ |
| Number of repetitions are given and explained to the athlete | ○○○ | ○○○ |
| Isokinetic test is administered and recorded/printed | ○○○ | ○○○ |

The psychomotor skill was performed completely and in the appropriate order    **0  1  2  3  4  5**

The tester had control of the subject and the situation (showed confidence)    **0  1  2  3  4  5**

Method of performing the skill allowed the tester the ability to determine:
severity, proper progression, and the *fit* in the overall picture (Oral)    **0  1  2  3  4  5**

In order for a grade of *minimum standard* to be given, the total must be ≥11    **TOTAL =**

I_____I_____I

**Not Acceptable**     **Meets Minimum Standards**     **Exceeds Minimum Standards**

**L:** Laboratory/Classroom Testing
**C:** Clinical/Field Testing
**P:** Practicum Testing
**A:** Assessment/Mock Exam Testing
**S:** Self-Reporting

**Positive Finding:** Isokinetic testing
**Involved Structure:** Knee: flexion/extension
**Special Considerations:** Print reports available from testing device
**Reference(s):** Adapted from Prentice
**Supplies Needed:** Isokinetic device

# OTHER TESTS
## (O-Test 28)

Skill Acquisition: _____     Practice Opportunities: _____

*Using the athlete as your partner, demonstrate how you would perform a type of* **plyometrics** *known as a* **medicine ball sit-up***. You have 3 minutes to complete this task.*

| Tester places athlete and limb in appropriate position | YES | NO |
|---|---|---|
| Seated on the floor | OOO | OOO |
| Sit-up position (knees bent, trunk flexed to 45 degrees) | OOO | OOO |
| Hands/arms in an outstretched position (waiting to receive the ball) | OOO | OOO |
| **Tester placed in proper position** | **YES** | **NO** |
| Standing in front of the athlete (holding the medicine ball) | OOO | OOO |
| Tester performs task according to accepted guidelines | OOO | OOO |
| **Tester throws the ball to the athlete** | **YES** | **NO** |
| Athlete: Catches the ball using both arms (eccentric phrase) | OOO | OOO |
| Athlete: Completes the amortization phase (time between moving down toward the floor and coming back up) | OOO | OOO |
| Athlete: Moves away from the floor and throws/pushes the ball back (concentric phase) | OOO | OOO |
| Tester: Receives the ball from the athlete and repeats | OOO | OOO |

| | |
|---|---|
| The psychomotor skill was performed completely and in the appropriate order | 0  1  2  3  4  5 |
| The tester had control of the subject and the situation (showed confidence) | 0  1  2  3  4  5 |
| Method of performing the skill allowed the tester the ability to determine: severity, proper progression, and the *fit* in the overall picture (Oral) | 0  1  2  3  4  5 |

In order for a grade of *minimum standard* to be given, the total must be ≥11     **TOTAL =**

I_____I_____I

**Not Acceptable**          **Meets Minimum Standards**     **Exceeds Minimum Standards**

**L:** Laboratory/Classroom Testing
**C:** Clinical/Field Testing
**P:** Practicum Testing
**A:** Assessment/Mock Exam Testing
**S:** Self-Reporting

**Positive Finding:** Develop power
**Involved Structure:** Rectus abdominis (abdominal muscles)
**Special Considerations:** N/A
**Reference(s):** Baechle et al
**Supplies Needed:** Medicine ball

## OTHER TESTS
# (O-Test 29)

Skill Acquisition: _____    Practice Opportunities: _____

*Please demonstrate the* **plyometric** *technique known at the* **medicine ball push-up**. *You have 2 minutes to complete this task.*

| Tester places athlete and limb in appropriate position | YES | NO |
|---|---|---|
| Prone on the floor | ○○○ | ○○○ |
| Push-up position | ○○○ | ○○○ |
| Hands on top of the medicine ball (elbows extended) | ○○○ | ○○○ |
| **Tester placed in proper position** | **YES** | **NO** |
| Standing (observation only) | ○○○ | ○○○ |
| **Tester performs task according to accepted guidelines** | **YES** | **NO** |
| Athlete: Drops the medicine ball (eccentric phase) | ○○○ | ○○○ |
| Athlete: Completes the amortization phase (time between eccentric phase and concentric phase) | ○○○ | ○○○ |
| Moving away from the floor and back to on top of the ball (concentric phase) | ○○○ | ○○○ |
| Landing and bouncing on the ball | ○○○ | ○○○ |

| | |
|---|---|
| The psychomotor skill was performed completely and in the appropriate order | 0  1  2  3  4  5 |
| The tester had control of the subject and the situation (showed confidence) | 0  1  2  3  4  5 |
| Method of performing the skill allowed the tester the ability to determine: severity, proper progression, and the *fit* in the overall picture (Oral) | 0  1  2  3  4  5 |

In order for a grade of *minimum standard* to be given, the total must be ≥11        **TOTAL =**

I_____I_____I

**Not Acceptable**        **Meets Minimum Standards**        **Exceeds Minimum Standards**

**L:** Laboratory/Classroom Testing
**C:** Clinical/Field Testing
**P:** Practicum Testing
**A:** Assessment/Mock Exam Testing
**S:** Self-Reporting

**Positive Finding:** Power
**Involved Structure:** Anterior shoulder/triceps
**Special Considerations:** N/A
**Reference(s):** Baechle et al
**Supplies Needed:** Medicine ball

# OTHER TESTS
# (O-Test 30)

Skill Acquisition: _____     Practice Opportunities: _____

*Please demonstrate the* **plyometric** *technique known as the* **triple double-leg vertical jump (triple vertical jump-double leg)**. *You have 3 minutes to complete this task.*

| Tester places athlete and limb in appropriate position | YES | NO |
|---|---|---|
| Standing | OOO | OOO |
| Feet shoulder width apart | OOO | OOO |
| Arms flexed to 90 degrees | OOO | OOO |
| **Tester placed in proper position** | **YES** | **NO** |
| Observation only | OOO | OOO |
| **Tester performs task according to accepted guidelines** | **YES** | **NO** |
| Instructs the athlete: | | |
|   To drop arms into hyperextension | OOO | OOO |
|   To flex knees, hip, and trunk | OOO | OOO |
|   To explosively jump up (vertical) | OOO | OOO |
|   To land on two feet (in the starting place and position) | OOO | OOO |
| Repeats (double) | OOO | OOO |
| Repeats (triple) | OOO | OOO |

The psychomotor skill was performed completely and in the appropriate order    0 1 2 3 4 5

The tester had control of the subject and the situation (showed confidence)    0 1 2 3 4 5

Method of performing the skill allowed the tester the ability to determine:
severity, proper progression, and the *fit* in the overall picture (Oral)    0 1 2 3 4 5

In order for a grade of *minimum standard* to be given, the total must be ≥11    **TOTAL =**

I_____I_____I
**Not Acceptable**     **Meets Minimum Standards**     **Exceeds Minimum Standards**

**L:** Laboratory/Classroom Testing
**C:** Clinical/Field Testing
**P:** Practicum Testing
**A:** Assessment/Mock Exam Testing
**S:** Self-Reporting

**Positive Finding:** Develop power
**Involved Structure:** Muscles of the lower body
**Special Considerations:** N/A
**Reference(s):** Baechle et al
**Supplies Needed:** N/A

## OTHER TESTS
## (O-Test 31)

Peer Review _____ Peer Review _____

Skill Acquisition: _____    Practice Opportunities: _____

*This task gives you the opportunity to develop a **functional test** using only "forward cutting," to help assure a safe return to participation for the **lower extremity**. You have 3 minutes to develop and complete this task.*

| Tester places athlete and limb in appropriate position | YES | NO |
|---|---|---|
| Standing | ○○○ | ○○○ |
| **Tester performs test according to accepted guidelines** | **YES** | **NO** |
| Instructs the athlete to warm up | ○○○ | ○○○ |
| Cutting activities progress from easy to difficult | ○○○ | ○○○ |
| Progression consists of speed: | | |
|   Progression: Half speed | ○○○ | ○○○ |
|   Progression: Three-quarter speed | ○○○ | ○○○ |
|   Progression: Full speed | ○○○ | ○○○ |
| Progression consists of direction: | | |
|   Progression: Activities to the left | ○○○ | ○○○ |
|   Progression: Activities to the right | ○○○ | ○○○ |
| Progression consists of angles/degrees: | | |
|   Progression: Running forward cutting at 15 degree angle | ○○○ | ○○○ |
|   Progression: Running forward cutting at 45 degree angle | ○○○ | ○○○ |
|   Progression: Running forward cutting at 90 degree angle | ○○○ | ○○○ |
| Progression consist of commands: | | |
|   Progression: Instructs the athlete to cut left or right at the cone (instructions given prior to the activity | ○○○ | ○○○ |
|   Progression: Instructs the athlete to cut left or right on the whistle (instructions given during the activity) | ○○○ | ○○○ |
| Progression consists of sport-specific activities: | | |
|   Progression (eg, catching, dribbling) | ○○○ | ○○○ |

The psychomotor skill was performed completely and in the appropriate order        0  1  2  3  4  5

The tester had control of the subject and the situation (showed confidence)        0  1  2  3  4  5

Method of performing the skill allowed the tester the ability to determine:
severity, proper progression, and the *fit* in the overall picture (Oral)        0  1  2  3  4  5

In order for a grade of *minimum standard* to be given, the total must be ≥11        **TOTAL =**

I_____I_____I
**Not Acceptable**        **Meets Minimum Standards**        **Exceeds Minimum Standards**

**L:** Laboratory/Classroom Testing
**C:** Clinical/Field Testing
**P:** Practicum Testing
**A:** Assessment/Mock Exam Testing
**S:** Self-Reporting

**Positive Finding:** Cutting progress
**Involved Structure:** Structures involved with running
**Special Considerations:** N/A
**Reference(s):** Adapted from Prentice
**Supplies Needed:** Cones, whistle, sport equipment

# OTHER TESTS
# (O-Test 32)

Peer Review _____  Peer Review _____

Skill Acquisition: _____    Practice Opportunities: _____

*Using a tennis ball, develop a* **functional test** *using only a "short toss," to help assure a safe return to participation for the* **upper extremity***. You have 3 minutes to develop and complete this task.*

| Tester places athlete and limb in appropriate position | YES | NO |
|---|---|---|
| Standing | ○○○ | ○○○ |
| **Tester performs test according to accepted guidelines** | **YES** | **NO** |
| Instructs the athlete to go through the motion of throwing and letting go of the tennis ball | ○○○ | ○○○ |
| Instructs the athlete to throw the ball so it hits a wall about 15 feet away | | |
|   Progression: Hits the wall and rolls back to the athlete | ○○○ | ○○○ |
|   Progression: Hits the wall, bounces once, then back to the athlete | ○○○ | ○○○ |
|   Progression: Hits the wall and comes back to the athlete in the air | ○○○ | ○○○ |
| Instructs the athlete to throw the ball to a partner 20 feet away | | |
|   Progression: 1 to 60 throws | ○○○ | ○○○ |
|   Progression: Increases velocity of the throws | ○○○ | ○○○ |
|   Progression: Uses a glove to catch the ball | ○○○ | ○○○ |
| Instructs the athlete to throw the ball to a partner 30 feet away | | |
|   Progression: 1 to 60 throws | ○○○ | ○○○ |

The psychomotor skill was performed completely and in the appropriate order    **0  1  2  3  4  5**

The tester had control of the subject and the situation (showed confidence)    **0  1  2  3  4  5**

Method of performing the skill allowed the tester the ability to determine:
severity, proper progression, and the *fit* in the overall picture (Oral)    **0  1  2  3  4  5**

In order for a grade of *minimum standard* to be given, the total must be ≥11    **TOTAL =**

I_____I_____I

**Not Acceptable**    **Meets Minimum Standards**    **Exceeds Minimum Standards**

**L:** Laboratory/Classroom Testing
**C:** Clinical/Field Testing
**P:** Practicum Testing
**A:** Assessment/Mock Exam Testing
**S:** Self-Reporting

**Positive Finding:** Throwing progression
**Involved Structure:** Throwing muscles
**Special Considerations:** N/A
**Reference(s):** Adapted from Prentice
**Supplies Needed:** Tennis ball, baseball, glove

## OTHER TESTS
# (O-Test 33)

Peer Review _____    Peer Review _____

Skill Acquisition: _____    Practice Opportunities: _____

*This task allows you the opportunity to demonstrate the measurement of **leg length (true/apparent)** for an athlete. You have 3 minutes to complete this task.*

| | YES | NO |
|---|---|---|
| **Tester places athlete and limb in appropriate position** | **YES** | **NO** |
| Supine with feet completely on the table | ○○○ | ○○○ |
| **Tester obtains measurements of true leg length** | **YES** | **NO** |
| Measures from ASIS to medial malleolus (tape measure) | ○○○ | ○○○ |
| Measures both extremities | ○○○ | ○○○ |
| Compares and records measurements | ○○○ | ○○○ |
| **Tester obtains measurements of apparent leg length** | **YES** | **NO** |
| Measures from naval to medial malleolus (tape measure) | ○○○ | ○○○ |
| Measures both extremities | ○○○ | ○○○ |
| Compares and records measurements | ○○○ | ○○○ |

The psychomotor skill was performed completely and in the appropriate order   **0 1 2 3 4 5**

The tester had control of the subject and the situation (showed confidence)   **0 1 2 3 4 5**

Method of performing the skill allowed the tester the ability to determine:
severity, proper progression, and the *fit* in the overall picture (Oral)   **0 1 2 3 4 5**

In order for a grade of *minimum standard* to be given, the total must be ≥11   **TOTAL =**

I_____I_____I

**Not Acceptable**          **Meets Minimum Standards**     **Exceeds Minimum Standards**

**L:** Laboratory/Classroom Testing
**C:** Clinical/Field Testing
**P:** Practicum Testing
**A:** Assessment/Mock Exam Testing
**S:** Self-Reporting

**Positive Finding:** Leg length
**Involved Structure:** Pelvis, legs
**Special Considerations:** May measure to the lateral malleolus
**Reference(s):** Magee
**Supplies Needed:** Table, tape measure, pencil/ paper

# OTHER TESTS
# (O-Test 34)

Peer Review _____ Peer Review _____

Skill Acquisition: _____     Practice Opportunities: _____

*This task allows you the opportunity to determine the **body composition** of an athlete using a **skinfold caliper**. You have 3 minutes to complete this task.*

| | YES | NO |
|---|---|---|
| **Tester places athlete and limb in appropriate position** | | |
| Standing | OOO | OOO |
| Disrobe to shorts (male) or shorts and a sports bra (female) | OOO | OOO |
| **Tester placed in proper position (possible landmarks)** | **YES** | **NO** |
| Triceps-vertical pinch at midline of posterior upper arm | OOO | OOO |
| Subscapular-oblique pinch below bottom tip of the scapula | OOO | OOO |
| Suprailiac-oblique pinch just above hip bone | OOO | OOO |
| Abdominal-vertical pinch 1 inch to the right of umbilicus | OOO | OOO |
| Quadriceps-vertical pinch at midthigh | OOO | OOO |
| **Tester performs task according to accepted guidelines** | **YES** | **NO** |
| All measures should be taken on the right side of the body | OOO | OOO |
| Grasps area with thumb and forefinger | OOO | OOO |
| Pulls skin and fat away from underlying muscular tissue | OOO | OOO |
| Pinches area with caliper | OOO | OOO |
| Reads caliper dial within 2 seconds of pinching area | OOO | OOO |
| Repeats measurement two to three times for each body site | OOO | OOO |
| Takes average of two to three measurements and records results | OOO | OOO |

The psychomotor skill was performed completely and in the appropriate order     0  1  2  3  4  5

The tester had control of the subject and the situation (showed confidence)     0  1  2  3  4  5

Method of performing the skill allowed the tester the ability to determine:
severity, proper progression, and the *fit* in the overall picture (Oral)     0  1  2  3  4  5

In order for a grade of *minimum standard* to be given, the total must be ≥11     **TOTAL =**

I_____I_____I

**Not Acceptable          Meets Minimum Standards          Exceeds Minimum Standards**

**L:** Laboratory/Classroom Testing
**C:** Clinical/Field Testing
**P:** Practicum Testing
**A:** Assessment/Mock Exam Testing
**S:** Self-Reporting

**Positive Finding:** Body composition
**Involved Structure:** Muscle/fat
**Special Considerations:** N/A
**Reference(s):** Manufacturer's recommendations
**Supplies Needed:** Caliper, pencil/paper

## OTHER TESTS
# (O-Test 35)

Skill Acquisition: _____          Practice Opportunities: _____

*This problem allows you the opportunity to demonstrate the measurement of **thigh girth** for an athlete. You have 3 minutes to complete this task.*

| | YES | NO |
|---|---|---|
| **Tester places athlete and limb in appropriate position** | YES | NO |
| Supine with feet completely on the table | ○○○ | ○○○ |
| **Tester prepares limb for measurement** | YES | NO |
| Marks superior pole of the patella with dot | ○○○ | ○○○ |
| Marks thigh at 2, 6, and 10 inches above patella with dot (may vary depending on the length of the leg) | ○○○ | ○○○ |
| **Tester measures girth of thigh in appropriate manner** | YES | NO |
| Encircles thigh with cloth tape measure at each mark on thigh | ○○○ | ○○○ |
| Instructs athlete to flex muscle (quadriceps set) | ○○○ | ○○○ |
| Records girth of thigh at each mark | ○○○ | ○○○ |
| Performs measurement bilaterally | ○○○ | ○○○ |

| | | |
|---|---|---|
| The psychomotor skill was performed completely and in the appropriate order | **0  1  2  3  4  5** | |
| The tester had control of the subject and the situation (showed confidence) | **0  1  2  3  4  5** | |
| Method of performing the skill allowed the tester the ability to determine: severity, proper progression, and the *fit* in the overall picture (Oral) | **0  1  2  3  4  5** | |
| In order for a grade of *minimum standard* to be given, the total must be ≥11 | **TOTAL =** | |

I_____I_____I

**Not Acceptable**          **Meets Minimum Standards**          **Exceeds Minimum Standards**

**L:** Laboratory/Classroom Testing
**C:** Clinical/Field Testing
**P:** Practicum Testing
**A:** Assessment/Mock Exam Testing
**S:** Self-Reporting

**Positive Finding:** Objective measurement
**Involved Structure:** Thigh (quadriceps)
**Special Considerations:** N/A
**Reference(s):** Starkey et al
**Supplies Needed:** Tape measure, dot, pencil/paper

# OTHER TESTS
# (O-Test 36)

Peer Review _____ Peer Review _____

Skill Acquisition: _____    Practice Opportunities: _____

*Please demonstrate how you would stretch the wrist flexors using* **PNF Contract/Relax (Agonist/Antagonist)**. *You have 2 minutes to complete this task.*

| Tester places athlete and limb in appropriate position | YES | NO |
|---|---|---|
| Seated | OOO | OOO |
| Wrist in full extension | OOO | OOO |
| **Tester performs test according to accepted guidelines** | **YES** | **NO** |
| Instructs the athlete on proper commands and sequence | OOO | OOO |
| Stabilizes the ulna/radius with one hand | OOO | OOO |
| Passively stretches the wrist flexors ("relax" command) | OOO | OOO |
| Holds stretch for 4 to 10 seconds (wrist passively stretched in as much extension as possible) | OOO | OOO |
| Passively moves the wrist from extension to flexion ("relax" command) | OOO | OOO |
| Resists wrist extension using the "push" command through the full ROM with the other hand (moves isotonically against maximal resistance) | OOO | OOO |
| Uses proper hand position for applying isotonic resistance | OOO | OOO |
| Repeats above steps | OOO | OOO |

The psychomotor skill was performed completely and in the appropriate order    0 1 2 3 4 5

The tester had control of the subject and the situation (showed confidence)    0 1 2 3 4 5

Method of performing the skill allowed the tester the ability to determine: severity, proper progression, and the *fit* in the overall picture (Oral)    0 1 2 3 4 5

In order for a grade of *minimum standard* to be given, the total must be ≥11    **TOTAL =**

I_____I_____I
**Not Acceptable**    **Meets Minimum Standards**    **Exceeds Minimum Standards**

**L:** Laboratory/Classroom Testing
**C:** Clinical/Field Testing
**P:** Practicum Testing
**A:** Assessment/Mock Exam Testing
**S:** Self-Reporting

**Positive Finding:** Increase flexibility
**Involved Structure:** Wrist flexors
**Special Considerations:** N/A
**Reference(s):** Prentice
**Supplies Needed:** N/A

## OTHER TESTS
# (O-Test 37)

Peer Review _____ Peer Review _____

Skill Acquisition: _____     Practice Opportunities: _____

*Please demonstrate how you would stretch the shoulder external rotators using* **PNF Hold/Relax (Agonist/Agonist)**. *You have 2 minutes to complete this task.*

| Tester places athlete and limb in appropriate position | YES | NO |
|---|---|---|
| Seated or supine | OOO | OOO |
| Upper arm supported (90/90 position) | OOO | OOO |
| Shoulder placed in full internal rotation | OOO | OOO |
| **Tester performs test according to accepted guidelines** | **YES** | **NO** |
| Instructs the athlete on proper commands and sequence | OOO | OOO |
| Stabilizes the humerus with one hand | OOO | OOO |
| Passively stretches the shoulder external rotators ("relax" command) | OOO | OOO |
| Holds stretch for 4 to 10 seconds (shoulder passively stretched in as much internal rotation as possible) | OOO | OOO |
| Passively moves the shoulder from full internal rotation about 20 degrees in the transverse plane toward external rotation ("relax" command) | OOO | OOO |
| Resists shoulder external rotation using the "hold" command with the other hand (isometric contraction against maximal resistance) | OOO | OOO |
| Holds isometric contraction for 4 to 10 seconds | OOO | OOO |
| Uses proper hand position for applying isometric resistance | OOO | OOO |
| Repeats above steps | OOO | OOO |

The psychomotor skill was performed completely and in the appropriate order    0 1 2 3 4 5

The tester had control of the subject and the situation (showed confidence)    0 1 2 3 4 5

Method of performing the skill allowed the tester the ability to determine:
severity, proper progression, and the *fit* in the overall picture (Oral)    0 1 2 3 4 5

In order for a grade of *minimum standard* to be given, the total must be ≥11    **TOTAL =**

I_____I_____I
**Not Acceptable**     **Meets Minimum Standards**     **Exceeds Minimum Standards**

**L:** Laboratory/Classroom Testing
**C:** Clinical/Field Testing
**P:** Practicum Testing
**A:** Assessment/Mock Exam Testing
**S:** Self-Reporting

**Positive Finding:** Increase flexibility
**Involved Structure:** External rotators
**Special Considerations:** N/A
**Reference(s):** Prentice
**Supplies Needed:** N/A

# OTHER TESTS
# (O-Test 38)

Peer Review _____ Peer Review _____

Skill Acquisition: _____        Practice Opportunities: _____

*Please demonstrate how you would strengthen the knee flexors using* **PNF Slow Reversal**. *You have 2 minutes to complete this task.*

| Tester places athlete and limb in appropriate position | YES | NO |
|---|---|---|
| Seated or prone | ○○○ | ○○○ |
| Knee in full extension | ○○○ | ○○○ |
| **Tester performs test according to accepted guidelines** | **YES** | **NO** |
| Instructs the athlete on proper commands and sequence | ○○○ | ○○○ |
| Stabilizes femur | ○○○ | ○○○ |
| Instructs the athlete to isotonically contract the hamstring—moving from extension to flexion ("pull" command) | ○○○ | ○○○ |
| Instructs the athlete to immediately reverse the direction, contracting the quadriceps moving from flexion to extension ("push" command) | ○○○ | ○○○ |
| Uses proper hand position for applying isotonic resistance | ○○○ | ○○○ |
| Repeats above steps | ○○○ | ○○○ |

| | |
|---|---|
| The psychomotor skill was performed completely and in the appropriate order | 0  1  2  3  4  5 |
| The tester had control of the subject and the situation (showed confidence) | 0  1  2  3  4  5 |
| Method of performing the skill allowed the tester the ability to determine: severity, proper progression, and the *fit* in the overall picture (Oral) | 0  1  2  3  4  5 |

In order for a grade of *minimum standard* to be given, the total must be ≥11        **TOTAL =**

I_____I_____I
**Not Acceptable**          **Meets Minimum Standards**          **Exceeds Minimum Standards**

**L:** Laboratory/Classroom Testing
**C:** Clinical/Field Testing
**P:** Practicum Testing
**A:** Assessment/Mock Exam Testing
**S:** Self-Reporting

**Positive Finding:** Muscle education/strengthening
**Involved Structure:** Hamstrings
**Special Considerations:** N/A
**Reference(s):** Prentice
**Supplies Needed:** N/A

# OTHER TESTS
# (O-Test 39)

Peer Review _____ Peer Review _____

Skill Acquisition: _____     Practice Opportunities: _____

*Please demonstrate how you would strengthen the ankle invertors using **PNF Slow Reversal-Hold**. You have 2 minutes to complete this task.*

| Tester places athlete and limb in appropriate position | YES | NO |
|---|---|---|
| Seated or supine | ○○○ | ○○○ |
| Ankle placed in full eversion | ○○○ | ○○○ |
| **Tester performs test according to accepted guidelines** | **YES** | **NO** |
| Instructs the athlete on proper commands and sequence | ○○○ | ○○○ |
| Stabilizes tibia | ○○○ | ○○○ |
| Instructs the athlete to isotonically contract the invertors—moving from eversion to inversion ("pull" command) | ○○○ | ○○○ |
| Instructs the athlete to isometrically contract the invertors at the end of the range ("hold" command) | ○○○ | ○○○ |
| Holds isometric contraction for 4 to 10 seconds | ○○○ | ○○○ |
| Instructs the athlete to reverse direction—isotonically contract the evertors, moving from inversion to eversion ("push" command) | ○○○ | ○○○ |
| Instructs the athlete to isometrically contract the evertors at the end of the range ("hold" command) | ○○○ | ○○○ |
| Holds isometric contraction for 4 to 10 seconds | ○○○ | ○○○ |
| Uses proper hand position for applying isotonic and isometric resistance | ○○○ | ○○○ |
| Repeats above steps | ○○○ | ○○○ |

The psychomotor skill was performed completely and in the appropriate order    0 1 2 3 4 5

The tester had control of the subject and the situation (showed confidence)    0 1 2 3 4 5

Method of performing the skill allowed the tester the ability to determine: severity, proper progression, and the *fit* in the overall picture (Oral)    0 1 2 3 4 5

In order for a grade of *minimum standard* to be given, the total must be ≥11    TOTAL =

I_____I_____I
**Not Acceptable**      **Meets Minimum Standards**      **Exceeds Minimum Standards**

**L:** Laboratory/Classroom Testing
**C:** Clinical/Field Testing
**P:** Practicum Testing
**A:** Assessment/Mock Exam Testing
**S:** Self-Reporting

**Positive Finding:** Muscle education/strengthening
**Involved Structure:** Tibialis anterior
**Special Considerations:** N/A
**Reference(s):** Prentice
**Supplies Needed:** N/A

# OTHER TESTS
## (O-Test 40)

Peer Review _____ Peer Review _____

Skill Acquisition: _____    Practice Opportunities: _____

*Please demonstrate how you would perform* **PNF Repeated Contraction** *for the ankle dorsiflexors. You have 2 minutes to complete this task.*

| Tester places athlete and limb in appropriate position | YES | NO |
|---|---|---|
| Supine or seated | ○○○ | ○○○ |
| Ankle placed in full plantar flexion | ○○○ | ○○○ |
| **Tester performs test according to accepted guidelines** | **YES** | **NO** |
| Stabilizes tibia | ○○○ | ○○○ |
| Resists dorsiflexion using the "pull command" through the full ROM with the other hand (moves isotonically against maximal resistance) | ○○○ | ○○○ |
| Repeats above step until fatigue is evident | ○○○ | ○○○ |
| Performs "quick stretch" at the weakest point of the motion (or at the end of dorsiflexion) | ○○○ | ○○○ |

| | |
|---|---|
| The psychomotor skill was performed completely and in the appropriate order | 0 1 2 3 4 5 |
| The tester had control of the subject and the situation (showed confidence) | 0 1 2 3 4 5 |
| Method of performing the skill allowed the tester the ability to determine: severity, proper progression, and the *fit* in the overall picture (Oral) | 0 1 2 3 4 5 |

In order for a grade of *minimum standard* to be given, the total must be ≥11          **TOTAL =**

I_____I_____I
**Not Acceptable**          **Meets Minimum Standards**          **Exceeds Minimum Standards**

**L:** Laboratory/Classroom Testing
**C:** Clinical/Field Testing
**P:** Practicum Testing
**A:** Assessment/Mock Exam Testing
**S:** Self-Reporting

**Positive Finding:** Strengthening
**Involved Structure:** Tibialis anterior
**Special Considerations:** N/A
**Reference(s):** Prentice
**Supplies Needed:** Table

## OTHER TESTS
# (O-Test 41)

Skill Acquisition: _____     Practice Opportunities: _____

*Please demonstrate how you would strengthen the shoulder horizontal flexors using* **PNF Rhythmic Stabilization.**
*You have 2 minutes to complete this task.*

| Tester places athlete and limb in appropriate position | YES | NO |
|---|---|---|
| Supine | ○○○ | ○○○ |
| Shoulder horizontally flexed to 90 degrees | ○○○ | ○○○ |
| **Tester performs test according to accepted guidelines** | **YES** | **NO** |
| Instructs the athlete on proper commands and sequence | ○○○ | ○○○ |
| Instructs the athlete to contract the muscles around the scapula | ○○○ | ○○○ |
| Instructs the athlete to isometrically contract the horizontal flexors ("hold" command) | ○○○ | ○○○ |
| Instructs the athlete to immediately reverse the direction, isometrically contracting the horizontal extensors ("hold" command) | ○○○ | ○○○ |
| Uses proper hand position for applying isometric resistance | ○○○ | ○○○ |
| Repeats above steps | ○○○ | ○○○ |

The psychomotor skill was performed completely and in the appropriate order    **0  1  2  3  4  5**

The tester had control of the subject and the situation (showed confidence)    **0  1  2  3  4  5**

Method of performing the skill allowed the tester the ability to determine:
severity, proper progression, and the *fit* in the overall picture (Oral)    **0  1  2  3  4  5**

In order for a grade of *minimum standard* to be given, the total must be ≥11    **TOTAL =**

I_____I_____I
**Not Acceptable**        **Meets Minimum Standards**    **Exceeds Minimum Standards**

**L:** Laboratory/Classroom Testing
**C:** Clinical/Field Testing
**P:** Practicum Testing
**A:** Assessment/Mock Exam Testing
**S:** Self-Reporting

**Positive Finding:** Muscle education/strengthening
Pectoralis major
**Involved Structure:** Posterior deltoid
**Special Considerations:** N/A
**Reference(s):** Prentice
**Supplies Needed:** N/A

## OTHER TESTS
# (O-Test 42)

Peer Review _____ Peer Review _____

Skill Acquisition: _____    Practice Opportunities: _____

*This task allows you the opportunity to demonstrate the assessment of **Romberg's Sign** on an athlete. You have 2 minutes to complete this task.*

| Tester places athlete and limb in appropriate position | YES | NO |
|---|---|---|
| Standing with feet together | OOO | OOO |
| **Tester performs test according to accepted guidelines** | **YES** | **NO** |
| Instructs athlete to close his or her eyes | OOO | OOO |
| Observes athlete's balance and behavior | OOO | OOO |

The psychomotor skill was performed completely and in the appropriate order    0 1 2 3 4 5

The tester had control of the subject and the situation (showed confidence)    0 1 2 3 4 5

Method of performing the skill allowed the tester the ability to determine: severity, proper progression, and the *fit* in the overall picture (Oral)    0 1 2 3 4 5

In order for a grade of *minimum standard* to be given, the total must be ≥11    **TOTAL =**

I_____I_____I

**Not Acceptable**　　　**Meets Minimum Standards**　　**Exceeds Minimum Standards**

**L:** Laboratory/Classroom Testing
**C:** Clinical/Field Testing
**P:** Practicum Testing
**A:** Assessment/Mock Exam Testing
**S:** Self-Reporting

**Positive Finding:** Loss of balance, swaying, inability to keep eyes closed
**Involved Structure:** Head/brain
**Special Considerations:** May be repeated using single leg stance
**Reference(s):** Arnheim et al; Konin et al
**Supplies Needed:** N/A

## OTHER TESTS
# (O-Test 43)

Peer Review _____ Peer Review _____

Skill Acquisition: _____    Practice Opportunities: _____

*The athlete is suspected of having a neck injury and is having difficulty breathing. Demonstrate your ability* **remove a facemask from a standard football helmet** *using any equipment on the supply table. Assume that a second member of the medical team is stabilizing the head. For this scenario, your only concern is the removal of the facemask. You have 2 minutes to complete this task.*

| Tester places athlete and limb in appropriate position | YES | NO |
|---|---|---|
| Supine on the floor | ○○○ | ○○○ |
| **Tester placed in proper position** | **YES** | **NO** |
| Kneeling on the side of the athlete | ○○○ | ○○○ |
| **Tester performs task according to accepted guidelines** | **YES** | **NO** |
| Selects the proper cutting tool | ○○○ | ○○○ |
| Removes the two side (lower) brackets first | ○○○ | ○○○ |
| Removes the two top (upper) brackets | ○○○ | ○○○ |

The psychomotor skill was performed completely and in the appropriate order    0  1  2  3  4  5

The tester had control of the subject and the situation (showed confidence)    0  1  2  3  4  5

Method of performing the skill allowed the tester the ability to determine: severity, proper progression, and the *fit* in the overall picture (Oral)    0  1  2  3  4  5

In order for a grade of *minimum standard* to be given, the total must be ≥11    **TOTAL =**

I_____I_____I
**Not Acceptable**        **Meets Minimum Standards**        **Exceeds Minimum Standards**

**L:** Laboratory/Classroom Testing
**C:** Clinical/Field Testing
**P:** Practicum Testing
**A:** Assessment/Mock Exam Testing
**S:** Self-Reporting

**Positive Finding:** Remove facemask
**Involved Structure:** N/A
**Special Considerations:** N/A
**Reference(s):** Starkey et al
**Supplies Needed:** Football helmet; proper cutters

# OTHER TESTS
# (O-Test 44)

Peer Review _____ Peer Review _____

Skill Acquisition: _____          Practice Opportunities: _____

*This problem allows you the opportunity to demonstrate your **palpation** skills. You have to locate and mark each of the following eight anatomical landmarks (see table for dots). You have 15 seconds to find each landmark. Time begins immediately after the landmark is read to you.*

|  | YES | NO |
|---|---|---|
| Head of the fourth metatarsal | ○○○ | ○○○ |
| Lateral femoral condyle | ○○○ | ○○○ |
| Deltoid tuberosity of the humerus | ○○○ | ○○○ |
| Gerdy's tubercle | ○○○ | ○○○ |
| Thenar eminence | ○○○ | ○○○ |
| Anatomical snuffbox | ○○○ | ○○○ |
| Popliteal fossa | ○○○ | ○○○ |
| Head of the fibula | ○○○ | ○○○ |

The psychomotor skill was performed completely and in the appropriate order       **0  1  2  3  4  5**

The tester had control of the subject and the situation (showed confidence)       **0  1  2  3  4  5**

Method of performing the skill allowed the tester the ability to determine:
severity, proper progression, and the *fit* in the overall picture (Oral)       **0  1  2  3  4  5**

In order for a grade of *minimum standard* to be given, the total must be ≥11       **TOTAL =**

I_____I_____I
**Not Acceptable**     **Meets Minimum Standards**     **Exceeds Minimum Standards**

**L:** Laboratory/Classroom Testing
**C:** Clinical/Field Testing
**P:** Practicum Testing
**A:** Assessment/Mock Exam Testing
**S:** Self-Reporting

**Findings:** Correct marking
**Reference(s):** Any anatomy/evaluation book
**Supplies Needed:** Dots, table

# OTHER TESTS
## (O-Test 45)

Peer Review _____ Peer Review _____

Skill Acquisition: _____    Practice Opportunities: _____

*This problem allows you the opportunity to demonstrate your **palpation** skills. You have to locate and mark each of the following eight anatomical landmarks (see table for dots). You have 15 seconds to find each landmark. Time begins immediately after the landmark is read to you.*

|  | YES | NO |
|---|---|---|
| Dorsal pedis artery (pulse) | ○○○ | ○○○ |
| Pes anserinus bursa | ○○○ | ○○○ |
| Acromion process | ○○○ | ○○○ |
| Greater trochanter | ○○○ | ○○○ |
| Head of the radius | ○○○ | ○○○ |
| Styloid process of the fifth metatarsal | ○○○ | ○○○ |
| Proximal attachment of pronator teres | ○○○ | ○○○ |
| Anterior talofibular ligament | ○○○ | ○○○ |

The psychomotor skill was performed completely and in the appropriate order       0  1  2  3  4  5

The tester had control of the subject and the situation (showed confidence)       0  1  2  3  4  5

Method of performing the skill allowed the tester the ability to determine:
severity, proper progression, and the *fit* in the overall picture (Oral)       0  1  2  3  4  5

In order for a grade of *minimum standard* to be given, the total must be ≥11       **TOTAL =**

I_____I_____I

**Not Acceptable**        **Meets Minimum Standards**        **Exceeds Minimum Standards**

**L:** Laboratory/Classroom Testing
**C:** Clinical/Field Testing
**P:** Practicum Testing
**A:** Assessment/Mock Exam Testing
**S:** Self-Reporting

**Findings:** Correct marking
**Reference(s):** Any anatomy/evaluation book
**Supplies Needed:** Dots, table

## OTHER TESTS
# (O-Test 46)

Peer Review _____ Peer Review _____

Skill Acquisition: _____    Practice Opportunities: _____

*This task allows you the opportunity to demonstrate the measurement of the **Q-angle** of an athlete. You have 3 minutes to complete this task.*

| Tester places athlete and limb in appropriate position | YES | NO |
|---|---|---|
| Supine with foot on the table | OOO | OOO |

| Tester obtains measurement in appropriate manner | YES | NO |
|---|---|---|
| Marks the ASIS | OOO | OOO |
| Draws an imaginary line from the ASIS to the midline of the patella (center point) | OOO | OOO |
| Draws a line between the tibial tubercle and midpoint of the patella | OOO | OOO |
| Uses the goniometer to measure the angle between lines that cross the patella | OOO | OOO |

The psychomotor skill was performed completely and in the appropriate order     **0  1  2  3  4  5**

The tester had control of the subject and the situation (showed confidence)     **0  1  2  3  4  5**

Method of performing the skill allowed the tester the ability to determine:
severity, proper progression, and the *fit* in the overall picture (Oral)     **0  1  2  3  4  5**

In order for a grade of *minimum standard* to be given, the total must be ≥11     **TOTAL =**

I_____I_____I

**Not Acceptable**          **Meets Minimum Standards**     **Exceeds Minimum Standards**

**L:** Laboratory/Classroom Testing
**C:** Clinical/Field Testing
**P:** Practicum Testing
**A:** Assessment/Mock Exam Testing
**S:** Self-Reporting

**Positive Finding:** Angle > 13 for male
Angle > 18 for female
**Involved Structure:** Lower limb
**Special Considerations:** May be done with the knee flexed
**Reference(s):** Starkey et al; Magee
**Supplies Needed:** Goniometer, pencil/paper, dots

## OTHER TESTS
# (O-Test 47)

Peer Review _____ Peer Review _____

Skill Acquisition: _____    Practice Opportunities: _____

*This problem allows you the opportunity to demonstrate* **wound care** *for a* **forearm laceration** *of an athlete. You have 3 minutes to complete this task.*

| | YES | NO |
|---|---|---|
| **Tester places athlete and limb in appropriate position** | **YES** | **NO** |
| Uses latex gloves | OOO | OOO |
| Avoids direct contact with blood and bodily fluids | OOO | OOO |
| **Tester evaluates injury and stops bleeding** | **YES** | **NO** |
| Checks laceration for foreign objects | OOO | OOO |
| Checks sensation near and distal to injury site | OOO | OOO |
| Applies direct pressure to control bleeding | OOO | OOO |
| Elevates injured area above the heart until bleeding is controlled | OOO | OOO |
| **Tester treats wound according to accepted guidelines** | **YES** | **NO** |
| Cleans wound with antiseptic | OOO | OOO |
| Applies antibiotic ointment | OOO | OOO |
| Applies sterile dressing over the wound | OOO | OOO |
| Secures dressing with bandage | OOO | OOO |
| Disposes of biohazardous materials appropriately | OOO | OOO |
| Cleans hands thoroughly (before and after) | OOO | OOO |

The psychomotor skill was performed completely and in the appropriate order     **0  1  2  3  4  5**

The tester had control of the subject and the situation (showed confidence)     **0  1  2  3  4  5**

Method of performing the skill allowed the tester the ability to determine:
severity, proper progression, and the *fit* in the overall picture (Oral)     **0  1  2  3  4  5**

In order for a grade of *minimum standard* to be given, the total must be ≥11     **TOTAL =**

I_____I_____I

**Not Acceptable          Meets Minimum Standards          Exceeds Minimum Standards**

**L:** Laboratory/Classroom Testing
**C:** Clinical/Field Testing
**P:** Practicum Testing
**A:** Assessment/Mock Exam Testing
**S:** Self-Reporting

**Positive Finding:** Wound care
**Involved Structure:** Involved structure
**Special Considerations:** N/A
**Reference(s):** Arnheim et al
**Supplies Needed:** Latex gloves, sterile dressing, roller gauze, antibiotic ointment, antiseptic

## OTHER TESTS
# (O-Test 48)

Peer Review _____ Peer Review _____

Skill Acquisition: _____    Practice Opportunities: _____

*This task allows you the opportunity to demonstrate the use of a* **sling psychrometer** *to measure heat and humidity. You have 2 minutes to complete this task.*

| | YES | NO |
|---|---|---|
| **Tester places measuring device in appropriate position** | | |
| Moistens web bulb | OOO | OOO |
| Slides instrument into measuring position | OOO | OOO |
| **Tester follows correct procedures for using measuring device** | YES | NO |
| Stands in the center of the practice area, out of shade | OOO | OOO |
| Twirls sling psychrometer for about 2 minutes | OOO | OOO |
| Slides instrument into in proper position to read | OOO | OOO |
| **Tester uses measurement according to accepted guidelines** | YES | NO |
| Records measurements correctly | OOO | OOO |

| | |
|---|---|
| The psychomotor skill was performed completely and in the appropriate order | 0 1 2 3 4 5 |
| The tester had control of the subject and the situation (showed confidence) | 0 1 2 3 4 5 |
| Method of performing the skill allowed the tester the ability to determine: severity, proper progression, and the *fit* in the overall picture (Oral) | 0 1 2 3 4 5 |

In order for a grade of *minimum standard* to be given, the total must be ≥11         **TOTAL =**

I_____I_____I
**Not Acceptable**       **Meets Minimum Standards**   **Exceeds Minimum Standards**

**L:** Laboratory/Classroom Testing
**C:** Clinical/Field Testing
**P:** Practicum Testing
**A:** Assessment/Mock Exam Testing
**S:** Self-Reporting

**Positive Finding:** Temperature/humidity
**Involved Structure:** N/A
**Special Considerations:** N/A
**Reference(s):** Manufacturer's recommendations
**Supplies Needed:** Sling psychrometer, water source, pencil/paper

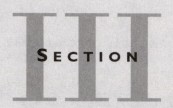

SECTION

# III

# MOCK PRACTICAL EXAM

## MOCK EXAM
## Student Questions

**Scenario 1 pertains to Manual Muscle Testing. This section of the mock practical exam is divided into three parts.**

*(MMT-L-Test 3)*
*Please demonstrate a manual muscle test for the* **soleus** *muscle. You have 2 minutes to complete this task.*

*(MMT-L-Test 4)*
*Please demonstrate a manual muscle test for the* **semitendinosus/semimembranosus** *muscles. You have 2 minutes to complete this task.*

*(MMT-U-Test 17)*
*This problem allows you the opportunity to demonstrate a manual muscle test for the* **pronator quadratus** *muscle. You have 2 minutes to complete this task.*

**Scenario 2 pertains to assessment of the cranial nerves. This section of the mock practical exam is divided into two parts.**

*(SST-U-Test 9)*
*Demonstrate how you would evaluate an athlete who is suspected of suffering a cranial nerve injury to the* **trigeminal nerve**. *This problem requires you to demonstrate assessment of both the sensory and motor functions of cranial nerve #5. You have 2 minutes to complete this task.*

*(SST-U-Test 6)*
*Please demonstrate how you would evaluate an athlete who is suspected of suffering a cranial nerve injury to the* **olfactory nerve (cranial nerve #1)**. *You have 2 minutes to complete this task.*

**Scenario 3 pertains to the utilization of Special Tests for assessment of an athlete. This section of the mock practical exam is divided into three parts.**

*(ST-L-Test 22)*
*This problem allows you the opportunity to demonstrate the* **Trendelenburg Test (Trendelenburg Sign)**. *You have 2 minutes to complete this task.*

*(ST-U-Test 10)*
*This problem allows you the opportunity to demonstrate the* **Neer Impingement Test (Shoulder Impingement Test)** *of the shoulder. You have 2 minutes to complete this task.*

*(ST-U-Test 19)*
*This problem allows you the opportunity to demonstrate **Finkelstein's Test** in order to help rule out de Quervain's disease or Hoffmann's disease. You have 2 minutes to complete this task.*

**Scenario 4 pertains to the assessment of your ability to palpate. This section of the mock practical exam has 10 anatomical landmarks.**

*(O-Test 44/45)*
*This problem allows you the opportunity to demonstrate your palpation skills. You have 10 landmarks to find and place a dot on the correct spot (see table for dots). You have 15 seconds to find each landmark. Your time begins immediately after the landmark is read to you.*
*1. Posterior tibial artery (pulse)*
*2. Navicular tubercle*
*3. Bicipital groove*
*4. Anterior superior iliac spine (ASIS)*
*5. Olecranon fossa*
*6. Head of the second metacarpal*
*7. Distal attachment of the peroneus brevis*
*8. Posterior tibiofibular ligament*
*9. Inferior angle of the scapula*
*10. Transverse process of C7*

**Scenario 5 pertains to the "Other/Miscellaneous" category. This section of the mock practical exam is divided into three parts.**

*(O-Test 28)*
*Using the model as your partner, demonstrate how you would perform a type of plyometrics known as a **medicine ball sit-up**. You have 2 minutes to complete this task.*

*(O-Test 13)*
*This problem allows you the opportunity to demonstrate the proper technique for performing a **supine straight leg raise**, incorporating a 5-lb cuff weight as fixed resistance. You have 2 minutes to complete this task.*

*(O-Test 18)*
*Using a 10-lb dumbbell, develop an endurance-based test in order to determine the **percent fatigue** of the middle deltoid muscle. This type of testing is also known as a "% Fatigue Test." You have 3 minutes to develop and administer this test.*

# MOCK EXAM
# Practical Exam Score Sheet

Name: _____     Final Score (50): _____

Date: _____

This is a mock practical exam. You are graded on what you do, not what you say. It is important that you demonstrate all aspects of the skill and make your intent clear to the examiner(s).

First, take a moment to examine the materials on the supply table. Any of these materials may be used during the exam. The model is only present for the purpose of demonstration. He or she will follow directions; however, the model will not respond to your questions. Please inform the examiners when you have completed each task. Do not move to the next scenario until you are instructed to do so.

## SCENARIO 1                                          TOTAL SCORE: (12)_____

Scenario 1 pertains to Manual Muscle Testing. This section of the mock practical exam is divided into three parts.

### (MMT-L-Test 3)

Please demonstrate a manual muscle test for the **soleus** muscle. You have 2 minutes to complete this task.

| Tester places athlete and limb in appropriate position | YES | NO |
|---|---|---|
| Prone (.5) | ○○○ | ○○○ |
| Knee flexed to 90 degrees (.5) | ○○○ | ○○○ |
| **Tester placed in proper position** | **YES** | **NO** |
| Supports the leg proximal to the ankle (.25) | ○○○ | ○○○ |
| Places the other hand on the calcaneus (.25) | ○○○ | ○○○ |
| **Tester performs test according to accepted guidelines** | **YES** | **NO** |
| Has the athlete actively plantar flex the ankle joint (without inversion and/or eversion) (1) | ○○○ | ○○○ |
| Applies resistance to the calcaneus; pulling the heel in the direction of dorsiflexion (1) | ○○○ | ○○○ |
| Holds resistance for 5 seconds (.25) | ○○○ | ○○○ |
| Performs assessment bilaterally (.25) | ○○○ | ○○○ |

**Reference(s):** Kendall                               SCORE: (4)_____
**Supplies Needed:** Table
**Comments:**

**(MMT-L-Test 4)**

*Please demonstrate a manual muscle test for the* **semitendinosus/semimembranosus** *muscles. You have 2 minutes to complete this task.*

| Tester places athlete and limb in appropriate position | YES | NO |
|---|---|---|
| Prone (1) | ○○○ | ○○○ |
| **Tester placed in proper position** | **YES** | **NO** |
| Holds the thigh firmly against the table (.25) | ○○○ | ○○○ |
| Places other hand against the distal tibia/fibula (posterior aspect) (.25) | ○○○ | ○○○ |
| **Tester performs test according to accepted guidelines** | **YES** | **NO** |
| Has athlete actively flex the knee between 50 and 70 degrees (.5) | ○○○ | ○○○ |
| Thigh and leg placed in medial rotation (.5) | ○○○ | ○○○ |
| Applies resistance to the leg proximal to the ankle, in the direction of knee extension (1) | ○○○ | ○○○ |
| Holds resistance for 5 seconds (.25) | ○○○ | ○○○ |
| Performs assessment bilaterally (.25) | ○○○ | ○○○ |

**Reference(s):** Kendall
**Supplies Needed:** Table
**Comments:**

SCORE: (4)_____

**(MMT-U-Test 17)**

*This problem allows you the opportunity to demonstrate a manual muscle test for the* **pronator quadratus** *muscle. You have 2 minutes to complete this task.*

| Tester places athlete and limb in appropriate position | YES | NO |
|---|---|---|
| Seated or supine (.25) | ○○○ | ○○○ |
| Elbow placed in full flexion (.25) | ○○○ | ○○○ |
| Elbow/forearm placed in full pronation (.25) | ○○○ | ○○○ |
| Elbow placed against athlete's side (avoiding shoulder abduction) (.25) | ○○○ | ○○○ |
| **Tester placed in proper position** | **YES** | **NO** |
| Stands to the side, facing the athlete (.25) | ○○○ | ○○○ |
| Stabilizes the elbow against the side with one hand (.25) | ○○○ | ○○○ |
| Places the other hand around the distal forearm (.25) | ○○○ | ○○○ |
| **Tester performs test according to accepted guidelines** | **YES** | **NO** |
| Instructs the athlete to hold the position (.5) | ○○○ | ○○○ |
| Applies resistance in a rotating motion against the distal forearm in the direction of supination (.5) | ○○○ | ○○○ |
| Holds resistance for 5 seconds (1) | ○○○ | ○○○ |
| Performs assessment bilaterally (.25) | ○○○ | ○○○ |

**Reference(s):** Kendall
**Supplies Needed:** N/A
**Comments:**

SCORE: (4)_____

**SCENARIO 2**                                                    **TOTAL SCORE: (8)**_____

Scenario 2 pertains to assessment of the cranial nerves. This section of the mock practical exam is divided into two parts.

**(SST-U-Test 9)**

*Demonstrate how you would evaluate an athlete who is suspected of suffering a cranial nerve injury to the* **trigeminal nerve**. *This problem requires you to demonstrate assessment of both the sensory and motor functions of cranial nerve #5. You have 2 minutes to complete this task.*

| Tester places athlete and limb in appropriate position | YES | NO |
|---|---|---|
| Seated or standing (.5) | OOO | OOO |
| **Tester performs test according to accepted guidelines** | **YES** | **NO** |
| Gives appropriate directions to the athlete (.5) | OOO | OOO |
| Instructs the athlete to close eyes (1) | OOO | OOO |
| Asks the athlete to recognize a light touch to the face (sensory) (1) | OOO | OOO |
| Asks the athlete to clench teeth together (motor) (1) | OOO | OOO |

**Reference(s):** Magee, Starkey et al                        **SCORE: (4)**_____
**Supplies Needed:** N/A
**Comments:**

**(SST-U-Test 6)**

*Please demonstrate how you would evaluate an athlete who is suspected of suffering a cranial nerve injury to the* **olfactory nerve** *(cranial nerve #1). You have 2 minutes to complete this task.*

| Tester places athlete and limb in appropriate position | YES | NO |
|---|---|---|
| Seated or standing (1) | OOO | OOO |
| **Tester performs test according to accepted guidelines** | **YES** | **NO** |
| Gives appropriate directions to the athlete (1) | OOO | OOO |
| Instructs the athlete to close eyes (1) | OOO | OOO |
| Asks the athlete to identify a familiar odor (1) | OOO | OOO |

**Reference(s):** Magee, Starkey et al                        **SCORE: (4)**_____
**Supplies Needed:** Something with a familiar odor
                    (eg, tape adhesive)
**Comments:**

**SCENARIO 3**                                                        **TOTAL SCORE: (13)**_____

Scenario 3 pertains to the utilization of Special Tests for assessment. This section of the mock practical exam is divided into three parts.

**(ST-L-Test 22)**

*This problem allows you the opportunity to demonstrate the* **Trendelenburg Test (Trendelenburg Sign)**. *You have 2 minutes to complete this task.*

| Tester places athlete and limb in appropriate position | YES | NO |
|---|---|---|
| Standing (.5) | OOO | OOO |
| **Tester placed in proper position** | **YES** | **NO** |
| Stands behind the athlete (observing only movement of the pelvis) (2) | OOO | OOO |
| **Tester performs test according to accepted guidelines** | **YES** | **NO** |
| Instructs the athlete to balance on one leg (10 seconds) (1) | OOO | OOO |
| Performs assessment bilaterally (.5) | OOO | OOO |

**Reference(s):** Konin, et al; Magee                              **SCORE: (4)**_____
**Supplies Needed:** N/A
**Comments:**

**(ST-U-Test 10)**

*This problem allows you the opportunity to demonstrate the* **Neer Impingement Test (Shoulder Impingement Test)** *of the shoulder. You have 2 minutes to complete this task.*

| Tester places athlete and limb in appropriate position | YES | NO |
|---|---|---|
| Standing or seated (.25) | OOO | OOO |
| Arms placed at the athlete's side (.5) | OOO | OOO |
| Shoulder internally rotated/elbow pronated (.5) | OOO | OOO |
| **Tester placed in proper position** | **YES** | **NO** |
| Stands to the side, facing the athlete (.25) | OOO | OOO |
| Places one hand against the scapula (.25) | OOO | OOO |
| Places the other hand under the elbow (supporting the arm) (.25) | OOO | OOO |
| **Tester performs test according to accepted guidelines** | **YES** | **NO** |
| Maintains relaxation of the limb (.25) | OOO | OOO |
| Pushes/jams the greater tuberosity into the border of the acromion (1.25) | OOO | OOO |
| Passively flex the shoulder through a full range of motion (1.25) | OOO | OOO |
| Performs assessment bilaterally (.25) | OOO | OOO |

**SCORE: (5)**_____

**Reference(s):** Konin et al; Magee
**Supplies Needed:** N/A
**Comments:**

**(ST-U-Test 19)**

*This problem allows you the opportunity to demonstrate* **Finkelstein's Test** *in order to help rule out de Quervain's disease or Hoffmann's disease. You have 2 minutes to complete this task.*

| Tester places athlete and limb in appropriate position | YES | NO |
|---|---|---|
| Standing or seated (.25) | ○○○ | ○○○ |
| Athlete is asked to form a fist around the thumb (fist with thumb inside) (1) | ○○○ | ○○○ |
| **Tester placed in proper position** | **YES** | **NO** |
| Stands in front, facing the athlete (.25) | ○○○ | ○○○ |
| Places hand under the forearm supporting the arm (.5) | ○○○ | ○○○ |
| Places the other hand around the fist (.5) | ○○○ | ○○○ |
| **Tester performs test according to accepted guidelines** | **YES** | **NO** |
| Maintains relaxation of the involved limb (.25) | ○○○ | ○○○ |
| Passively deviates the wrist toward the ulna (ulnar deviation) (1) | ○○○ | ○○○ |
| Performs assessment bilaterally (.25) | ○○○ | ○○○ |

SCORE: (4)_____

**Reference(s):** Konin, et al; Magee
**Supplies Needed:** N/A
**Comments:**

**SCENARIO 4**                    TOTAL SCORE: (5)_____

Scenario 4 pertains to the assessment of your ability to palpate. This section of the mock practical exam has 10 anatomical points.

**(O-Test 44/45)**

*This problem allows you the opportunity to demonstrate your* **palpation skills**. *You have 10 landmarks to find and place a dot on the correct spot (see table for dots). You have 15 seconds to find each landmark. Your time begins immediately after the landmark is read to you.*

| | YES | NO |
|---|---|---|
| Posterior tibial artery (pulse) (.5) | ○○○ | ○○○ |
| Navicular tubercle (.5) | ○○○ | ○○○ |
| Bicipital groove (.5) | ○○○ | ○○○ |
| Anterior superior iliac spine (ASIS) (.5) | ○○○ | ○○○ |
| Olecranon fossa (.5) | ○○○ | ○○○ |
| Head of the second metacarpal (.5) | ○○○ | ○○○ |
| Distal attachment of peroneus brevis (.5) | ○○○ | ○○○ |
| Posterior tibiofibular ligament (.5) | ○○○ | ○○○ |
| Inferior angle of the scapula (.5) | ○○○ | ○○○ |
| Transverse process of C7 (.5) | ○○○ | ○○○ |

SCORE: (5)_____

**Reference(s):** Any anatomy/evaluation book
**Supplies Needed:** Dots, table
**Comments:**

**SCENARIO 5**                                         **TOTAL SCORE: (12)_____**

Scenario 5 pertains to the "Other/Miscellaneous" category. This section of the mock practical exam is divided into three parts.

**(O-Test 28)**

*Using the model as your partner, demonstrate how you would perform a type of plyometrics known as a* **medicine ball sit-up**. *You have 2 minutes to complete this task.*

| Tester places athlete and limb in appropriate position | YES | NO |
|---|---|---|
| Seated on the floor (.25) | ○○○ | ○○○ |
| Sit-up position (knees bent, trunk flexed to 45 degrees) (.25) | ○○○ | ○○○ |
| Hands/arms in an outstretched position (waiting to receive the ball) (.25) | ○○○ | ○○○ |
| **Tester placed in proper position** | **YES** | **NO** |
| Standing in front of the athlete (holding the medicine ball) (.25) | ○○○ | ○○○ |
| **Tester performs task according to accepted guidelines** | **YES** | **NO** |
| Tester: Throws the ball to the athlete (.5) | ○○○ | ○○○ |
| Athlete: Catches the ball using both arms (eccentric phrase) (.5) | ○○○ | ○○○ |
| Athlete: Completes the amortization phase (time between moving down toward the floor and coming back up) (1) | ○○○ | ○○○ |
| Athlete: Moves away from the floor and throws/pushes the ball back (concentric phase) (.5) | ○○○ | ○○○ |
| Tester: Receives the ball from the athlete and repeats (.5) | ○○○ | ○○○ |

**SCORE: (4)_____**

            **Reference(s):** Baechle et al
**Supplies Needed:** Medicine ball
         **Comments:**

**(O-Test 13)**

*This problem allows you the opportunity to demonstrate the proper technique for performing a* **supine straight leg raise**, *incorporating a 5-lb cuff weight as fixed resistance. You have 2 minutes to complete this task.*

| Tester places athlete and limb in appropriate position | YES | NO |
|---|---|---|
| Supine (.25) | ○○○ | ○○○ |
| Hip/knee placed in anatomical position (heels on the table) (.25) | ○○○ | ○○○ |
| Attaches cuff weight securely to the involved limb (.5) | ○○○ | ○○○ |
| **Tester performs test according to accepted guidelines** | **YES** | **NO** |
| Tightens involved quadriceps (hold) (.5) | ○○○ | ○○○ |
| Lifts involved limb off the table (6 to 8 inches) (.5) | ○○○ | ○○○ |
| Retightens involved quadriceps (hold) (.5) | ○○○ | ○○○ |
| Lowers involved limb slowly (.5) | ○○○ | ○○○ |
| Allows the calf (gastrocnemius) muscle to make contact with the table first, not the heel (1) | ○○○ | ○○○ |

**SCORE: (4)_____**

          **Reference(s):** Prentice
**Supplies Needed:** 5-lb cuff weight
          **Comments:**

**(O-Test 18)**

*Using a 10-lb dumbbell, develop an endurance-based test in order to determine the **percent fatigue** of the middle deltoid muscle. This type of testing is also known as a "% Fatigue Test." You have 3 minutes to develop and administer this test.*

| Tester places athlete and limb in appropriate position | YES | NO |
|---|---|---|
| Standing or seated (.25) | ○○○ | ○○○ |
| Arms hanging to the side (.25) | ○○○ | ○○○ |

| Tester performs test according to accepted guidelines | YES | NO |
|---|---|---|
| Instructs the athlete to hold a 10-lb dumbbell with the uninvolved limb (.5) | ○○○ | ○○○ |
| Instructs the athlete to fully abduct the shoulder (slow, controlled pace) (1) | ○○○ | ○○○ |
| Continues until the athlete cannot complete the next repetition or for 1 minute continuously (count the number of repetitions completed) (1) | ○○○ | ○○○ |
| Repeats the above three steps with the involved limb (.5) | ○○○ | ○○○ |
| Compares the number of repetitions completed (determines deficit) (.5) | ○○○ | ○○○ |

**SCORE: (4)_____**

**Reference(s):** Adapted from Baechle
**Supplies Needed:** 10-lb dumbbell
**Comments:**

# BIBLIOGRAPHY

Anderson MK, Hall SJ. *Sports Injury Management*. Baltimore, Md: Williams & Wilkins; 1995.

Arnheim DD, Prentice WE. *Principles of Athletic Training*. Boston, Mass: McGraw Hill; 2000.

Baechle TR, Earle RW. *Essentials of Strength Training and Conditioning*. Champaign, Ill: Human Kinetics; 2000.

Bickley LS. *Bates' Guide to Physical Examination and History Taking*. Philadelphia, Pa: Lippincott; 1999.

Cecil, RL, Goldman L, Bennett JC . *Cecil Textbook of Medicine*. Philadelphia, Pa: WB Saunders; 2000.

Edmond SL. *Manipulation Mobilization*. St. Louis, Mo: Mosby; 1993.

Hillman SK. *Introduction to Athletic Training*. Champaign, Ill: Human Kinetics; 2000.

Hoppenfeld S. *Physical Examination of the Spine and Extremities*. Norwalk, Conn: Appleton-Century-Crofts; 1976.

Houglum PA. *Therapeutic Exercise for Athletic Injuries*. Champaign, Ill: Human Kinetics; 2001.

Kendall FP, McCreary EK, Provance PG. *Muscle Testing and Function*. 4th ed. Baltimore, Md: Williams & Wilkins; 1993.

Konin JG, Wiksten DL, Isear JA. *Special Tests for Orthopedic Examination*. Thorofare, NJ: SLACK Incorporated; 1997.

Magee DJ. *Orthopedic Physical Assessment*. 3rd ed. Philadelphia, Pa: WB Saunders; 1997.

NATA. *Athletic Training Educational Competencies*. 3rd ed. Dallas, Tex: NATA; 1999.

NATABOC. Informational material. Available at: http://www.nataboc.org. Accessed January 7, 2002.

NATABOC. *Study Guide for the NATA Board of Certification, Inc: Entry-Level Athletic Trainer Certification Examination*. 2nd ed (rev). Philadelphia, Pa: FA Davis; 1993.

NATABOC. *Examiner Training Program Home Study Workbook: For NATABOC Practical Examiners*. Omaha, Neb: NATABOC; 1999.

Norkin CC, White DJ. *Measurement of Joint Motion: A guide to Goniometry*. Philadelphia, Pa: FA Davis; 1985.

O'Connor DP. *Clinical Pathology for Athletic Trainers: Recognizing Systemic Disease*. Thorofare, NJ: SLACK Incorporated; 2001.

Perrin DH. *Athletic Taping and Bracing*. Champaign, Ill: Human Kinetics; 1995.

*Physician's Desk Reference*. 54th ed. Montvale, NJ: Medical Economics Co; 2000.

Prentice WE. *Rehabilitation Techniques in Sports Medicine*. Boston Mass: McGraw Hill; 1999.

Shultz SJ, Houglum PA, Perrin DH. *Assessment of Athletic Injuries*. Champaign, Ill: Human Kinetics; 2000.

Starkey C, Ryan K. *Evaluation of Orthopedic and Athletic Injuries*. Philadelphia, Pa: FA Davis; 2002.

Street SA, Runkle D. *Athletic Protective Equipment: Care, Selection, and Fitting*. Boston, Mass: McGraw Hill; 2000.

Van Ost L, Manfre' K. *Athletic Training: Student Guide to Success*. Thorofare, NJ: SLACK Incorporated; 2000.

Wright KE, Whitehill WR. *The Comprehensive Manual of Taping and Wrapping Techniques*. Gardner, Kan: Cramer Products Inc; 1996.